Household Safety Sourcebook

Hypertension Sourcebook

Immune System Disorders Sourcebook

Infant & Toddler Health Sourcebook

Infectious Diseases Sourcebook

Injury & Trauma Sourcebook

Kidney & Urinary Tract Diseases & Disorders Sourcebook

Learning Disabilities Sourcebook, 2nd Edition

Leukemia Sourcebook

Liver Disorders Sourcebook

Lung Disorders Sourcebook

Medical Tests Sourcebook, 2nd Edition

Men's Health Concerns Sourcebook, 2nd Edition

Mental Health Disorders Sourcebook, 3rd Edition

Mental Retardation Sourcebook

Movement Disorders Sourcebook

Muscular Dystrophy Sourcebook

Obesity Sourcebook

Osteoporosis Sourcebook

Pain Sourcebook, 2nd Edition

Pediatric Cancer Sourcebook

Physical & Mental Issues in Aging Sourcebook

Podiatry Sourcebook

Pregnancy & Birth Sourcebook, 2nd Edition

Prostate Cancer

Public Health Sourcebook

Reconstructive & Cosmetic Surgery Sourcebook

Rehabilitation Sourcebook

Respiratory Diseases & Disorders Sourcebook

Sexually Transmitted Diseases Sourcebook, 2nd Edition

Skin Disorders Sourcebook

Sleep Disorders Sourcebook, 2nd Edition

Smoking Concerns Sourcebook

Sports Injuries Sourcebook, 2nd Edition

Stress-Related Disorders Sourcebook

Stroke Sourcebook

Substance Abuse Sourcebook

Surgery Sourcebook

Thyroid Sourcebook

Transplantation Sourcebook

Traveler's Health Sourcebook

Vegetarian Sourcebook

Women's Health Concerns Sourcebook, 2nd Edition

Workplace Health & Safety Sourcebook

Worldwide Health Sourcebook

Teen Health Series

Alcohol Information for Teens

Asthma Information for Teens

Cancer Information for Teens

Diet Information for Teens

Drug Information for Teens

Eating Disorders Information for Teens

Fitness Information for Teens

Mental Health Information for Teens

Sexual Health Information for Teens

Skin Health Information for Teens

Sports Injuries Information for Teens

Suicide Information for Teens

Diet and Nutrition
SOURCEBOOK

Third Edition

Health Reference Series

Third Edition

Diet and Nutrition SOURCEBOOK

*Basic Consumer Health Information about Dietary
Guidelines and the Food Guidance System,
Recommended Daily Nutrient Intakes, Serving
Proportions, Weight Control, Vitamins and Supplements,
Nutrition Issues for Different Life Stages and Lifestyles,
and the Needs of People with Specific Medical Concerns,
Including Cancer, Celiac Disease, Diabetes, Eating
Disorders, Food Allergies, and Cardiovascular Disease*

*Along with Facts about Federal Nutrition Support
Programs, a Glossary of Nutrition and Dietary Terms,
and Directories of Additional Resources for More
Information about Nutrition*

Edited by
Joyce Brennfleck Shannon

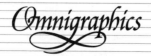

Omnigraphics

615 Griswold Street • Detroit, MI 48226

Bibliographic Note

Because this page cannot legibly accommodate all the copyright notices, the Bibliographic Note portion of the Preface constitutes an extension of the copyright notice.

Edited by Joyce Brennfleck Shannon

Health Reference Series

Karen Bellenir, *Managing Editor*
David A. Cooke, M.D., *Medical Consultant*
Elizabeth Barbour, *Research and Permissions Coordinator*
Cherry Stockdale, *Permissions Assistant*
Dawn Matthews, *Verification Assistant*
Laura Pleva Nielsen, *Index Editor*
EdIndex, Services for Publishers, *Indexers*

* * *

Omnigraphics, Inc.

Matthew P. Barbour, *Senior Vice President*
Kay Gill, *Vice President—Directories*
Kevin Hayes, *Operations Manager*
Leif Gruenberg, *Development Manager*
David P. Bianco, *Marketing Director*

* * *

Peter E. Ruffner, *Publisher*

Frederick G. Ruffner, Jr., *Chairman*

Copyright © 2006 Omnigraphics, Inc.

ISBN 0-7808-0800-2

Library of Congress Cataloging-in-Publication Data

Diet and nutrition sourcebook : basic consumer health information about dietary guidelines and the food guidance system, recommended daily nutrient intakes, serving proportions, weight control, vitamins and supplements, nutrition issues for different life stages and lifestyles, and the needs of people with specific medical concerns, including cancer, celiac disease, diabetes, eating disorders, food allergies, and cardiovascular disease : along with facts about federal nutrition support programs, a glossary of nutrition and dietary terms, and directories of additional resources for more information about nutrition / edited by Joyce Brennfleck Shannon. -- 3rd ed.
  p. ; cm. -- (Health reference series)
  Includes bibliographical references and index.
  Summary: "Provides basic consumer health information about diet,nutrition, and related medical diseases and conditions. Includes index, glossary of related terms, and other resources" --Provided by publisher.
  ISBN 0-7808-0800-2 (hardcover : alk. paper)
  1. Nutrition--Popular works. 2. Diet--Popular works. 3. Health--Popular works. 4. Consumer education. I. Shannon, Joyce Brennfleck.
  II. Series: Health reference series (Unnumbered)
  [DNLM: 1. Nutrition--Popular Works. 2. Nutrition--Resource Guides.
3. Public Health--Popular Works. 4. Public Health--Resource Guides.
QU 145 D5652 2006]
RA784.D542 2006
613.2--dc22
                                                                    2005031842

Table of Contents

Visit www.healthreferenceseries.com to view *A Contents Guide to the Health Reference Series*, a listing of more than 10,000 topics and the volumes in which they are covered.

Part II: Nutrition Intake and Proportions

Part III: Life Stage Nutrition Issues

Part VI: Supplements

Part VII: Nutrition for People with Specific Medical Concerns

Part VIII: National Government Nutrition Support Programs

Part IX: Additional Help and Information

Preface

About This Book

Nutrition impacts every aspect of life, including energy levels, physical well-being, and mental performance, but figuring out how to eat a healthy balance of nutritious foods in amounts appropriate for the number of calories expended—especially in the presence of an abundant food supply, sedentary lifestyles, and time pressures—is an overwhelming challenge for many people. Statistics from the National Center for Health Statistics suggest that nearly two-thirds of American adults are overweight or obese. In addition, the U.S. Department of Agriculture's Center for Nutrition Policy and Promotion reports that 74% of Americans need to amend their eating habits to reduce the risk of heart disease, stroke, diabetes, osteoporosis, certain cancers, and other ailments.

Diet and Nutrition Sourcebook, Third Edition can help people sort through the abundant, and often confusing, information about nutrition. It contains facts about the recently updated *Dietary Guidelines for Americans* and offers suggestions for people at all stages of life and in various lifestyles, from infants to seniors and including singles, families, vegetarians, and athletes. It also discusses weight control, dining out, dietary supplements, and nutrition support programs. Nutrition advice for people with specific medical concerns—including cancer, celiac disease, diabetes, food allergies, and heart disease—is included, along with a glossary, suggestions for further reading, and directories of online resources and organizations able to provide additional help and information.

How to Use This Book

This book is divided into parts and chapters. Parts focus on broad areas of interest. Chapters are devoted to single topics within a part.

Part I: General Nutrition Information describes the revised *Dietary Guidelines for Americans* and the new MyPyramid food guidance graphic. It explains the specific components of a healthy diet and offers individual chapters on protein, calcium, carbohydrates, fiber, fruits and vegetables, fats, vitamins, sodium, fluids, additives, and sugar. Cautions about nutrition misinformation and nutrition myths are also included.

Part II: Nutrition Intake and Proportions explains necessary and discretionary calorie allowances, the differences between servings and portions, and the use of Nutrition Facts labels in making food choices.

Part III: Life Stage Nutrition Issues presents information about age- and gender-related nutrition concerns. It describes infants' needs and explains how to help children and teens develop good eating habits. Issues related to nutrition during pregnancy, menopause, and aging are also considered.

Part IV: Lifestyle and Nutrition offers guidelines for incorporating healthy eating into different situations, including eating alone, eating with a family, or dining out. It also describes lifestyle preferences with dietary implications and addresses the connection between physical activity and nutrient requirements.

Part V: Weight Control offers information about the health risks associated with excess weight. It describes the elements of safe and successful weight loss diets, explains the components of several popular diets, and discusses dieting practices that may pose health risks.

Part VI: Supplements describes the use and regulation of dietary supplements, including their safety and possible adverse health effects. It also describes the supplements that are commonly used to combat the effects of aging, prevent heart disease, and control cholesterol. A separate chapter highlights concerns associated with supplements sometimes used in an effort to enhance athletic performance.

Part VII: Nutrition for People with Specific Medical Concerns offers nutrition guidelines for people with concerns related to chronic diseases and disorders, including cancer, celiac disease, cystic fibrosis, diabetes, eating disorders, food allergies, heart disease, kidney disease, epilepsy, and congenital disorders of metabolism.

Part VIII: National Government Nutrition Support Programs describes the federal food stamp program, Women, Infants, and Children (WIC) Supplemental Program, and school and senior adult nutrition programs.

Part IX: Additional Help and Information includes a glossary of dietary and nutrition terms, a guide to finding useful nutrition information on the internet, a list of nutrition resources, and a directory of organizations able to provide more information.

Bibliographic Note

This volume contains documents and excerpts from publications issued by the following U.S. government agencies: Administration on Aging (AOA); Centers for Disease Control and Prevention (CDC); National Cancer Institute (NCI); National Center for Complementary and Alternative Medicine (NCCAM); National Heart, Lung, and Blood Institute (NHLBI); National Institute of Allergy and Infectious Diseases (NIAID); National Institute of Child Health and Human Development (NICHD); National Institute of Diabetes and Digestive and Kidney Diseases (NIDDK); National Institute of Mental Health (NIMH); National Institutes of Health Clinical Center; National Institute on Aging (NIA); National Institute on Alcohol Abuse and Alcoholism (NIAAA); National Institute on Drug Abuse (NIDA); National Institutes of Health Office of Dietary Supplements; U.S. Department of Agriculture (USDA); U.S. Department of Health and Human Services (HHS); U.S. Environmental Protection Agency (EPA); and the U.S. Food and Drug Administration (FDA).

In addition, this volume contains copyrighted documents from the following organizations: Academy for Eating Disorders; A.D.A.M., Inc.; American Academy of Family Physicians (AAFP); American Association for Clinical Chemistry; American Dietetic Association; American Heart Association; American Institute for Cancer Research; Brown University Medical School–Center for Gerontology and Health Care; Case Nutrition Consulting; Center for Science in the Public Interest; Colorado State University Cooperative Extension; Cystic Fibrosis Foundation; Harvard School of Public Health–Department of Nutrition; International Food Information Council Foundation; Medical College of Wisconsin HealthLink; National Center for Education in

Maternal and Child Health; Nemours Center for Children's Health Media; Northwestern University–Feinberg School of Medicine; Partnership for Essential Nutrition; Pennsylvania State University College of Agricultural Sciences; and Stanford University.

Full citation information is provided on the first page of each chapter. Every effort has been made to secure all necessary rights to reprint the copyrighted material. If any omissions have been made, please contact Omnigraphics to make corrections for future editions.

Acknowledgements

In addition to the listed organizations, agencies, and individuals who have contributed to this *Sourcebook*, special thanks go to managing editor Karen Bellenir, research and permissions coordinator Liz Barbour, verification assistant Dawn Matthews, and document engineer Bruce Bellenir for their help and support.

About the Health Reference Series

The *Health Reference Series* is designed to provide basic medical information for patients, families, caregivers, and the general public. Each volume takes a particular topic and provides comprehensive coverage. This is especially important for people who may be dealing with a newly diagnosed disease or a chronic disorder in themselves or in a family member. People looking for preventive guidance, information about disease warning signs, medical statistics, and risk factors for health problems will also find answers to their questions in the *Health Reference Series*. The *Series*, however, is not intended to serve as a tool for diagnosing illness, in prescribing treatments, or as a substitute for the physician/patient relationship. All people concerned about medical symptoms or the possibility of disease are encouraged to seek professional care from an appropriate health care provider.

Locating Information within the Health Reference Series

The *Health Reference Series* contains a wealth of information about a wide variety of medical topics. Ensuring easy access to all the fact sheets, research reports, in-depth discussions, and other material contained within the individual books of the *Series* remains one of our highest priorities. As the *Series* continues to grow in size and scope, however, locating the precise information needed by a reader may become more challenging.

A Contents Guide to the Health Reference Series was developed to direct readers to the specific volumes that address their concerns. It presents an extensive list of diseases, treatments, and other topics of general interest compiled from the Tables of Contents and major index headings. To access *A Contents Guide to the Health Reference Series*, visit www.healthreferenceseries.com.

Medical Consultant

Medical consultation services are provided to the *Health Reference Series* editors by David A. Cooke, M.D. Dr. Cooke is a graduate of Brandeis University, and he received his M.D. degree from the University of Michigan. He completed residency training at the University of Wisconsin Hospital and Clinics. He is board-certified in Internal Medicine. Dr. Cooke currently works as part of the University of Michigan Health System and practices in Ann Arbor, MI. In his free time, he enjoys writing, science fiction, and spending time with his family.

Our Advisory Board

We would like to thank the following board members for providing guidance to the development of this *Series*:

- Dr. Lynda Baker,
  Associate Professor of Library and Information Science,
  Wayne State University, Detroit, MI

- Nancy Bulgarelli,
  William Beaumont Hospital Library, Royal Oak, MI

- Karen Imarisio,
  Bloomfield Township Public Library, Bloomfield Township, MI

- Karen Morgan,
  Mardigian Library, University of Michigan-Dearborn,
  Dearborn, MI

- Rosemary Orlando,
  St. Clair Shores Public Library, St. Clair Shores, MI

Health Reference Series *Update Policy*

The inaugural book in the *Health Reference Series* was the first edition of *Cancer Sourcebook* published in 1989. Since then, the *Series* has been enthusiastically received by librarians and in the medical community. In order to maintain the standard of providing high-quality health information for the layperson the editorial staff at Omnigraphics felt it was necessary to implement a policy of updating volumes when warranted.

Medical researchers have been making tremendous strides, and it is the purpose of the *Health Reference Series* to stay current with the most recent advances. Each decision to update a volume is made on an individual basis. Some of the considerations include how much new information is available and the feedback we receive from people who use the books. If there is a topic you would like to see added to the update list, or an area of medical concern you feel has not been adequately addressed, please write to:

Editor
Health Reference Series
Omnigraphics, Inc.
615 Griswold Street
Detroit, MI 48226
E-mail: editorial@omnigraphics.com

Part One

General Nutrition Information

Chapter 1

Dietary Guidelines for Americans: Keys to a Healthy Lifestyle

Feel Better Today, Stay Healthy for Tomorrow

The food and physical activity choices you make every day affect your health—how you feel today, tomorrow, and in the future. The science-based advice of the *Dietary Guidelines for Americans, 2005* highlights how to make smart choices from every food group; find your balance between food and physical activity; and get the most nutrition out of your calories.

You may be eating plenty of food, but not eating the right foods that give your body the nutrients you need to be healthy. You may not be getting enough physical activity to stay fit and burn those extra calories. This chapter is a starting point for finding your way to a healthier you.

Eating right and being physically active are not just a diet or a program—they are keys to a healthy lifestyle. With healthful habits, you may reduce your risk of many chronic diseases such as heart disease, diabetes, osteoporosis, and certain cancers, and increase your chances for a longer life. The sooner you start the better for you, your family, and your future.

"Finding Your Way to a Healthier You: Based on the *Dietary Guidelines for Americans 2005*," U.S. Department of Health and Human Services (HHS) and U.S. Department of Agriculture (USDA), HHS Pub. No. HHS-ODPHP-2005-01-DGA-B, April 5, 2005. Also, "How to Use the Nutrition Facts Label," from *We Can! Families Finding the Balance: A Parent Handbook*, National Heart, Lung, and Blood Institute, NIH Publication No. 05–5273, June 2005.

Make Smart Choices from Every Food Group

The best way to give your body the balanced nutrition it needs is by eating a variety of nutrient-packed foods every day. Just be sure to stay within your daily calorie needs.

A healthy eating plan is one that:

- emphasizes fruits, vegetables, whole grains, and fat-free or low-fat milk and milk products;

- includes lean meats, poultry, fish, beans, eggs, and nuts; and

- is low in saturated fats, trans fats, cholesterol, salt (sodium), and added sugars.

Don't give in when you eat out and are on the go. It is important to make smart food choices and watch portion sizes wherever you are—at the grocery store, at work, in your favorite restaurant, or running errands. Try these tips:

- At the store, plan ahead by buying a variety of nutrient-rich foods for meals and snacks throughout the week.

- When grabbing lunch, have a sandwich on whole grain bread and choose low-fat/fat-free milk, water, or other drinks without added sugars.

- In a restaurant, opt for steamed, grilled, or broiled dishes instead of those that are fried or sautéed.

- On a long commute or shopping trip, pack some fresh fruit, cut-up vegetables, string cheese sticks, or a handful of unsalted nuts—to help you avoid impulsive, less healthful snack choices.

Mix Up Your Choices within Each Food Group

- **Focus on fruits.** Eat a variety of fruits—whether fresh, frozen, canned, or dried—rather than fruit juice for most of your fruit choices. For a 2,000-calorie diet, you will need 2 cups of fruit each day (for example, 1 small banana, 1 large orange, and ¼ cup of dried apricots or peaches).

- **Vary your veggies.** Eat more dark green vegetables such as broccoli, kale, and other dark leafy greens; orange vegetables such as carrots, sweet potatoes, pumpkin, and winter squash; and beans and peas such as pinto beans, kidney beans, black beans, garbanzo beans, split peas, and lentils.

- **Get your calcium-rich foods.** Everyday get 3 cups of low-fat or fat-free milk—or an equivalent amount of low-fat yogurt and/or low-fat cheese (1½ ounces of cheese equals 1 cup of milk)—for kids aged 2 to 8, it is 2 cups of milk. If you do not or cannot consume milk, choose lactose-free milk products and/or calcium-fortified foods and beverages.

- **Make half your grains whole.** Eat at least 3 ounces of whole grain cereals, breads, crackers, rice, or pasta every day. One ounce is about 1 slice of bread, 1 cup of breakfast cereal, or ½ cup of cooked rice or pasta. Look to see that grains such as wheat, rice, oats, or corn are referred to as whole in the list of ingredients.

- **Go lean with protein.** Choose lean meats and poultry. Bake it, broil it, or grill it, and vary your protein choices—with more fish, beans, peas, nuts, and seeds.

- **Know the limits on fats, salt, and sugars.** Read the Nutrition Facts label on foods. Look for foods low in saturated fats and trans fats. Choose and prepare foods and beverages with little salt (sodium) and/or added sugars (caloric sweeteners).

Find Your Balance between Food and Physical Activity

Becoming a healthier you is not just about eating healthy—it is also about physical activity. Regular physical activity is important for your overall health and fitness. It also helps you control body weight by balancing the calories you take in as food with the calories you expend each day.

- Be physically active for at least 30 minutes most days of the week.

- Increasing the intensity or the amount of time that you are physically active can have even greater health benefits and may be needed to control body weight. About 60 minutes a day may be needed to prevent weight gain.

- Children and teenagers should be physically active for 60 minutes every day, or most every day.

Consider this: If you eat 100 more food calories a day than you burn, you will gain about 1 pound in a month, or about 10 pounds in a year. The bottom line is that to lose weight, it is important to reduce calories and increase physical activity.

Get the Most Nutrition Out of Your Calories

There is a right number of calories for you to eat each day. This number depends on your age, activity level, and whether you are trying to gain, maintain, or lose weight (2,000 calories is the value used as a general reference on the food label). You could use up the entire amount on a few high-calorie items, but chances are you would not get the full range of vitamins and nutrients your body needs to be healthy.

Choose the most nutritionally rich foods you can from each food group each day—those packed with vitamins, minerals, fiber, and other nutrients, and lower in calories. Pick foods like fruits, vegetables, whole grains, and fat-free or low-fat milk and milk products more often.

Nutrition: To Know the Facts, Use the Label

Most packaged foods have a Nutrition Facts label. For a healthier you, use this tool to make smart food choices quickly and easily. Try these tips:

- Keep these low—saturated fats, trans fats, cholesterol, and sodium.
- Get enough of these—potassium, fiber, vitamins A and C, calcium, and iron.
- Use the % Daily Value (DV) column when possible—5% DV or less is low, 20% DV or more is high.

Check servings and calories. Look at the serving size and how many servings you are actually consuming. If you double the servings you eat, you double the calories and nutrients, including the % DVs.

Make your calories count. Look at the calories on the label and also compare them with the nutrients you are getting to decide whether the food is worth eating. When one serving of a single food item has over 400 calories per serving, it is high in calories.

Do not sugarcoat it. Since sugars contribute calories with few, if any, nutrients, look for foods and beverages low in added sugars. Read the ingredient list and make sure that added sugars are not one of the first few ingredients. Some names for added sugars (caloric sweeteners) include sucrose, glucose, high fructose corn syrup, corn syrup, maple syrup, and fructose.

Know your fats. Look for foods low in saturated fats, trans fats, and cholesterol to help reduce the risk of heart disease (5% DV or less is low, 20% DV or more is high). Most of the fats you eat should be polyunsaturated and monounsaturated fats. Keep total fat intake between 20% to 35% of daily calories.

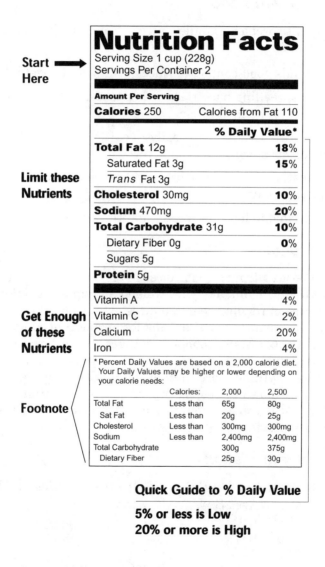

Figure 1.1. Nutrition Facts Label

Reduce sodium (salt), increase potassium. Research shows that eating less than 2,300 milligrams of sodium (about 1 teaspoon of salt) per day may reduce the risk of high blood pressure. Most of the sodium people eat comes from processed foods, not from the salt-shaker. Also, look for foods high in potassium, which counteracts some of sodium's effects on blood pressure.

Play It Safe with Food

Know how to prepare, handle, and store food safely to keep you and your family safe:

- Clean hands, food-contact surfaces, fruits, and vegetables.

- To avoid spreading bacteria to other foods, meat and poultry should not be washed or rinsed.

- Separate raw, cooked, and ready-to-eat foods while shopping, preparing, or storing.

- Cook meat, poultry, and fish to safe internal temperatures to kill microorganisms.

- Chill perishable foods promptly and thaw foods properly.

About Alcohol

If you choose to drink alcohol, do so in moderation. Moderate drinking means up to 1 drink a day for women and up to 2 drinks for men. Twelve ounces of regular beer, 5 ounces of wine, or 1½ ounces of 80-proof distilled spirits count as a drink for purposes of explaining moderation. Remember that alcoholic beverages have calories and are low in nutritional value.

Generally, anything more than moderate drinking can be harmful to your health. And some people, or people in certain situations, should not drink at all. If you have questions or concerns, talk to your doctor or healthcare provider.

Additional Information

U.S. Department of Health and Human Services (HHS)
200 Independence Ave., S.W.
Washington, DC 20201
Toll-Free: 877-696-6775
Phone: 202-619-6775
Website: http://www.healthierus.gov/dietaryguidelines

Chapter 2

Food Guide Pyramid

Anatomy of MyPyramid

MyPyramid symbolizes a personalized approach to healthy eating and physical activity. The symbol has been designed to be simple. It has been developed to remind consumers to make healthy food choices and to be active every day. The different parts of the symbol include:

- **Activity,** represented by the steps and the person climbing them, as a reminder of the importance of daily physical activity.

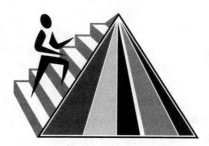

Figure 2.1. *MyPyramid.gov: Steps to a Healthier You*

This chapter includes the following U.S. Department of Agriculture information: "Anatomy of MyPyramid," 2005; excerpts from "Frequently Asked Questions: Food Guidance System," June 2005; and the "MyPyramid Symbol," 2005.

- **Moderation,** represented by the narrowing of each food group from bottom to top. The wider base stands for foods with little or no solid fats or added sugars. These should be selected more often. The narrower top area stands for foods containing more added sugars and solid fats. Individuals who are more active may allow more sugar and solid fat in their diets.

- **Personalization,** shown by the person on the steps, the slogan, and the website address.

- **Proportionality,** shown by the different widths of the food group bands. The widths suggest how much food a person should choose from each group. The widths are just a general guide, not exact proportions.

- **Variety,** symbolized by the 6 color bands representing the 5 food groups and oils. This illustrates that foods from all groups are needed each day for good health.

- **Gradual improvement,** encouraged by the slogan. It suggests that individuals can benefit from taking small steps to improve their diet and lifestyle each day.

Frequently Asked Questions about the Food Guidance System

What is the original Food Guide Pyramid?

Developed in 1992, the original Pyramid was an educational tool used to help Americans select healthful diets. The original Pyramid translated nutrition recommendations for consumers, from the *Dietary Guidelines* and the *Recommended Dietary Allowances (RDA's)* published in 1989, into the kinds and amounts of food to eat each day. Now MyPyramid, is replacing the original Food Guide Pyramid. The MyPyramid symbol in its simplest form has no foods pictured in it.

What is the relationship between the Dietary Guidelines and MyPyramid?

The *Dietary Guidelines for Americans* represent federal nutrition policy. MyPyramid is the educational tool designed to help consumers make healthier food and physical activity choices for a healthy lifestyle that are consistent with the guidelines. The U.S. Departments of Agriculture (USDA) and Health and Human Services (HHS) jointly publish the *Dietary Guidelines for Americans,* first released in 1980 and revised in 1985, 1990, 1995, 2000, and January 2005. MyPyramid translates the principles of the 2005 *Dietary Guidelines for Americans* and other nutritional standards to assist consumers in making healthier food and physical activity choices. MyPyramid was developed and issued by USDA.

How will consumers know what to eat?

One symbol cannot carry all the nutrition guidance. The new symbol was designed to be simple. It reminds consumers to make healthy food choices and to be physically active every day.

Why doesn't the new graphic illustrate trans fatty acids, water, or other items?

In the original 1992 Food Guide Pyramid graphic, it was not possible to incorporate all nutrition guidance in one graphic, so several key messages were selected for illustration. When revising USDA's food guidance, the choice was to either to further complicate the graphic by adding more concepts or to simplify the graphic. USDA chose to reduce the graphic's complexity and develop stronger supporting tools that provide clear guidance for consumers.

Why revise the original Pyramid?

USDA has been providing nutrition guidance for over 100 years. USDA released the original Food Guide Pyramid in 1992. MyPyramid reflects the most current science, and is designed for ease of use by consumers.

What are the goals for MyPyramid?

The primary goal for MyPyramid is to encourage dietary and physical activity behavior change among American consumers. Although most consumers recognize the original Pyramid, only a small percentage of them follow it in its entirety.

What's different about MyPyramid?

The MyPyramid symbol is one part of the food guidance system, an update to the Food Guide Pyramid. The new MyPyramid offers consumers a more personalized approach to healthy eating and physical activity.

What are the shortfalls of the American diet?

The American diet is not in balance. On average, Americans don't eat enough dark greens, orange vegetables, legumes, fruits, whole grains, or low-fat milk products. They eat too many fats and added sugars. To bring the diet into balance, MyPyramid recommends eating more of the under-consumed foods, and less of foods rich in solid fats, added sugars, and caloric sweeteners.

What are the benefits of the new Food Guidance System?

- It enables the use of a symbol as a stand-alone visual to represent the overall food guidance system without being cluttered by specific messages.

- It more effectively teaches consumers what and how much to eat through clear, tailored nutrition messages and diet personalization.

- It helps combat obesity by encouraging healthier eating patterns.

- It helps to improve the overall health and well-being of Americans.

- It more effectively reaches consumers through the use of multiple channels including the Internet.

Additional Information

USDA Center for Nutrition Policy and Promotion
3101 Park Center Dr., Room 1034
Alexandria, VA 22302-1594
Website: http://www.mypyramid.gov
E-mail: support@cnpp.usda.gov

Chapter 3

Your Digestive System and How It Works

The digestive system is a series of hollow organs joined in a long, twisting tube from the mouth to the anus. Inside this tube is a lining called the mucosa. In the mouth, stomach, and small intestine, the mucosa contains tiny glands that produce juices to help digest food.

Two solid organs, the liver and the pancreas, produce digestive juices that reach the intestine through small tubes. In addition, parts of other organ systems (for instance, nerves and blood) play a major role in the digestive system.

Why Is Digestion Important?

When we eat such things as bread, meat, and vegetables, they are not in a form that the body can use as nourishment. Our food and drink must be changed into smaller molecules of nutrients before they can be absorbed into the blood and carried to cells throughout the body. Digestion is the process by which food and drink are broken down into their smallest parts so that the body can use them to build and nourish cells and to provide energy.

How Is Food Digested?

Digestion involves the mixing of food, its movement through the digestive tract, and the chemical breakdown of the large molecules

"Your Digestive System and How It Works," National Institute of Diabetes and Digestive and Kidney Diseases (NIDDK), NIH Publication No. 04-2681, May 2004.

of food into smaller molecules. Digestion begins in the mouth with chewing and swallowing, and is completed in the small intestine. The chemical process varies somewhat for different kinds of food.

Movement of Food through the System

The large, hollow organs of the digestive system contain muscle that enables their walls to move. The movement of organ walls can propel food and liquid and also can mix the contents within each organ. Typical movement of the esophagus, stomach, and intestine is

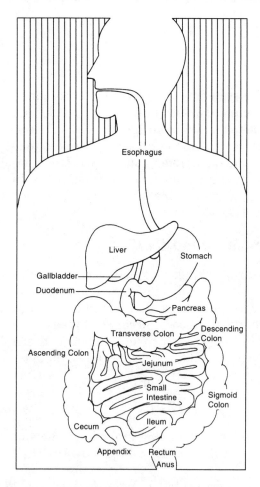

Figure 3.1. The Digestive System

14

called peristalsis. The action of peristalsis looks like an ocean wave moving through the muscle. The muscle of the organ produces a narrowing and then propels the narrowed portion slowly down the length of the organ. These waves of narrowing push the food and fluid in front of them through each hollow organ.

The first major muscle movement occurs when food or liquid is swallowed. Although we are able to start swallowing by choice, once the swallow begins, it becomes involuntary and proceeds under the control of the nerves.

The esophagus is the organ into which the swallowed food is pushed. It connects the throat above with the stomach below. At the junction of the esophagus and stomach, there is a ring-like valve closing the passage between the two organs. However, as the food approaches the closed ring, the surrounding muscles relax and allow the food to pass.

The food then enters the stomach, which has three mechanical tasks to do. First, the stomach must store the swallowed food and liquid. This requires the muscle of the upper part of the stomach to relax and accept large volumes of swallowed material. The second job is to mix up the food, liquid, and digestive juice produced by the stomach. The lower part of the stomach mixes these materials by its muscle action. The third task of the stomach is to empty its contents slowly into the small intestine.

Several factors affect emptying of the stomach, including: the nature of the food (mainly its fat and protein content), the degree of muscle action of the emptying stomach, and the next organ to receive the contents (the small intestine). As the food is digested in the small intestine and dissolved into the juices from the pancreas, liver, and intestine, the contents of the intestine are mixed and pushed forward to allow further digestion.

Finally, all of the digested nutrients are absorbed through the intestinal walls. The waste products of this process include undigested parts of the food, known as fiber, and older cells that have been shed from the mucosa. These materials are propelled into the colon, where they remain, usually for a day or two, until the feces are expelled by a bowel movement.

Production of Digestive Juices

The glands that act first—the salivary glands—are in the mouth. Saliva produced by these glands contains an enzyme that begins to digest the starch from food into smaller molecules.

The next set of digestive glands is in the stomach lining. They produce stomach acid and an enzyme that digests protein. One of the unsolved puzzles of the digestive system is why the acid juice of the stomach does not dissolve the tissue of the stomach itself. In most people, the stomach mucosa is able to resist the juice, although food and other tissues of the body cannot.

After the stomach empties the food and juice mixture into the small intestine, the juices of two other digestive organs mix with the food to continue the process of digestion. One of these organs is the pancreas. It produces a juice that contains a wide array of enzymes to break down the carbohydrate, fat, and protein in food. Other enzymes that are active in the process come from glands in the wall of the intestine or even a part of that wall.

The liver produces yet another digestive juice—bile. The bile is stored between meals in the gallbladder. At mealtime, it is squeezed out of the gallbladder into the bile ducts to reach the intestine and mix with the fat in our food. The bile acids dissolve the fat into the watery contents of the intestine, much like detergents that dissolve grease from a frying pan. After the fat is dissolved, it is digested by enzymes from the pancreas and the lining of the intestine.

Absorption and Transport of Nutrients

Digested molecules of food, as well as water and minerals from the diet, are absorbed from the cavity of the upper small intestine. Most absorbed materials cross the mucosa into the blood and are carried off in the bloodstream to other parts of the body for storage or further chemical change. This part of the process varies with different types of nutrients.

Carbohydrates. It is recommended that about 55 to 60 percent of total daily calories be from carbohydrates. Some of the most common foods contain mostly carbohydrates. Examples are bread, potatoes, legumes, rice, spaghetti, fruits, and vegetables. Many of these foods contain both starch and fiber.

The digestible carbohydrates are broken into simpler molecules by enzymes in the saliva, in juice produced by the pancreas, and in the lining of the small intestine. Starch is digested in two steps: First, an enzyme in the saliva and pancreatic juice breaks the starch into molecules called maltose; then an enzyme in the lining of the small intestine (maltase) splits the maltose into glucose molecules that can be absorbed into the blood. Glucose is carried through the bloodstream to the liver, where it is stored or used to provide energy for the work of the body.

Table sugar is another carbohydrate that must be digested to be useful. An enzyme in the lining of the small intestine digests table sugar into glucose and fructose, each of which can be absorbed from the intestinal cavity into the blood. Milk contains yet another type of sugar, lactose, which is changed into absorbable molecules by an enzyme called lactase, also found in the intestinal lining.

Protein. Foods such as meat, eggs, and beans consist of giant molecules of protein that must be digested by enzymes before they can be used to build and repair body tissues. An enzyme in the juice of the stomach starts the digestion of swallowed protein. Further digestion of the protein is completed in the small intestine. Here, several enzymes from the pancreatic juice and the lining of the intestine carry out the breakdown of huge protein molecules into small molecules called amino acids. These small molecules can be absorbed from the hollow of the small intestine into the blood and then can be carried to all parts of the body to build the walls and other parts of cells.

Fats. Fat molecules are a rich source of energy for the body. The first step in digestion of a fat such as butter is to dissolve it into the watery content of the intestinal cavity. The bile acids produced by the liver act as natural detergents to dissolve fat in water and allow the enzymes to break the large fat molecules into smaller molecules, some of which are fatty acids and cholesterol. The bile acids combine with the fatty acids and cholesterol and help these molecules to move into the cells of the mucosa. In these cells the small molecules are formed back into large molecules, most of which pass into vessels near the intestine. These small vessels carry the reformed fat to the veins of the chest, and the blood carries the fat to storage depots in different parts of the body.

Vitamins. Another vital part of our food that is absorbed from the small intestine is the class of chemicals called vitamins. The two different types of vitamins are classified by the fluid in which they can be dissolved: water-soluble vitamins (all the B vitamins and vitamin C) and fat-soluble vitamins (vitamins A, D, and K).

Water and salt. Most of the material absorbed from the cavity of the small intestine is water in which salt is dissolved. The salt and water come from swallowed food and liquid and the juices secreted by the many digestive glands.

How Is the Digestive Process Controlled?

Hormone Regulators

A fascinating feature of the digestive system is that it contains its own regulators. The major hormones that control the functions of the digestive system are produced and released by cells in the mucosa of the stomach and small intestine. These hormones are released into the blood of the digestive tract, travel back to the heart through the arteries, and return to the digestive system where they stimulate digestive juices and cause organ movement.

The hormones that control digestion are gastrins, secretin, and cholecystokinin (CCK):

- **Gastrins** cause the stomach to produce an acid for dissolving and digesting some foods, and is necessary for the normal growth of the lining of the stomach, small intestine, and colon.

- **Secretin** causes the pancreas to send out a digestive juice that is rich in bicarbonate. It stimulates the stomach to produce pepsin, an enzyme that digests protein, and it also stimulates the liver to produce bile.

- **Cholecystokinin** (CCK) causes the pancreas to grow and to produce the enzymes of pancreatic juice, and it causes the gallbladder to empty.

Additional hormones in the digestive system regulate appetite:

- **Ghrelin** is produced in the stomach and upper intestine in the absence of food in the digestive system and stimulates appetite.

- **Peptide YY** is produced in the GI tract in response to a meal in the system and inhibits appetite.

Both of these hormones work on the brain to help regulate the intake of food for energy.

Nerve Regulators

Two types of nerves help to control the action of the digestive system. Extrinsic (outside) nerves come to the digestive organs from the unconscious part of the brain or from the spinal cord. They release a chemical called acetylcholine and another called adrenaline. Acetylcholine causes the muscle of the digestive organs to squeeze with more force and increase the push of food and juice through the digestive tract. Acetylcholine also causes the stomach and pancreas to produce more digestive juice. Adrenaline relaxes the muscle of the stomach and intestine and decreases the flow of blood to these organs.

Even more important, though, are the intrinsic (inside) nerves, which make up a very dense network embedded in the walls of the esophagus, stomach, small intestine, and colon. The intrinsic nerves are triggered to act when the walls of the hollow organs are stretched by food. They release many different substances that speed up or delay the movement of food and the production of juices by the digestive organs.

Additional Information

National Digestive Diseases Information Clearinghouse
2 Information Way
Bethesda, MD 20892-3570
Toll-Free: 800-891-5389
Fax: 703-738-4929
Website: http://www.digestive.niddk.nih.gov
E-mail: nddic@info.niddk.nih.gov

Chapter 4

Protein and Amino Acids

Protein

The building blocks of human proteins are twenty amino acids that may be consumed from both plant and animal sources. Of these 20 amino acids, 9 are considered to be essential because their carbon skeletons cannot be synthesized by human enzymes. The remaining nonessential amino acids can be synthesized endogenously with transfer of amino groups to carbon compounds that are formed as intermediates of glucose (glucogenic amino acids) and lipid (ketogenic amino acids) metabolism.

Protein is the basic structural material of all cells. Biologically active proteins include enzymes, immunoglobulins, hormones, neurotransmitters, nutrient transport and storage compounds, and cell membrane receptors. Plasma proteins (e.g., albumin) contribute to oncotic pressure that directs the flow of fluid and metabolic waste from the intracellular compartment into the capillary venules. These proteins (e.g., hemoglobin) also contribute to plasma buffering capacity and oxygen-carbon dioxide transport (e.g., hemoglobin, myoglobin). Acute phase reactant proteins (e.g., ferritin, prealbumin) secreted by

"Protein," reprinted with permission from the Department of Preventative Medicine, Northwestern University Feinberg School of Medicine, © 2002 Northwestern University. Also, "Meat and Beans: Tips to Help You Make Wise Choices from the Meat & Beans Group," U.S. Department of Agriculture (USDA), April 2005.

the liver bind minerals such as iron and zinc, rendering them unavailable to support microbial proliferation.

Biological Value

Biological value of a dietary protein is determined by the amount and proportion of essential amino acids it provides. If any one of the essential amino acids is not available in sufficient amounts or is present in excessive amounts relative to other essential amino acids, protein synthesis will not be supported. Under these circumstances, labile body proteins such as plasma albumin will be catabolized to provide the limiting amino acid so that protein synthesis may continue.

Protein from animal sources (meat, fish, dairy products, and egg white) is considered high biological value protein, or a complete protein, because all nine essential amino acids are present in these proteins. An exception to this rule is collagen-derived gelatin which is lacking in tryptophan.

Plant sources of protein (grains, legumes, nuts, and seeds) generally do not contain sufficient amounts of one or more of the essential amino acids. Thus protein synthesis can occur only to the extent that the limiting amino acids are available. These proteins are considered to have intermediate biological value, or to be partially complete because, although consumed alone, they do not meet the requirements for essential amino acids, but they can be combined to provide amounts and proportions of essential amino acids equivalent to high biological proteins from animal sources.

Plants that are entirely lacking in essential amino acids are considered incomplete proteins or sources of low biological value protein. These sources include most fruits and vegetables. A low biological value means that it is difficult or impossible to compensate for insufficient amounts of essential amino acids by combining different sources as with partially complete proteins.

Deficiency

If protein needs are not adequately met by dietary sources, an imbalance may develop. This imbalance is reflected by levels of urinary nitrogen which exceed the amounts being consumed from dietary protein. This increase in urinary nitrogen is due to the catabolism of visceral proteins and lean body mass to provide the essential amino acids that are not available in adequate amounts from dietary sources.

Negative nitrogen balance may result from consumption of insufficient quantity of high biological protein, consumption of poor quality dietary protein of any quantity, or consumption of intermediate quality protein sources that are not appropriately mixed because the quantities of essential amino acids consumed will not be sufficient to support demand for synthesis of vital proteins. In addition to appropriate quantity and quality of protein consumed, sufficient energy must also be consumed to support protein metabolism or negative nitrogen balance will develop regardless of the quality or quantity of protein consumed.

Protein malnutrition, or kwashiorkor, is the clinical consequence of uncorrected negative nitrogen balance. Protein deficiencies rarely occur when energy intake is adequate except in impoverished areas where adequate quality or quantity of protein is not consumed due to high costs of protein sources. The most common cause of protein deficiency is insufficient energy intake, which is exacerbated when demand for both protein and energy is high. Protein-energy malnutrition (PEM), or marasmus, may develop clinically from malabsorption syndrome, with excessive protein losses from burns, wound exudates, or fistula drainage, or with losses in urine from renal disease. Risk of PEM is also increased under conditions of metabolic stress such as infection, trauma, burns, acquired immunodeficiency syndrome (AIDS),

Table 4.1. Classification of Amino Acids

Essential Amino Acids	Nonessential Amino Acids
1. Histidine	1. Alanine
2. Isoleucine	2. Arginine*
3. Leucine	3. Aspartic acid
4. Lysine	4. Cysteine*
5. Methionine	5. Cystine
6. Phenylalanine	6. Glutamic acid
7. Threonine	7. Glutamine*
8. Tryptophan	8. Glycine
9. Valine	9. Proline
	10. Serine
	11. Tyrosine

*These amino acids, along with taurine, may be considered conditionally essential in that their requirements are increased during periods of catabolic stress.

and surgery, where high levels of catabolic hormones increase protein catabolism. Clinical features of PEM include weight loss, diarrhea, loss of lean body mass, muscle weakness, depigmented hair and skin, pressure sores, and depressed immune function.

Toxicity

Dietary protein consumed in excess of requirements is not stored, but is deaminated followed by oxidation of the carbon skeleton through pathways of glucose or fat metabolism, or its storage as glycogen or fat, depending upon the specific amino acid and the energy balance at the time. The nitrogen waste generated is excreted in the urine as either urea or ammonia.

High protein intakes can increase urinary calcium excretion, but the effect on calcium balance is controversial since amino acids also increase the efficiency of intestinal absorption. Other health effects of high protein intakes are less clear including the relationship of long-term high protein intakes to risk of renal disease or of diabetic nephropathy.

The effect of exercise on protein requirements is not as much as commonly believed. Endurance athletes actually have a higher requirement than body-builders due to catabolic losses of lean body mass following aerobic exercise. Nevertheless, this increased requirement can be readily met without supplementation when the high energy intakes required by athletes are consumed. Use of amino acid supplements may actually interfere with synthesis of body protein by creating imbalances. Since amino acids compete for absorption, presentation of large quantities of free amino acids to the intestinal mucosal surface reduces the amount that can be absorbed from the available supply.

Requirements

Approximately 10–15% of total daily energy intake should be consumed as protein. Protein needs for sedentary adults average about 50 grams. Growth, pregnancy, lactation, and exercise increase protein needs as indicated in Table 4.2.

Dietary Sources of Protein

Meat, poultry, and fish are rich sources of high biological value protein. Plant sources of protein (legumes, nuts, and seeds) contribute additional amounts of protein.

Meat and Beans: Tips for Making Wise Choices

Go Lean with Protein

Start with a lean choice:

* The leanest beef cuts include: round steaks, roasts (round eye, top round, bottom round, round tip) top loin, top sirloin, and chuck, shoulder, and arm roasts.

Table 4.2. Protein Requirements

Infants (0–6 months) grams/pound (g/lb)	1.0
Infants (6–12 months) g/lb	0.72
Children (1–3 years) g/lb	0.55
Children (4–6 years) g/lb	0.50
Children (7–10 years) g/lb	0.45
Adolescence (11–14 years)	
total g/day females	46
total g/day males	45
Adolescence (15–18 years)	
total g/day females	44
total g/day males	59
Young adults (19–24 years)	
total g/day females	46
total g/day males	58
Pregnancy total g/day	60
Lactation total g/day	65
Sedentary Adult g/lb	0.4
Recreational Activity g/lb	0.5–0.75
Competitive Athletics g/lb	0.6–0.9
Muscle Building g/lb	0.7–0.9
Maximum Usable Amount	
Adults g/lb	1.0

References:

Mahan, L.K. and Escott-Stump, S. *Krause's Food, Nutrition & Diet Therapy,* 10th ed., 2000.

Rosenbloom, Christine. *Sports Nutrition. A Guide for Working Professionals,* 3rd ed., 2000.

- The leanest pork choices include pork loin, tenderloin, center loin, and ham.

- Choose extra lean ground beef. The label should say at least 90% lean. You may be able to find ground beef that is 93% or 95% lean.

- Buy skinless chicken parts, or take off the skin before cooking.

- Boneless, skinless chicken breasts and turkey cutlets are the leanest poultry choices.

- Choose lean turkey, roast beef, ham, or low-fat luncheon meats for sandwiches instead of luncheon meats with more fat such as regular bologna or salami.

Keep it lean:

- Trim away all of the visible fat from meats and poultry before cooking.

- Broil, grill, roast, poach, or boil meat, poultry, or fish, instead of frying.

- Drain off any fat that appears during cooking.

- Skip or limit the breading on meat, poultry, or fish. Breading adds fat and calories. It will also cause the food to soak up more fat during frying.

- Prepare dry beans and peas without added fats.

- Choose and prepare foods without high fat sauces or gravies.

Vary Your Protein Choices

Choose fish more often for lunch or dinner. Look for fish rich in omega-3 fatty acids, such as salmon, trout, and herring. Some ideas include these dishes:

- Salmon steak or filet
- Salmon loaf
- Grilled or baked trout

Choose dry beans or peas as a main dish or part of a meal often. The following examples are some possible choices:

- Chili with kidney or pinto beans

Table 4.3. Dietary Sources of Protein

Food	Protein (grams)
Dairy	
Skim milk, 1 cup	8.3
Whole milk, 1 cup	8.0
Ice cream, regular, 1 cup	5.0
Yogurt, low-fat, 1 cup	10.7
Cottage cheese, 1% fat, 1 cup	28.0
American cheese, 1 oz	7.0
Egg, 1 large	6.3
Meat Substitutes	
Tofu, 3 oz	6.9
Veggie burger, 3 oz	25.7
Peanut butter, 2 Tbsp	8.1
Almonds, 1 oz	5.4
Sesame seeds, 1 oz	7.5
Black beans, ½ cup	7.5
Pinto beans, ½ cup	7.0
Garbanzo beans, ½ cup	7.3
Fish, Meat, and Poultry	
Tuna, 3 oz drained	21.7
Salmon, 3 oz cooked	16.8
Ground beef, 3 oz, cooked	25.7
Beef, round steak, 3 oz cooked	27.0
Pork chop, 3 oz cooked	24.5
Ham, 1 oz	5.9
Chicken breast, 3 oz	18.9
Chicken, dark meat, 3 oz	23.6
Turkey breast, 3 oz	25.7
Turkey, dark meat, 3 oz	24.3
Fruits	
Banana, 1 medium	1.2
Apple, large	0
Orange, large	1.7
Vegetables	
Corn, cooked, ½ cup	2.2
Carrots, cooked, ½ cup	0.8
Green beans, cooked, ½ cup	1.0
Green peas, cooked, ½ cup	4.1
Potatoes, white, ½ cup	1.2

- Stir-fried tofu
- Split pea, lentil, minestrone, or white bean soups
- Baked beans
- Black bean enchiladas
- Garbanzo or kidney beans on a chef's salad
- Rice and beans
- Veggie burgers or garden burgers
- Hummus (chickpeas) spread on pita bread

Choose nuts as a snack, on salads, or in main dishes. Use nuts to replace meat or poultry, not in addition to these items:

- Use pine nuts in pesto sauce for pasta.
- Add slivered almonds to steamed vegetables.
- Add toasted peanuts or cashews to a vegetable stir fry instead of meat.
- Sprinkle a few nuts on top of low-fat ice cream or frozen yogurt.
- Add walnuts or pecans to a green salad instead of cheese or meat.

What to Look for on the Food Label

- Check the Nutrition Facts label for the saturated fat, trans fat, cholesterol, and sodium content of packaged foods.
- Processed meats such as hams, sausages, frankfurters, and luncheon or deli meats have added sodium. Check the ingredient and Nutrition Facts label to help limit sodium intake.
- Fresh chicken, turkey, and pork that have been enhanced with a salt-containing solution also have added sodium. Check the product label for statements such as "self-basting" or "contains up to __% of __."
- Lower fat versions of many processed meats are available. Look on the Nutrition Facts label to choose products with less fat and saturated fat.

Keep It Safe to Eat

- Separate raw, cooked, and ready-to-eat foods.

- Do not wash or rinse meat or poultry.

- Wash cutting boards, knives, utensils, and counter tops in hot soapy water after preparing each food item and before going on to the next one.

- Store raw meat, poultry, and seafood on the bottom shelf of the refrigerator so juices do not drip onto other foods.

- Cook foods to a safe temperature to kill microorganisms. Use a meat thermometer, which measures the internal temperature of cooked meat and poultry, to make sure that the meat is cooked all the way through.

- Chill (refrigerate) perishable food promptly and defrost foods properly. Refrigerate or freeze perishables, prepared food, and leftovers within two hours.

- Plan ahead to defrost foods. Never defrost food on the kitchen counter at room temperature. Thaw food by placing it in the refrigerator, submerging air-tight packaged food in cold tap water, or defrosting on a plate in the microwave.

- Avoid raw or partially cooked eggs, foods containing raw eggs, and raw or undercooked meat and poultry.

- Women who may become pregnant, pregnant women, nursing mothers, and young children should avoid some types of fish and eat types lower in mercury.

Chapter 5

Calcium: Sources, Consumption, and Absorption

Calcium: What Is It?

Calcium, the most abundant mineral in the human body, has several important functions. More than 99% of total body calcium is stored in the bones and teeth where it functions to support their structure. The remaining 1% is found throughout the body in blood, muscle, and the fluid between cells. Calcium is needed for muscle contraction, blood vessel contraction and expansion, the secretion of hormones and enzymes, and sending messages through the nervous system. A constant level of calcium is maintained in body fluid and tissues so that these vital body processes function efficiently.

Bone undergoes continuous remodeling, with constant resorption (breakdown of bone) and deposition of calcium into newly deposited bone (bone formation). The balance between bone resorption and deposition changes as people age. During childhood there is a higher amount of bone formation and less breakdown. In early and middle adulthood, these processes are relatively equal. In aging adults, particularly among postmenopausal women, bone breakdown exceeds its formation, resulting in bone loss, which increases the risk for osteoporosis (a disorder characterized by porous, weak bones).

Excerpts from "Dietary Supplement Fact Sheet: Calcium," National Institutes of Health–Office of Dietary Supplements, updated April 27, 2005; and "Milk: Tips to Help You Make Wise Choices," U.S. Department of Agriculture (USDA), April 5, 2005.

What is the recommended intake for calcium?

Recommendations for calcium are provided in the Dietary Reference Intake (DRI) developed by the Institute of Medicine (IOM) of the National Academy of Sciences. Dietary Reference Intake (DRI) is the general term for a set of reference values used for planning and assessing nutrient intakes of healthy people. Three important types of reference values included in the DRI are Recommended Dietary Allowance (RDA), Adequate Intake (AI), and Tolerable Upper Intake Level (UL). The RDA recommends the average daily intake that is sufficient to meet the nutrient requirements of nearly all (97–98%) healthy individuals in each age and gender group. An AI is set when there is insufficient scientific data available to establish a RDA. AI meets or exceeds the amount needed to maintain a nutritional state of adequacy in nearly all members of a specific age and gender group. The UL, on the other hand, is the maximum daily intake unlikely to result in adverse effects.

For calcium, the recommended intake is listed as an Adequate Intake (AI), which is a recommended average intake level based on observed or experimentally determined levels. Table 5.1 contains the current recommendations for calcium for infants, children, and adults.

Many Americans are not meeting their recommended intake for calcium including the following groups:

- 44% boys and 58% girls ages 6–11
- 64% boys and 87% girls ages 12–19
- 55% men and 78% of women ages 20+

Table 5.1. Recommended Adequate Intake by the IOM for Calcium

Male and Female Age	Calcium (milligrams/day)	Pregnancy and Lactation
0 to 6 months	210	N/A
7 to 12 months	270	N/A
1 to 3 years	500	N/A
4 to 8 years	800	N/A
9 to 13 years	1300	N/A
14 to 18 years	1300	1300
19 to 50 years	1000	1000
51+ years	1200	N/A

What foods provide calcium?

In the United States (U.S.), milk, yogurt, and cheese are the major contributors of calcium in the typical diet. The inadequate intake of dairy foods may explain why some Americans are deficient in calcium since dairy foods are the major source of calcium in the diet. The U.S. Department of Agriculture's Food Guide Pyramid recommends that individuals two years and older eat 2–3 servings of dairy products per day. A serving is equal to these amounts:

- 1 cup (8 fl oz) of milk
- 8 oz of yogurt
- 1.5 oz of natural cheese (such as Cheddar)
- 2.0 oz of processed cheese (such as American)

A variety of non-fat and reduced fat dairy products that contain the same amount of calcium as regular dairy products are available in the U.S. today for individuals concerned about saturated fat content from regular dairy products.

Although dairy products are the main source of calcium in the U.S. diet, other foods also contribute to overall calcium intake. Individuals with lactose intolerance (those who experience symptoms such as bloating and diarrhea because they cannot completely digest the milk sugar lactose) and those who are vegan (people who consume no animal products) tend to avoid or completely eliminate dairy products from their diets. Thus, it is important for these individuals to meet their calcium needs with alternative calcium sources. Foods such as Chinese cabbage, kale, and broccoli are other alternative calcium sources. Although most grains are not high in calcium (unless fortified), they do contribute calcium to the diet because they are consumed frequently. Additionally, there are several calcium-fortified food sources presently available, including fruit juices, fruit drinks, tofu, and cereals.

Portion sizes of various foods provide the same amount of calcium in one cup of milk. Calcium absorption varies among foods. Certain plant-based foods such as some vegetables contain substances which can reduce calcium absorption. Calcium content of 8 fluid ounces of milk is equal to the following amounts:

- 1 cup of yogurt
- 1½ ounces of Cheddar cheese
- 1½ cups of cooked kale

- 2¼ cups of cooked broccoli
- 8 cups of cooked spinach

What affects calcium absorption and excretion?

Calcium absorption refers to the amount of calcium that is absorbed from the digestive tract into our body's circulation. Calcium absorption can be affected by the calcium status of the body, vitamin D status, age, pregnancy, and plant substances in the diet. The amount of calcium consumed at one time such as in a meal can also affect absorption. For example, the efficiency of calcium absorption decreases as the amount of calcium consumed at a meal increases.

- **Age:** Net calcium absorption can be as high as 60% in infants and young children, when the body needs calcium to build strong bones. Absorption slowly decreases to 15–20% in adulthood and even more as one ages. Because calcium absorption declines with age, recommendations for dietary intake of calcium are higher for adults ages 51 and over.

- **Vitamin D:** Vitamin D helps improve calcium absorption. Your body can obtain vitamin D from food and it can also make vitamin D when your skin is exposed to sunlight. Thus, adequate vitamin D intake from food and sun exposure is essential to bone health.

- **Pregnancy:** Current calcium recommendations for non-pregnant women are also sufficient for pregnant women because intestinal calcium absorption increases during pregnancy. For this reason, the calcium recommendations established for pregnant women are not different than the recommendations for women who are not pregnant.

- **Plant substances:** Phytic acid and oxalic acid, which are found naturally in some plants, may bind to calcium and prevent it from being absorbed optimally. These substances affect the absorption of calcium from the plant itself, not the calcium found in other calcium-containing foods eaten at the same time. Examples of foods high in oxalic acid are spinach, collard greens, sweet potatoes, rhubarb, and beans. Foods high in phytic acid include whole grain bread, beans, seeds, nuts, grains, and soy isolates. Although soybeans are high in phytic acid, the calcium present in soybeans is still partially absorbed. Fiber, particularly from wheat bran, could also prevent calcium absorption because of its content of phytate. However, the effect of fiber on calcium absorption is

Table 5.2. Selected Food Sources of Calcium

Food	Calcium (mg)	Percent Daily Value (%DV)
Yogurt, plain, low fat, 8 oz.	415	42%
Yogurt, fruit, low fat, 8 oz.	245–384	25%–38%
Sardines, canned in oil, with bones, 3 oz.	324	32%
Cheddar cheese, 1½ oz., shredded	306	31%
Milk, non-fat, 8 fl oz.	302	30%
Milk, reduced fat (2% milk fat), no solids, 8 fl oz.	297	30%
Milk, whole (3.25% milk fat), 8 fl oz.	291	29%
Milk, buttermilk, 8 fl oz.	285	29%
Milk, lactose reduced, 8 fl oz.*	285–302	29%–30%
Mozzarella, part skim 1½ oz.	275	28%
Tofu, firm, made w/calcium sulfate, ½ cup**	204	20%
Orange juice, calcium fortified, 6 fl oz.	200–260	20%–26%
Salmon, pink, canned, solids with bone, 3 oz.	181	18%
Pudding, chocolate, instant, made with 2% milk, ½ cup	153	15%
Cottage cheese, 1% milk fat, 1 cup unpacked	138	14%
Tofu, soft, made w/calcium sulfate, ½ cup**	138	14%
Spinach, cooked, ½ cup	120	12%
Instant breakfast drink, various flavors and brands, powder prepared with water, 8 fl oz.	105–250	10%–25%
Frozen yogurt, vanilla, soft serve, ½ cup	103	10%
Ready to eat cereal, calcium fortified, 1 cup	100–1000	10%–100%
Turnip greens, boiled, ½ cup	99	10%
Kale, cooked, 1 cup	94	9%
Kale, raw, 1 cup	90	9%
Ice cream, vanilla, ½ cup	85	8.5%
Soy beverage, calcium fortified, 8 fl oz.	80–500	8–50%
Chinese cabbage, raw, 1 cup	74	7%
Tortilla, corn, ready to bake/fry, 1 medium	42	4%
Tortilla, flour, ready to bake/fry, one 6" diameter	37	4%
Sour cream, reduced fat, cultured, 2 Tbsp	32	3%
Bread, white, 1 oz.	31	3%
Broccoli, raw, ½ cup	21	2%
Bread, whole wheat, 1 slice	20	2%
Cheese, cream, regular, 1 Tbsp	12	1%

*Content varies slightly according to fat content; average =300 mg calcium

**Calcium values are only for tofu processed with a calcium salt. Tofu processed with a non-calcium salt will not contain significant amounts of calcium.

more of a concern for individuals with low calcium intakes. The average American tends to consume much less fiber per day than the level that would be needed to affect calcium absorption.

Calcium excretion refers to the amount of calcium eliminated from the body in urine, feces, and sweat. Calcium excretion can be affected by many factors including dietary sodium, protein, caffeine, and potassium.

- **Sodium and protein:** Typically, dietary sodium and protein increase calcium excretion as the amount of their intake is increased. However, if a high protein, high sodium food also contains calcium, this may help counteract the loss of calcium.

- **Potassium:** Increasing dietary potassium intake (such as from 7–8 servings of fruits and vegetables per day) in the presence of a high sodium diet (greater than 5100 mg/day, which is more than twice the Tolerable Upper Intake Level of 2300 mg for sodium per day) may help decrease calcium excretion particularly in postmenopausal women.

- **Caffeine:** Caffeine has a small effect on calcium absorption. It can temporarily increase calcium excretion and may modestly decrease calcium absorption, an effect easily offset by increasing calcium consumption in the diet. One cup of regular, brewed coffee causes a loss of only 2–3 mg of calcium easily offset by adding a tablespoon of milk. Moderate caffeine consumption, (1 cup of coffee or 2 cups of tea per day), in young women who have adequate calcium intakes has little to no negative effects on their bones.

- **Phosphorus:** The effect of dietary phosphorus on calcium is minimal. Some researchers speculate that the detrimental effects of consuming foods high in phosphate, such as carbonated soft drinks, is due to the replacement of milk with soda rather than the phosphate level itself.

- **Alcohol:** Alcohol can affect calcium status by reducing the intestinal absorption of calcium. It can also inhibit enzymes in the liver that help convert vitamin D to its active form which in turn reduces calcium absorption. However, the amount of alcohol required to affect calcium absorption is unknown. Evidence is currently conflicting whether moderate alcohol consumption is helpful or harmful to bone.

When can a calcium deficiency occur?

Inadequate calcium intake, decreased calcium absorption, and increased calcium loss in urine can decrease total calcium in the body, with the potential of producing osteoporosis and the other consequences of chronically low calcium intake. If an individual does not consume enough dietary calcium or experiences rapid losses of calcium from the body, calcium is withdrawn from their bones in order to maintain calcium levels in the blood.

Mineral oil and stimulant laxatives can both decrease dietary calcium absorption. Furthermore, glucocorticoids (for example: prednisone) can cause calcium depletion and eventually osteoporosis when used for more than a few weeks.

Who may need extra calcium to prevent a deficiency?

Post-Menopausal Women: Menopause often leads to increases in bone loss with the most rapid rates of bone loss occurring during the first five years after menopause.

Amenorrheic Women and the Female Athlete Triad: Amenorrhea results from decreases in circulating estrogen, which then negatively affect calcium balance. Studies comparing healthy women with normal menstrual cycles to amenorrheic women with anorexia nervosa (a type of disordered eating) found decreased levels of calcium absorption, a higher urinary calcium excretion, and a lower rate of bone formation in women with anorexia.

The condition "female athlete triad" refers to the combination of disordered eating, amenorrhea, and osteoporosis. Exercise-induced amenorrhea has been shown to result in decreases in bone mass. In female athletes, low bone mineral density, menstrual irregularities, dietary factors, and a history of prior stress fractures are associated with an increased risk of future stress fractures.

Lactose Intolerant Individuals: Lactose maldigestion (or lactase non-persistence) describes the inability of an individual to completely digest lactose, the naturally occurring sugar in milk. Lactose intolerance refers to the symptoms that occur when the amount of lactose exceeds the ability of an individual's digestive tract to break down lactose. In the U.S., approximately 25% of all adults have a limited ability to digest lactose.

Symptoms of lactose intolerance include bloating, flatulence, and diarrhea after consuming large amounts of lactose (such as the amount in 1 quart of milk). Individuals who experience lactose maldigestion may be at risk for calcium deficiency, not due to an inability to absorb calcium, but rather from the avoidance of dairy products.

If an individual experiences lactose maldigestion and chooses to avoid dairy products, it is important for them to include non-dairy sources of calcium in their daily diet or consider taking a calcium supplement to help meet their recommended calcium needs.

Vegetarians: There are several types of vegetarian eating practices. Calcium absorption may be reduced in vegetarians because they eat more plant foods containing oxalic and phytic acids, compounds which interfere with calcium absorption. However, vegetarian diets that contain less protein may reduce calcium excretion. Yet, vegans may be at increased risk for inadequate intake of calcium because of their lack of consumption of dairy products. Therefore, it is important for vegans to include adequate amounts of non-dairy sources of calcium in their daily diet, or consider taking a calcium supplement to meet their recommended calcium intake. Furthermore, while early studies found vegetarian diets to be beneficial for bone health, more recent studies have found no benefits or even the opposite effect.

Is there a health risk of too much calcium?

The Tolerable Upper Limit (UL) is the highest level of daily intake of calcium from food, water, and supplements that is likely to pose no risks of adverse health effects to almost all individuals in the general population. The UL for children and adults ages 1 year and older (including pregnant and lactating women) is 2500 mg/day. It was not possible to establish a UL for infants under the age of 1 year.

While low intakes of calcium can result in deficiency and undesirable health conditions, excessively high intakes of calcium can also have adverse effects. Adverse conditions associated with high calcium intakes are hypercalcemia (elevated levels of calcium in the blood), impaired kidney function, and decreased absorption of other minerals. Another concern with high calcium intakes is the potential for calcium to interfere with the absorption of other minerals, iron, zinc, magnesium, and phosphorus.

Most Americans should consider their intake of calcium from all foods including fortified ones before adding supplements to their diet to help avoid the risk of reaching levels at or near the UL for calcium (2500 mg). If you need additional assistance regarding your calcium needs, consider checking with a physician or registered dietitian.

Milk: Tips for Making Wise Choices

- Include milk as a beverage at meals. Choose fat-free or low-fat milk.

- If you usually drink whole milk, switch gradually to fat-free milk, to lower saturated fat and calories. Try milk that is reduced fat (2%), then low-fat (1%), and finally fat-free (skim).

- If you drink cappuccinos or lattes—ask for them with fat-free (skim) milk.

- Add fat-free or low-fat milk instead of water to oatmeal and hot cereals.

- Use fat-free or low-fat milk when making condensed cream soups (such as cream of tomato).

- Have fat-free or low-fat yogurt as a snack.

- Make a dip for fruits or vegetables from yogurt.

- Make fruit and yogurt smoothies in the blender.

- For dessert, make chocolate or butterscotch pudding with fat-free or low-fat milk.

- Top fruit with flavored yogurt for a quick dessert.

- Top casseroles, soups, stews, or vegetables with shredded low-fat cheese.

- Top a baked potato with fat-free or low-fat yogurt.

Here are some tips for those who choose not to consume milk products:

- If you avoid milk because of lactose intolerance, the most reliable way to get the health benefits of milk is to choose lactose-free alternatives within the milk group, such as cheese, yogurt, or lactose-free milk, or to consume the enzyme lactase before consuming milk products.

- Calcium choices for those who do not consume milk products include:

  - Calcium fortified juices, cereals, breads, soy beverages, or rice beverages.

  - Canned fish (sardines, salmon with bones), soybeans and other soy products (soy-based beverages, soy yogurt, tempeh), some other dried beans, and some leafy greens (collard and turnip greens, kale, or bok choy). The amount of calcium that can be absorbed from these foods varies.

Chapter 6

Carbohydrates: What They Are and Why We Need Them

The Skinny on Carbohydrates

For too many Americans, carbohydrates—or carbs—have become something to avoid in the daily diet. But as nutrition experts know, carbohydrate is an essential macronutrient that provides fuel for the brain and muscles and contains the fiber needed for proper gut function. Moreover, many foods primarily composed of carbohydrates have been demonstrated through numerous scientific studies to lower the risk for certain cancers, stroke, heart disease, and high blood pressure. In addition, these foods play an important role in the control of body weight, especially when combined with exercise, which is why the leading medical and nutrition authorities recommend weight loss programs that are rich in foods containing carbohydrate, such as from whole grains, fruits, vegetables, and low-fat dairy products.

What exactly are carbohydrates, where are they found and why do our bodies need them? This chapter provides an explanation of this essential macronutrient and its role in the functioning of the body and in improved health.

This chapter includes: "The Skinny on Carbohydrates," reprinted with permission from http://www.essentialnutrition.org. © 2004 The Partnership for Essential Nutrition. Also, excerpts from "Carbohydrates," from *Dietary Guidelines for Americans 2005*, U.S. Department of Health and Human Services (HHS) and U.S. Department of Agriculture (USDA); and an excerpt titled, "Nomenclature for Carbohydrates," from *Report of the Dietary Guidelines Advisory Committee on the Dietary Guidelines for Americans, 2005*, HHS and USDA.

What Are Carbohydrates?

Carbohydrates are in a wide variety of foods and are one of the three major macronutrients that supply the body with energy—fat and protein being the others. But unlike fat and protein, carbohydrates are efficiently converted into glucose, which is used directly by the muscles and brain. That is why the Institute of Medicine (IOM), part of the National Academy of Sciences, recently issued a recommendation that children and adults get a minimum of 130 grams of carbohydrate a day to maintain maximum brain function.[1] This amount is more than six times what the initial phase of the Atkins Diet allows (20 grams of carbohydrate a day).

Besides being the most easily accessible energy source for muscles and organs of the body, carbohydrates play an important role in the construction and maintenance of the body's tissues, organs, and cells including nerve cells. At the same time, carbohydrates are found in a wide range of foods that bring a variety of other important nutrients to the diet, such as vitamins and minerals, phytochemicals, antioxidants, and dietary fiber. A diet high in these nutrients has been associated with a lower risk for certain cancers, cardiovascular disease, stroke, and diabetes.

Carbohydrates are grouped into two main categories: 1) simple carbohydrates, which contain simple sugars, such as glucose and fructose, found in fruits, berries, some vegetables, table sugar and honey; and 2) complex carbohydrates, found in many plant-based foods, whole grains, and low-fat dairy products. For optimal health, nutrition and public health authorities recommend consuming a wide range of carbohydrate-containing foods with an emphasis on fruits, vegetables, whole grains, and low-fat dairy products. For both weight control and good health, experts advise caution in over-consuming processed foods where sugar is added, such as soft drinks, pastries, and other sweets.

Carbohydrates and Improved Health

There have been major advances in the understanding of how carbohydrates influence nutrition and promote better health. Of special significance is the role that carbohydrates play in gut function, disease prevention, and body weight regulation.

Because many carbohydrates contain dietary fiber, one of the most important benefits of eating carbohydrates is the health effects associated with consuming fiber-rich foods. Commonly called roughage, fiber is an indigestible complex carbohydrate found in plants and has no calories because the body cannot absorb it. Fiber-containing carbohydrates come in two forms—water-insoluble and water-soluble—based on their physical characteristics and effects on the body. Each form functions differently and provides different health benefits.

Although most consumers just associate fiber with preventing constipation, a high fiber diet has been linked with a lower risk of heart disease in a large number of studies that have followed people for many years. In a Harvard study of more than 40,000 male health professionals, researchers found that a high fiber intake reduced the risk of coronary heart disease by 40 percent, compared to a low fiber intake.[2] Fiber has also been linked with a reduced risk of diabetes, diverticular disease, and may be protective against colon cancer.[3] Moreover, fibers called cellulose and hemicelluloses take up space in the gastrointestinal (GI) tract without yielding calories, promoting the feeling of fullness, which is helpful to those watching their weight.

Carbohydrates prevent disease in other ways besides being the sole source of fiber. Packaged along with fiber in fruits and vegetables—which are primarily carbohydrates—they are rich in antioxidants and contain a number of phytochemicals that have been linked to a lower risk of certain cancers, stroke, heart disease, and high blood pressure.[4] Based on an extensive review of more than 4,500 research studies around the world, in 1997, the American Institute for Cancer Research (AICR) and the World Cancer Research Fund issued the expert report, *Food, Nutrition and the Prevention of Cancer: a global perspective*, which concluded that, "a simple change, such as eating the recommended five servings of fruit and vegetables each day, could by itself reduce cancer rates more than 20 percent."[5] According to the research conducted to date, carotenoids and other antioxidants and various phytochemicals that are packaged in carbohydrate-containing foods are key players in reducing cancer risk, and more likely, it is the combination of these compounds that confer protection.

Besides protecting against cancer, researchers have also found that diets rich in fruits and vegetables can lower the risk of heart disease and stroke. One large Harvard study of both men and women found that those who ate eight or more servings of fruits and vegetables a day had a 20 percent lower risk of heart disease than those who ate fewer than three servings daily.[6] Another Harvard study of nearly 80,000 women and 40,000 men found that people who ate five servings of fruits and vegetables a day had a 30 percent lower risk of ischemic stroke, the most common type of stroke.[7]

The other important health benefit associated with carbohydrates is regulating body weight, an area of research that seems to have gotten lost in the low carbohydrate craze. According to the recent report from the World Health Organization (WHO) and the Food and Agriculture Organization of the United Nations, *Carbohydrates in Human Nutrition*, people eating a diet high in fruits, vegetables, whole grains, and low-fat dairy products are less likely to accumulate body fat than those following a low carbohydrate, high fat diet.[8] The WHO report lists three possible reasons:

- High carbohydrate diets have lower energy density than their counterparts, meaning that carbohydrates have less calories weight for weight than fat.

- Studies have found that both in the form of starch and sugars, carbohydrates aid satiety, which leads people to eat less.

- Research also shows that very little dietary carbohydrate is converted to body fat mainly because it is a less efficient process for the body. Instead, most carbohydrates are burnt for fuel while the fiber in carbohydrate foods is not digested at all.

How Much Do We Need?

Recognizing the many health benefits associated with carbohydrates—and especially diets rich in fruits, vegetables, whole grains, and low-fat dairy foods—the Dietary Reference Intakes Report issued by the Institute of Medicine in 2002 recommended that Americans get the majority of their calories a day from carbohydrates.[9] Specifically, the IOM report states that:

- adults should get 45 percent to 65 percent of their calories from carbohydrates, 20 percent to 35 percent from fat, and 10 percent to 25 percent from protein.

- the minimum amount of carbohydrate that children and adults need for proper brain function is 130 grams a day.

- added sugars should comprise no more than 25 percent of total calories consumed. The IOM report was designed for normal weight individuals; overweight people need far less.

- for adults 50 years and younger, the recommended total intake for dietary fiber is 38 grams for men and 25 grams for women. For those over 50, it is 30 grams and 21 grams respectively.

Summing It Up

For maintaining good health and weight control, nutrition and public health authorities agree that the bulk of a person's calories should come from carbohydrates, especially from fruits, vegetables, whole grains, and low-fat dairy products. Of equal importance, experts stress the importance of variety so that people will have access to all the essential nutrients and fiber available through carbohydrate-containing foods.

References

1. Institute of Medicine; *Dietary Reference Intakes for Macronutrients*, National Academies Press, Washington DC 2002.

2. Harvard School of Public Health fact sheet on fiber, *Fiber—Start Roughing It!* Nutrition Source, 2004 President and Fellows of Harvard College.

3. *Ibid.*

4. Harvard School of Public Health fact sheet on fruits and vegetables, *Fruits and Vegetables*, Nutrition Source, 2004 President and Fellows of Harvard College.

5. WCRF/AICR; *Food, Nutrition and the Prevention of Cancer: a global perspective*, 1997; page 540.

6. Harvard School of Public Health fact sheet on fruits and vegetables, *Fruits and Vegetables*, Nutrition Source, 2004 President and Fellows of Harvard College.

7. *Ibid.*

8. FAO/WHO 1998. Carbohydrates in Human Nutrition: Report of a Joint FAO/WHO Expert Consultation, 14-18 April 1997, Rome. *FAO Food and Nutrition Paper No. 66.* Rome.

9. Institute of Medicine; *Daily Reference Intakes for Macronutrients*, National Academies Press, Washington DC, 2002.

Key Recommendations for Carbohydrate Use from Dietary Guidelines for Americans

Choose Fiber-Rich Fruits, Vegetables, and Whole Grains

- The recommended dietary fiber intake is 14 grams per 1,000 calories consumed. Initially, some Americans will find it challenging to achieve this level of intake. However, making fiber-rich food choices more often will move people toward this goal and is likely to confer significant health benefits.

- The majority of servings from the fruit group should come from whole fruit (fresh, frozen, canned, dried) rather than juice. Increasing the proportion of fruit that is eaten in the form of whole fruit rather than juice is desirable to increase fiber intake. However, inclusion of some juice, such as orange juice, can help meet recommended levels of potassium intake.

- Legumes—such as dry beans and peas—are especially rich in fiber and should be consumed several times per week. They are considered part of both the vegetable group and the meat and beans group as they contain nutrients found in each of these food groups.

- Consuming at least half the recommended grain servings as whole grains is important, for all ages, at each calorie level, to meet the fiber recommendation. Consuming at least 3 ounce-equivalents of whole grains per day can reduce the risk of coronary heart disease, may help with weight maintenance, and may lower risk for other chronic diseases. Thus, at lower calorie levels, adults should consume more than half (specifically, at least 3 ounce-equivalents) of whole grains per day, by substituting whole grains for refined grains.

Choose and Prepare Foods and Beverages with Little Added Sugars or Caloric Sweeteners

- Individuals who consume food or beverages high in added sugars tend to consume more calories than those who consume food or beverages low in added sugars; they also tend to consume lower amounts of micronutrients. Although more research is needed, available prospective studies show a positive association between the consumption of sweetened beverages and weight gain. For this reason, decreased intake of such foods, especially beverages with caloric sweeteners, is recommended to reduce calorie intake and help achieve recommended nutrient intakes and weight control.

- Total discretionary calories should not exceed the allowance for any given calorie level. The discretionary calorie allowance covers all calories from added sugars, alcohol, and the additional fat found in even moderate fat choices from the milk and meat group.

For example, the 2,000-calorie pattern includes only about 267 discretionary calories. At 29 percent of calories from total fat (including 18 g of solid fat), if no alcohol is consumed, then only 8 teaspoons (32 g) of added sugars can be afforded. This is less than the amount in a typical 12-ounce sweetened soft drink. If fat is decreased to 22 percent of calories, then 18 teaspoons (72 g) of added sugars is allowed. If fat is increased to 35 percent of calories, then no allowance remains for added sugars, even if alcohol is not consumed.

- In some cases, small amounts of sugars added to nutrient-dense foods, such as breakfast cereals and reduced-fat milk products, may increase a person's intake of such foods by enhancing the palatability of these products, thus improving nutrient intake without contributing excessive calories.

- The Nutrition Facts Panel on the food label provides the amount of total sugars but does not list added sugars separately. People should examine the ingredient list to find out whether a food contains added sugars. The ingredient list is usually located under the Nutrition Facts Panel or on the side of a food label. Ingredients are listed in order of predominance, by weight—the ingredient with the greatest contribution to the product weight is listed first and the ingredient contributing the least amount is listed last.

Practice Good Oral Hygiene and Consume Less Sugar- and Starch-Containing Foods to Reduce Incidence of Dental Caries

- Sugars and starches contribute to dental caries by providing substrate for bacterial fermentation in the mouth. Thus, the frequency and duration of consumption of starches and sugars can be important factors because they increase exposure to cariogenic substrates. Drinking fluoridated water and/or using fluoride-containing dental hygiene products help reduce the risk of dental caries. Most bottled water is not fluoridated. With the increase in consumption of bottled water, there is concern that Americans may not be getting enough fluoride for maintenance of oral health. A combined approach of reducing the frequency and duration of exposure to fermentable carbohydrate intake and optimizing oral hygiene practices, such as drinking fluoridated water and brushing and flossing teeth, is the most effective way to reduce incidence of dental caries.

Names for Added Sugars That Appear on Food Labels

Some of the names for added sugars that may be in processed foods and listed on the label ingredients list include the following:

- Brown sugar
- Invert sugar
- Corn sweetener
- Lactose
- Corn syrup
- Maltose
- Dextrose
- Malt syrup
- Fructose

- Molasses
- Fruit juice concentrates
- Raw sugar
- Glucose
- Sucrose
- High-fructose corn syrup
- Sugar
- Honey
- Syrup

Considerations for Specific Population Groups

Older Adults: Dietary fiber is important for normal digestive and bowel function. Since constipation may affect up to 20 percent of people over 65 years of age, older adults should choose to consume foods rich in dietary fiber. Other causes of constipation among this age group may include drugs and lack of appropriate hydration.

Children: Carbohydrate intakes of children need special considerations with regard to obtaining sufficient amounts of fiber, avoiding excessive amounts of calories from added sugars, and preventing dental caries. Several cross-sectional surveys on U.S. children and adolescents have found inadequate dietary fiber intakes, which could be improved by increasing consumption of whole fruits, vegetables, and whole-grain products. Sugars can improve the palatability of foods and beverages that otherwise might not be consumed. This may explain why the consumption of sweetened dairy foods and beverages and presweetened cereals is positively associated with nutrient intake of children and adolescents. However, beverages with caloric sweeteners, sugars and sweets, and other sweetened foods that provide little or no nutrients are negatively associated with diet quality and can contribute to excessive energy intakes, affirming the importance of reducing added sugar intake substantially from current levels. Most of the studies of preschool children suggest a positive association between sucrose consumption and dental caries, though other factors (particularly infrequent brushing or not using fluoridated toothpaste) are more predictive of caries outcome than is sugar consumption.

Nomenclature for Carbohydrates

The nomenclature for carbohydrates is somewhat confusing. Sugars can be one sugar unit (monosaccharides) such as glucose, fructose, and galactose; and they can be two sugar units linked together (disaccharides) such as sucrose, lactose, and maltose. A further distinction is sometimes made between intrinsic and extrinsic sugars. The term intrinsic sugar means those sugars that are naturally occurring within a food, whereas extrinsic sugars are those that are added to foods. The U.S. Department of Agriculture (USDA) has defined added sugars as sugars and syrups that are added to foods during processing or preparation, and also includes sugars and syrups added at the table. There is no difference in the molecular structure of sugar molecules, whether they are naturally occurring in the food or added to the food.

Starches are many glucose units linked together (polysaccharide). Although most starch can be broken down by human enzymes into glucose for absorption, some starch does not undergo digestion in the small intestine and is called resistant starch, which is found in plant foods such as legumes, pasta, and refrigerated cooked potatoes.

Fibers, like starches, are polysaccharides made up mostly of glucose units (in the case of cellulose) or other combinations of monosaccharides. However, the monosaccharides in fibers are bonded to each other differently than they are in starches, and human enzymes cannot break the bonds in the fibers. Thus, fibers are not absorbed from the small intestine and pass relatively intact into the large intestine, as do resistant starches.

Chapter 7

Fabulous Fruits and Versatile Vegetables

Putting the Dietary Guidelines for Americans into Practice

Fruits and vegetables are key parts of your daily diet. Everyone needs 5 to 9 daily servings of fruits and vegetables for the nutrients they contain and for general health. Nutrition and health may be reasons you eat certain fruits and vegetables, but there are many other reasons why you choose the ones you do. Perhaps it is because of taste, or physical characteristics such as crunchiness, juiciness, or bright colors. You may eat some fruits and vegetables because of fond memories—like watermelon or corn at cookouts, your mom's green bean casserole, or tomatoes your dad brought in from the backyard garden. Or you may simply like them because most are quick to prepare and easy to eat. The important thing is that you eat them and encourage children to do the same.

Fruits and vegetables give you many of the nutrients that you need: vitamins, minerals, dietary fiber, water, and healthful phytochemicals. Some are sources of vitamin A, while others are rich in vitamin C, folate, or potassium. Almost all fruits and vegetables are naturally low in fat and calories and none have cholesterol. All of these healthful

---

The information in this chapter is from the following U.S. Department of Agriculture (USDA) documents: "Fabulous Fruits and Versatile Vegetables," June 2003; "How Many Vegetables Are Needed Daily or Weekly?" 2005; "Tips to Help You Eat Vegetables," 2005; "How Much Fruit Is Needed Daily?" 2005; and "Tips to Help You Eat Fruits," 2005.

51

characteristics may protect you from getting chronic diseases, such as heart disease, stroke, and some types of cancer.

Fruits

Fruits taste great and they're bright and colorful, easy to find, and easy to prepare and eat. Fruits are available in many different forms—fresh, frozen, canned, dried, and as juice. All are good ways to get the recommended servings of fruit a day.

Vegetables

For some of us, summertime just wouldn't be the same without fresh produce. Maybe you garden or take trips to a local farmers market. Even your grocery store may have more fruit and vegetables in the summer. With vegetables, you and your family are getting delicious food and, nutritionally, you are getting many of the nutrients needed for good health vitamins, minerals, and dietary fiber.

Like fruits, vegetables are available not only fresh, but frozen, canned, dried, and as juice. You can eat them raw, steamed, boiled, stir-fried, grilled, microwaved, or baked. Aim for 3 to 5 servings of vegetables a day. Here are some ways you can jazz up vegetables to make them even more flavorful to help you eat the servings you need.

Spice it!

- Top corn or black beans with salsa or a dash of hot sauce.
- Add garlic to mashed potatoes.
- Add a dash of nutmeg to spinach dishes.

Slice it!

- Add cooked, chopped onions to cooked peas.
- Add sliced or diced vegetables to meatloaf, stews, or scrambled eggs.
- Make a grated carrot salad.

Mix it!

- Cook zucchini and stewed tomatoes together.
- Mix green beans, Italian dressing, and almonds together.
- Stir-fry broccoli with chicken or beef.

Zap it!

- Microwave broccoli and sprinkle it with Parmesan cheese.
- Microwave a sweet potato topped with ground cloves or cinnamon.
- Heat frozen, mixed vegetables for a last-minute side dish.

Choose a Variety of Fruits and Vegetables

Fruits and vegetables are available in a rainbow of colors. Try to eat a variety, including some from each of the following categories.

Dark-green/leafy: Bok choy, broccoli, collard greens, endive, kale, mustard greens, romaine, spinach, turnip greens.

Citrus and berries: Blueberries, cranberries, grapefruit, kiwi fruit, oranges, raspberries, strawberries, tangerines.

Orange/deep-yellow: Acorn squash, apricots, butternut squash, cantaloupe, carrots, mango, pumpkin, sweet potatoes.

Dry beans and peas: Adzuki beans, baked beans, black beans (turtle beans), black-eyed peas, chickpeas (garbanzo beans), cranberry beans, dark- and light-red kidney beans (Mexican beans), Great Northern beans (white beans), green and red lentils, soybeans, kidney beans, lentils, lima beans, navy beans (pea beans), pink beans, pinto beans, small red beans (Mexican red beans), split peas, Tofu (soybean curd), yellow-eyed beans.

More Choices: Apples, asparagus, avocados, bananas, bean sprouts, cabbage, cauliflower, celery, corn, cucumbers, grapes, green beans, green peas, lettuce, mushrooms, onions, papaya, peaches, pears, peppers, plums, potatoes, raisins, sprouts, tomatoes, watermelon, zucchini.

Health Benefits of Fruits and Vegetables

Fruits and vegetables differ in the nutrients they contain. To promote health, include some from each category regularly.

Citrus fruits are rich in vitamin C, but did you know that strawberries, mangoes, red peppers, and tomatoes are also sources of vitamin C? Vitamin C helps heal cuts and wounds and also keeps your gums healthy.

Carrots are good for your eyesight because carrots contain carotenoids (beta-carotene, for example) that form vitamin A—a vitamin that helps keep your eyes healthy. Broccoli, spinach, pumpkin, winter squash, and sweet potatoes are also sources of carotenoids—so are tomatoes, apricots, and cantaloupe. In addition to your eyes, vitamin A is good for your skin and also helps protect you against infections.

Research suggests that dietary fiber is important for proper bowel function by keeping us regular. But what exactly is dietary fiber? It is the part of plants that the human digestive tract cannot break down. As a result, dietary fiber keeps waste moving through our intestines. Most of us do not eat enough dietary fiber, and health experts suggest we eat more. Dry beans and peas are the best sources of fiber. There are a wide variety of these tasty foods in different sizes, shapes, flavors, and colors. Cooked, dry beans and peas are good sources of dietary fiber and protein. They are low in fat, cholesterol-free, and provide magnesium, iron, zinc, and folate. Often, Americans do not get enough of these nutrients.

In addition to dry beans and peas, many fruits and vegetables provide fiber. Be fiber smart. Some forms of a food are better sources of fiber than others. For example, a medium, raw apple with skin contains 3.6 grams of fiber, ½ cup of applesauce has 1.5 grams of fiber, and ¾ cup of apple juice has only 0.2 grams of fiber.

Table 7.1. Daily Recommendations for Vegetable Consumption

Category	Age	Amount of Vegetables
Children	2–3 years old	1 cup
	4–8 years old	1½ cups
Girls	9–13 years old	2 cups
	14–18 years old	2½ cups
Boys	9–13 years old	2½ cups
	14–18 years old	3 cups
Women	19–30 years old	2½ cups
	31–50 years old	2½ cups
	51+ years old	2 cups
Men	19–30 years old	3 cups
	31–50 years old	3 cups
	51+ years old	2½ cups

Note: These amounts are appropriate for individuals who get less than 30 minutes per day of moderate physical activity, beyond normal daily activities. Those who are more physically active may be able to consume more while staying within calorie needs.

Source: USDA 2005.

Tips to Help You Eat Vegetables

General Information

- Buy fresh vegetables in season. They cost less and are likely to be at their peak flavor.

- Stock up on frozen vegetables for quick and easy cooking in the microwave.

- Buy vegetables that are easy to prepare. Purchase pre-washed bags of salad greens and add baby carrots or grape tomatoes for a salad in minutes. Buy packages of baby carrots or celery sticks for quick snacks.

- Use a microwave to prepare vegetables. White or sweet potatoes can be baked quickly this way.

- Vary veggie choices to keep meals interesting.

- Try crunchy vegetables, raw or lightly steamed.

Nutritional Value

- Select potassium-rich vegetables often, such as sweet potatoes, white potatoes, white beans, tomato products (paste, sauce, and juice), beet greens, soybeans, lima beans, winter squash, spinach, lentils, kidney beans, and split peas.

- Sauces or seasonings can add calories, fat, and sodium to vegetables. Use the Nutrition Facts label to compare the calories and % Daily Value for fat and sodium in plain and seasoned vegetables.

- Prepare more foods from fresh ingredients to lower sodium intake. Most sodium in the food supply comes from packaged or processed foods.

- Buy canned vegetables labeled "no salt added." If you want to add a little salt, it will likely be less than the amount in the regular canned product.

Vegetables with Meals

- Plan some meals around a vegetable main dish, such as a vegetable stir-fry or soup. Then add other foods to complement it.

- Try a main dish salad for lunch. Go light on the salad dressing.

- Include a green salad with your dinner every night.

- Shred carrots or zucchini into meatloaf, casseroles, quick breads, and muffins.

- Include chopped vegetables in pasta sauce or lasagna.

- Order a veggie pizza with toppings like mushrooms, green peppers, or onions, and ask for extra veggies.

- Use pureed, cooked vegetables such as potatoes to thicken stews, soups, and gravies. These add flavor, nutrients, and texture.

- Grill vegetable kabobs as part of a barbecue meal. Try tomatoes, mushrooms, green peppers, and onions.

Make Vegetables Appealing

- Many vegetables taste great with a dip or dressing. Try a low-fat salad dressing with raw broccoli, red and green peppers, celery sticks, and cauliflower.

- Add color to salads by adding baby carrots, shredded red cabbage, or spinach leaves. Include seasonal vegetables for variety throughout the year.

- Include cooked dry beans or peas in flavorful mixed dishes, such as chili or minestrone soup.

- Decorate plates or serving dishes with vegetable slices.

- Keep a bowl of cut-up vegetables in a see-through container in the refrigerator. Carrot and celery sticks are traditional, but consider broccoli florets, cucumber slices, or red or green pepper strips.

Vegetable Tips for Children

- Set a good example for children by eating vegetables with meals and as snacks.

- Let children decide on the dinner vegetables or what goes into salads.

- Depending on their age, children can help select, clean, peel, or cut vegetables.

- When shopping, allow children to pick a new vegetable to try.

- Use cut vegetables as part of afternoon snacks.

- Children often prefer foods served separately. So, rather than mixed vegetables, try serving two vegetables separately.

Keep It Safe

- Wash vegetables before preparing or eating them. Under clean, running water, rub vegetables briskly with your hands to remove dirt and surface microorganisms. Dry after washing.

- Keep vegetables separate from raw meat, poultry, and seafood while shopping, preparing, or storing.

Tips to Help You Eat Fruits

General Tips

- Keep a bowl of whole fruit on the table, counter, or in the refrigerator.

- Refrigerate cut fruit for later use.

Table 7.2. Daily Recommendations for Fruit Consumption

Category	Age	Amount of Fruit
Children	2–3 years old	1 cup
	4–8 years old	1 to 1½ cups
Girls	9–13 years old	1½ cups
	14–18 years old	1½ cups
Boys	9–13 years old	1½ cups
	14–18 years old	2 cups
Women	19–30 years old	2 cups
	31–50 years old	1½ cups
	51+ years old	1½ cups
Men	19–30 years old	2 cups
	31–50 years old	2 cups
	51+ years old	2 cups

Note: These amounts are appropriate for individuals who get less than 30 minutes per day of moderate physical activity, beyond normal daily activities. Those who are more physically active may be able to consume more while staying within calorie needs.

Source: USDA 2005.

- Buy fresh fruit in season when it may be less expensive and at peak flavor.

- Buy fruit that is dried, frozen, or canned (in water or juice), as well as fresh, so that you always have a supply on hand.

- Consider convenience when shopping. Buy pre-cut packages of fruit (such as melon or pineapple chunks) for a healthy snack in seconds. Choose packaged fruit that does not have added sugars.

Nutritional Value

- Make most of your choices whole or cut fruit rather than juice, for the benefits dietary fiber provides.

- Select potassium-rich fruits often, such as bananas, prunes and prune juice, dried peaches, apricots, cantaloupe, honeydew melon, and orange juice.

- When choosing canned fruit, select fruit canned in 100% fruit juice or water rather than syrup.

- Vary your fruit choices. Fruits differ in nutrient content.

Fruit with Meals

- At breakfast, top your cereal with bananas or peaches; add blueberries to pancakes; drink 100% orange or grapefruit juice. Try a fruit mixed with low-fat or fat-free yogurt.

- At lunch, pack a tangerine, banana, or grapes to eat, or choose fruit from a salad bar. Individual containers of fruit like peaches or applesauce are easy and convenient.

- At dinner, add crushed pineapple to coleslaw, or include mandarin oranges or grapes in a tossed salad.

- Make a Waldorf salad, with apples, celery, walnuts, and dressing.

- Try meat dishes that incorporate fruit, such as chicken with apricots or mango chutney.

- Add fruit, such as pineapple or peaches, to kabobs as part of a barbecue meal.

- For dessert, have baked apples, pears, or a fruit salad.

Snacks

- Cut fruit makes a great snack. Either cut it yourself, or buy pre-cut packages of fruit pieces like pineapples or melons. Try whole fresh berries or grapes.

- Dried fruit also makes a great snack. It is easy to carry and stores well. Because it is dried, ¼ cup is equivalent to ½ cup of other fruit.

- Keep a package of dried fruit in your desk or bag. Some dried fruit that is available includes: apricots, apples, pineapple, bananas, cherries, figs, dates, cranberries, blueberries, prunes (dried plums), and raisins (dried grapes).

- As a snack, spread peanut butter on apple slices or top frozen yogurt with berries or slices of kiwi fruit.

- Frozen juice bars (100% juice) make healthy alternatives to high-fat snacks.

Make Fruit Appealing

- Many fruits taste great with a dip or dressing. Try low-fat yogurt or pudding as a dip for fruits like strawberries or melons.

- Make a fruit smoothie by blending fat-free or low-fat milk or yogurt with fresh or frozen fruit. Try bananas, peaches, strawberries, or other berries.

- Try applesauce as a fat-free substitute for some of the oil when baking cakes.

- Try different textures of fruit. For example, apples are crunchy, bananas are smooth and creamy, and oranges are juicy.

- For fresh fruit salads, mix apples, bananas, or pears with acidic fruit like oranges, pineapple, or lemon juice to keep them from turning brown.

Fruit Tips for Children

- Set a good example for children by eating fruit everyday with meals or as snacks.

- Offer children a choice of fruits for lunch.

- Depending on their age, children can help select, clean, peel, or cut fruit.

- While shopping, allow children to select a new fruit to try later.

- Decorate plates or serving dishes with fruit slices.

- Top off a bowl of cereal with some berries. Or, make a smiley face with sliced bananas for eyes, raisins for a nose, and an orange slice for a mouth.

- Offer raisins or other dried fruit instead of candy.

- Make fruit kabobs using pineapple chunks, bananas, grapes, and berries.

- Pack a juice box (100% juice) versus soda or other sugar-sweetened beverages.

- Choose fruit options, such as sliced apples, mixed fruit cup, or 100% fruit juice, that are available in some fast food restaurants.

- Offer fruit pieces and 100% fruit juice to children. There is often little fruit in fruit-flavored beverages or chewy fruit snacks.

Food Safety

- Wash fruit before preparing or eating it. Under clean, running water, rub fruit briskly with your hands to remove dirt and surface microorganisms. Dry after washing.

- Keep fruit separate from raw meat, poultry, and seafood while shopping, preparing, or storing.

Chapter 8

Dietary Fiber

Filling Up on Fiber

What Is Fiber?

Fiber is found in fruits, vegetables, grains, nuts, seeds, dried beans, split peas, and lentils. It is the part of plants that the body cannot digest easily. Fiber includes plant cell walls (cellulose) and other substances, such as pectin and gums. There is no dietary fiber in meat or dairy products.

We need to eat fiber for good health. A high fiber diet may lower the risks for certain cancers, heart disease, and even obesity. Most Americans' diets contain, on the average, about 10 grams of fiber. Try to choose foods that add up to 20–30 grams of fiber per day. Table 8.1 will help you figure how much fiber is in foods.

Remember that a diet too high in fiber (more than 35 grams per day) is not recommended. As is true of other nutrients, some fiber is needed—but too much can unbalance your diet.

This chapter includes: "Filling Up on Fiber," prepared by Katherine Cason, Associate Professor of Food Science. Revised by Julie A. Haines, Assistant Director, Nutrition Links Program. © 2004 The Pennsylvania State University. Also, excerpts from "Will 2005 Be the Year of the Whole Grain?" *Amber Waves*, June 2005, U.S. Department of Agriculture (USDA); an excerpt titled, "What Is the Relationship between Whole Grain Intake and Health?" from *Report of the Dietary Guidelines Advisory Committee on the Dietary Guidelines for Americans*, 2005; and "Tips to Help You Eat Whole Grains," USDA, 2005.

Adding Fiber

The U.S. Food and Drug Administration (FDA) has defined a high-fiber food to equal 5 grams of fiber per serving. A good source of fiber equals 2.5 grams to 4.9 grams of fiber per serving.

There are many ways to add fiber to your diet:

- Add sliced fresh fruit to cereal, yogurt, or cottage cheese.

- Use whole grain breads (which contain at least 3 grams of fiber per serving) in place of white bread.

- Choose whole grain crackers.

- Use fresh fruit and vegetables every day. Eat fruit at every meal and snack on fresh or dried fruit, raw vegetables, or low-fat popcorn.

- Use more beans and peas in meals. Try split pea or lentil soup, brown rice and beans, or chili.

- Choose high-fiber cereals (5 grams of fiber or more per serving) for breakfast in place of refined, sugary cereals.

- Eat potatoes with the skin.

- When cooking vegetables, steam or stir-fry until they are tender but still crisp.

- Use sunflower seeds, sesame seeds, or wheat germ for toppings on casseroles, or add them to baked goods like quick breads and cookies.

How Much Fiber Did You Eat Today?

Adults need 20–30 grams of fiber each day for good health. Consult Table 8.1 to check how much fiber you ate today. Read food labels to find the amount of dietary fiber in each product.

How Much Fiber Do Children Need?

Experts in children's nutrition agree it is important to teach children healthful eating habits when they are young. But what about fiber? We have not heard much about its benefits for children.

We are beginning to understand fiber's importance in children's diets. It has key health benefits in promoting regularity. Fiber not only helps to maintain good health as children grow, it helps them establish

Table 8.1. Grams of Fiber in Common Foods (continued on next page)

Food	Amount	Grams of Fiber
Fruits		
Apple	1 medium	3.7
Apple juice	¾ cup	0
Banana	1 medium	1.8
Cantaloupe	¼ melon	1.0
Orange	1 medium	3.6
Orange juice	¾ cup	0.4
Peach	1 medium	1.4
Raisins	¼ cup	2.0
Strawberries	½ cup	2.0
Vegetables		
Broccoli, cooked	½ cup	3.6
Cabbage, raw	½ cup	1.0
Carrot	1 medium	2.3
Corn	½ cup	2.0
Green beans	½ cup	1.0
Onion, cooked	1 medium	0.8
Peas, green	½ cup	3.0
Potato, with skin	1 medium	3.0
Potatoes, French fried	10 strips	1.6
Tomato	1 medium	1.6
Tomato juice	¾ cup	1.4
Breads and Cereals		
Bran flakes	¾ cup	4.2
Bread, white	1 slice	0.5
Bread, whole wheat	1 slice	2.0
Corn flakes	1 cup	0.5
Crisp rice cereal	1 cup	0.1
Oatmeal, cooked	½ cup	2.3
Popcorn	1 cup	1.2
Rice, white, cooked	½ cup	1.0
Spaghetti and macaroni	½ cup	1.0
Tortilla, corn	1 medium	1.5
Oat bran muffin	1 medium	13.1

Table 8.1. Grams of Fiber in Common Foods (continued)

Food	Amount	Grams of Fiber
Nuts		
Peanuts	¼ cup	3.2
Peanut butter	2 Tbsp	3.4
Walnuts	¼ cup	2.0
Legumes		
Baked beans	½ cup	9.8
Kidney beans	½ cup	6.5
Lima beans	½ cup	6.5
Navy beans	½ cup	5.0
Pinto beans	½ cup	6.4

eating patterns that may assist in reducing their risk of developing heart disease and some types of cancer later in life.

The Dietary Guidelines for Americans recommend that after children are two years old, the fat in their diets should be lowered gradually until it reaches the level recommended for adults, around age five. As fat is lowered, more foods rich in fiber, vitamins, and minerals need to be provided.

Care must be taken in the amount of fiber given to children. High-fiber diets can reduce the amount of calories children get because foods high in fiber tend to be bulky and low in calories. Fiber can also bind minerals so that they are not available for the child to absorb. But most children currently do not get enough fiber.

Dietary fiber should be increased gradually. Caution is especially prudent for groups that may not be getting enough calories or minerals, such as preschool children, adolescents with mineral-deficient diets, children with inadequate nutrition, and some vegetarian children who have nutritionally inadequate diets. The best way to add fiber is by increasing the amounts of fruits, vegetables, legumes, cereals, and other grain products consumed. It is also important for anyone who is eating more fiber to drink extra liquids, including water, juice, or milk.

So how much fiber should children eat? Until recently there were no formal guidelines geared for children's needs and their developmental cycle. Now there is a fiber recommendation for children ages 3–18. The new formula is the child's age plus 5. For example, a five-year-old child needs about 10 grams of fiber, 5 + 5 = 10. This formula allows for the greater need for fiber as the child grows. Children should eat fruits and vegetables every day.

Whole Grain Consumption

For the first time, the Dietary Guidelines have specific recommendations for whole grain consumption separate from those for refined grains. The Guidelines, released in January 2005, encourage all Americans over 2 years old to eat at least three 1-ounce-equivalent servings of whole grains each day, or roughly half of their recommended 5 to 10 daily servings of grains, depending on calorie needs.

The goal of this new recommendation is to improve Americans' health by raising awareness of whole grains and their role in nutritious diets. The Guidelines could also, however, have big impacts on

Table 8.2. Some Fiber-Containing Foods in Portions Consumed by Children

Food	Amount	Grams of Fiber
Grains		
Raisin bran cereal	1 cup	7
Whole wheat biscuit cereal	1 cup	6
Bran waffle	2 rounds	4
Oatmeal	1 cup	4
Whole wheat bread	1 slice	2
Bran muffin	1 small	2
Fruit-filled cereal bar	1	1
Vegetables		
Cooked green peas	1/2 cup	3
Cooked broccoli	1/2 cup	3.5
Cooked carrots	1/2 cup	2
Cooked corn	1/2 cup	2
Fruits		
Apple, with peel	1 medium	3
Orange	1 medium	3.5
Raisins	1/4 cup	2
Banana	1/2 medium	1

farmers and farm production. How big depends on consumers' and manufacturers' responses.

Will Consumers Follow the Guidelines?

Historical eating trends, and the popularity of diets, demonstrate that consumers do modify their food choices in response to diet and health information. For example, in response to health warnings about consuming too much saturated fat, per capita consumption of whole milk declined by 70 percent between 1970 and 2003, while consumption of lower fat and skim milk increased by 140 percent. However, trends in overall fat consumption suggest that some dietary advice is ignored. Total per capita consumption of added fats and oils has risen 63 percent since 1970, despite widespread health warnings.

The new whole grain recommendations are ambitious, given Americans' current eating patterns. Though Americans have been eating more grain products, they consume few whole grains. According to the USDA Economic Research Service (ERS) food availability data, Americans were eating, on average, 10 servings of grains a day in 2003—only 1 of which was whole grain. Whole grain data are incomplete, as information on some whole grains, such as buckwheat and quinoa, are not available.

Whether consumers embrace whole grains involves weighing their attributes—taste, convenience, availability, price, and perceived health benefits—relative to other food choices. For most consumers, taste is the deciding factor, as shown by years of survey data from the Food Marketing Institute. Whole grain products that fail to pass the consumer taste test will have difficulty competing against refined products that do.

Convenience may also be an issue for some consumers. Many whole grains require longer preparation and cooking time than refined grains. For example, brown rice takes 25 minutes longer to cook than white. For some consumers, availability may also hinder whole grain consumption, though less so now that whole grain products are increasingly plentiful in places other than health food stores and mail-order companies.

Cost is another consideration. Historically, some whole grain products were more expensive because they were specialty items produced in smaller quantities. An ERS analysis puts the average cost of whole grain/whole wheat bread at $1.99 per pound in 2003, versus $1.66 per pound for white bread. Where they exist, price spreads above industry wide thin profit margins may provide an unexpected benefit to food manufacturers who produce whole grain products. However, any price spread will likely be short-lived as more manufacturers join the whole grain market.

Consumers Confused about Labels and Serving Sizes

For consumers who follow the Guidelines and decide to eat more whole grains, constraints may remain. Even motivated consumers may have difficulty meeting dietary recommendations because it is often difficult to tell which products contain whole grains. There is no universally accepted definition of whole grain foods, and labels may be hard to understand. Labels of wheat bread, stone-ground, and seven-grain bread do not guarantee that the food contains whole grains. Color is not a good indicator of whole grains either because foods may be darker simply because of added molasses.

The difficulty consumers have in identifying whole grains makes it harder to meet the dietary requirements. According to a Natural Marketing Institute report, 71 percent of consumers think that they are already consuming enough whole grains. Data based on consumers' recalling their intake from the previous day, however, indicate that nearly 40 percent of Americans consume no whole grains. Consumers who mistakenly think that they are already consuming enough whole grains will not make the effort to increase their intake.

Once consumers identify whole grain products, they may still struggle with getting recommended amounts of whole grain into their diets. Most consumers are unclear on what a serving of whole grains is, particularly in an era where oversized food portions are common. In general, a serving of grains is an ounce-equivalent of food, such as a slice of bread; a half cup of cooked cereal, rice, or pasta; or about 1 cup of dry cereal (¼ cup for dense, granola cereals to 1½ cups for some unsweetened puffed cereals). Consumers who do not have a good sense of a serving size may have difficulty judging how their daily consumption tallies up against serving recommendations.

In the short run, consumers will probably not meet the goal of three ounce-equivalents of whole grains per day. However, as knowledge of the Guidelines grows and as consumers learn more about the health benefits of whole grains, consumption patterns will likely change. Consumers, however, are only one side of the equation; manufacturers will play their part in supplying whole grain alternatives.

What Are Whole Grain Foods?

There is no universally accepted definition of whole grains. The new Dietary Guidelines uses the American Association of Cereal Chemists' definition, which is "foods made from the entire grain seed, usually called the kernel, which consists of the bran, germ, and endosperm. If the kernel has been cracked, crushed, or flaked, it must retain nearly the same relative proportions of bran, germ, and endosperm as the original grain in order to be called whole grain." The U.S. Food and Drug Administration (FDA) requires foods that bear the whole grain health claim to: (1) contain 51 percent or more whole grain ingredients by weight per reference amount and (2) be low in fat.

Whole grains can be consumed either as a single food, such as wild rice and popcorn, or as a food ingredient, as in some multigrain breads. Whole grains are good sources of fiber and other nutrients, such as calcium, magnesium, and potassium. Refined grains are the product of a process that removes most of the bran and some of the germ. During this process, some dietary fiber, vitamins, minerals, and other natural plant compounds are lost.

Almost all refined grains are enriched before being further processed into foods, a step taken by many grain companies since the 1940s. In order to conform to FDA's standards of identity, enriched foods were required to be fortified with thiamine, riboflavin, niacin, and iron. In 1998, the FDA required that folic acid be added to the enrichment mixture. Currently, enrichment is not required for whole grain foods.

What Is the Relationship between Whole Grain Intake and Health?

Consuming at least 3 servings (equivalent to 3 ounces) of whole grains per day can reduce the risk of diabetes, some cancers, coronary heart disease (CHD), and help with weight maintenance. Thus, daily intake of 3 ounces of whole grains per day is recommended, preferably by substituting whole grains for refined grains.

Tips to Help You Eat Whole Grains

At Meals

- To eat more whole grains, substitute a whole grain product for a refined product—such as eating whole wheat bread instead of white bread, or brown rice instead of white rice. It is important to substitute the whole grain product for the refined one, rather than adding the whole grain product.

- For a change, try brown rice or whole wheat pasta. Try brown rice stuffing in baked green peppers, or tomatoes and whole wheat macaroni in macaroni and cheese.

- Use whole grains in mixed dishes, such as barley in vegetable soup or stews, and bulgur wheat in casserole or stir-fries.

- Create a whole grain pilaf with a mixture of barley, wild rice, brown rice, broth, and spices. For a special touch, stir in toasted nuts or chopped dried fruit.

- Experiment by substituting whole wheat or oat flour for up to half of the flour in pancake, waffle, muffin or other flour-based recipes. They may need a bit more leavening.

- Use whole grain bread or cracker crumbs in meatloaf.

- Try rolled oats or a crushed, unsweetened whole grain cereal as breading for baked chicken, fish, veal cutlets, or eggplant parmesan.

- Try an unsweetened, whole grain ready-to-eat cereal as croutons in salad or in place of crackers with soup.

- Freeze leftover cooked brown rice, bulgur, or barley. Heat and serve it later as a quick side dish.

As Snacks

- Snack on ready-to-eat, whole grain cereals such as toasted oat cereal.

- Add whole grain flour or oatmeal when making cookies or other baked treats.

- Try a whole grain snack chip, such as baked tortilla chips.

- Popcorn, a whole grain, can be a healthy snack with little or no added salt and butter.

What to Look for on the Food Label

Choose foods that name one of the following whole grain ingredients first on the label's ingredient list:

- brown rice
- bulgur
- graham flour
- oatmeal
- whole grain corn

- whole oats
- whole rye
- whole wheat
- wild rice

Foods labeled with the words multi-grain, stone-ground, 100% wheat, cracked wheat, seven-grain, or bran are usually not whole grain products. Color is not an indication of a whole grain. Bread can be brown because of molasses or other added ingredients. Read the ingredient list to see if it is a whole grain.

Use the Nutrition Facts label and choose products with a higher % Daily Value (% DV) for fiber—the % DV for fiber is a good clue to the amount of whole grain in the product. Read the food label's ingredient list. Look for terms that indicate added sugars (sucrose, high-fructose corn syrup, honey, and molasses) and oils (partially hydrogenated vegetable oils) that add extra calories. Choose foods with fewer added sugars, fats, or oils.

Most sodium in the food supply comes from packaged foods. Similar packaged foods can vary widely in sodium content, including breads. Use the Nutrition Facts label to choose foods with a lower % DV for sodium. Foods with less than 140 milligrams (mg) sodium per serving can be labeled as low sodium foods. Claims such as "low in sodium" or "very low in sodium" on the front of the food label can help you identify foods that contain less salt (or sodium).

Whole Grain Tips for Children

- Set a good example for children by eating whole grains with meals or as snacks.

- Let children select and help prepare a whole grain side dish.

- Teach older children to read the ingredient list on cereals or snack food packages and choose those with whole grains at the top of the list.

Chapter 9

Saturated Fat, Trans Fat, and Cholesterol

Information about Fats from the Dietary Guidelines for Americans

Fats and oils are part of a healthful diet, but the type of fat makes a difference to heart health, and the total amount of fat consumed is also important. High intake of saturated fats, *trans* fats, and cholesterol increases the risk of unhealthy blood lipid levels, which, in turn, may increase the risk of coronary heart disease. A high intake of fat (greater than 35 percent of calories) generally increases saturated fat intake and makes it more difficult to avoid consuming excess calories. A low intake of fats and oils (less than 20 percent of calories) increases the risk of inadequate intakes of vitamin E and of essential fatty acids and may contribute to unfavorable changes in high-density lipoprotein (HDL) blood cholesterol and triglycerides.

Key Recommendations

*   Consume less than 10 percent of calories from saturated fatty acids and less than 300 milligrams (mg)/day of cholesterol, and keep *trans* fatty acid consumption as low as possible.

This chapter includes excerpts from "Fats," from *Dietary Guidelines for Americans, 2005*, U.S. Department of Health and Human Services (HHS) and the U.S. Department of Agriculture (USDA); "What Are Oils?" USDA, 2005; excerpts from "Revealing Trans Fats," *FDA Consumer*, May 2004, U.S. Food and Drug Administration (FDA); and an excerpt titled "How Fat Relates to Health," from *Report of the Dietary Guidelines Advisory Committee on the Dietary Guidelines for Americans, 2005*, HHS and USDA.

- Keep total fat intake between 20 to 35 percent of calories, with most fats coming from sources of polyunsaturated and monounsaturated fatty acids such as fish, nuts, and vegetable oils.

- When selecting and preparing meat, poultry, dry beans, and milk or milk products, make choices that are lean, low-fat, or fat-free.

- Limit intake of fats and oils high in saturated and/or *trans* fatty acids, and choose products low in such fats and oils.

Key Recommendations for Specific Population Groups

- *Children and adolescents.* Keep total fat intake between 30 to 35 percent of calories for children 2 to 3 years of age and between 25 to 35 percent of calories for children and adolescents 4 to 18 years of age, with most fats coming from sources of polyunsaturated and monounsaturated fatty acids such as fish, nuts, and vegetable oils.

Fats supply energy and essential fatty acids and serve as a carrier for the absorption of the fat-soluble vitamins A, D, E, and K and carotenoids. Fats serve as building blocks of membranes and play a key regulatory role in numerous biological functions. Dietary fat is found in foods derived from both plants and animals.

Table 9.1 indicates the maximum gram amounts of saturated fat that can be consumed to keep saturated fat intake below 10 percent of total calorie intake for selected calorie levels. This table may be useful when combined with label-reading guidance.

Table 9.1. Maximum Daily Amounts of Saturated Fat to Keep Saturated Fat Below 10 Percent of Total Calorie Intake

Total Calorie Intake	Limit on Saturated Fat Intake
1,600	18 grams (g) or less
2,000[a]	20 g or less
2,200	24 g or less
2,500[a]	25 g or less
2,800	31 g or less

[a] Percent Daily Values on the Nutrition Facts Panel of food labels are based on a 2,000-calorie diet. Values for 2,000 and 2,500 calories are rounded to the nearest 5 grams to be consistent with the Nutrition Facts Panel.

Table 9.2 shows a few practical examples of the differences in the saturated fat content of different forms of commonly consumed foods. Comparisons are made between foods in the same food group (e.g., regular cheddar cheese and low-fat cheddar cheese), illustrating that choices of lower saturated fat can be made within the same food group.

Table 9.2. Differences in Saturated Fat and Calorie Content of Commonly Consumed Foods

Food Category	Portion	Saturated Fat Content (grams)	Calories
Cheese			
Regular cheddar cheese	1 oz	6.0	114
Low-fat cheddar cheese	1 oz	1.2	49
Ground beef			
Regular ground beef (25% fat)	3 oz (cooked)	6.1	236
Extra lean ground beef (5% fat)	3 oz (cooked)	2.6	148
Milk			
Whole milk (3.24%)	1 cup	4.6	146
Low-fat (1%) milk	1 cup	1.5	102
Breads			
Croissant (med)	1 medium	6.6	231
Bagel, oat bran (4")	1 medium	0.2	227
Frozen desserts			
Regular ice cream	1/2 cup	4.9	145
Frozen yogurt, low-fat	1/2 cup	2.0	110
Table spreads			
Butter	1 tsp	2.4	34
Soft margarine with zero trans	1 tsp	0.7	25
Chicken			
Fried chicken (leg with skin)	3 oz (cooked)	3.3	212
Roasted chicken (breast no skin)	3 oz (cooked)	0.9	140
Fish			
Fried fish	3 oz	2.8	195
Baked fish	3 oz	1.5	129

Source: ARS Nutrient Database for Standard Reference, Release 17.

What Are Oils?

Oils are fats that are liquid at room temperature, like the vegetable oils used in cooking. Oils come from many different plants and from fish. Some common oils are:

- canola oil
- corn oil
- cottonseed oil
- sunflower oil
- safflower oil
- soybean oil
- olive oil

Some oils are used mainly as flavorings, such as walnut oil and sesame oil. A number of foods are naturally high in oils including:

- nuts
- some fish
- olives
- avocados

Foods that are mainly oil include mayonnaise, certain salad dressings, and soft (tub or squeeze) margarine with no *trans* fats. Check the Nutrition Facts label to find margarines with 0 grams of *trans* fat. Amounts of *trans* fat are required on labels.

Most oils are high in monounsaturated or polyunsaturated fats, and low in saturated fats. Oils from plant sources (vegetable and nut oils) do not contain any cholesterol. In fact, no foods from plant sources contain cholesterol. A few plant oils, however, including coconut oil and palm kernel oil, are high in saturated fats and for nutritional purposes should be considered to be solid fats.

Solid fats are fats that are solid at room temperature such as butter and shortening. Solid fats come from many animal foods and can be made from vegetable oils through a process called hydrogenation. The following are examples of some common solid fats:

- butter
- stick margarine
- pork fat (lard)
- chicken fat
- beef fat (tallow, suet)
- shortening

Revealing Trans Fats

Basically, *trans* fat is made when manufacturers add hydrogen to vegetable oil—a process called hydrogenation. Hydrogenation increases the shelf life and flavor stability of foods containing these fats.

Trans fat can be found in vegetable shortenings, some margarines, crackers, cookies, snack foods, and other foods made with or fried in partially hydrogenated oils. Unlike other fats, the majority of *trans* fat is formed when food manufacturers turn liquid oils into solid fats like shortening and hard margarine. A small amount of *trans* fat is found naturally, primarily in dairy products, some meat, and other animal-based foods.

Trans fat, like saturated fat and dietary cholesterol, raises the LDL cholesterol that increases your risk for coronary heart disease (CHD). Americans consume on average 4 to 5 times as much saturated fat as *trans* fat in their diets. Although saturated fat is the main dietary culprit that raises LDL, *trans* fat and dietary cholesterol also contribute significantly.

What Can You Do about Saturated Fat, Trans Fat, and Cholesterol?

When comparing foods, look at the Nutrition Facts panel, and choose foods with the lower amounts of saturated fat, *trans* fat, and cholesterol. Health experts recommend that you keep your intake of saturated fat, *trans* fat, and cholesterol as low as possible while consuming a nutritionally adequate diet. However, these experts recognize that eliminating these three components entirely from your diet is not practical because they are unavoidable in ordinary diets.

Where Can You Find Trans Fat on the Food Label?

You will find *trans* fat listed on the Nutrition Facts panel directly under the line for saturated fat.

How Do Your Choices Stack Up?

You can review your food choices and see how they stack up. Table 9.3 illustrates total fat, saturated fat, *trans* fat, and cholesterol content per serving for selected food products.

Do not assume similar products are the same. Be sure to check the Nutrition Facts panel because even similar foods can vary in calories, ingredients, nutrients, and the size and number of servings in a package.

How Can You Use the Label to Make Heart-Healthy Food Choices?

The Nutrition Facts panel can help you choose foods lower in saturated fat, *trans* fat, and cholesterol. Compare similar foods and choose the food with the lower combined saturated and *trans* fats and the lower amount of cholesterol.

Although the updated Nutrition Facts panel lists the amount of *trans* fat in a product, it will not show a Percent Daily Value (%DV).

Table 9.3. Total Fat, Saturated Fat, *Trans* Fat, and Cholesterol Content Per Serving*

Product	Common Serving Size	Total Fat g	Saturated Fat g	Percent Daily Value (% DV) for Saturated Fat	*Trans* Fat g	Combined Saturated and *Trans* Fat g	Cholesterol mg	% DV for Cholesterol
French Fried Potatoes[a] (Fast Food)	Medium (147 g)	27	7	35%	8	15	0	0%
Butter**	1 Tbsp	11	7	35%	0	7	30	10%
Margarine, stick[t]	1 Tbsp	11	2	10%	3	5	0	0%
Margarine, tub[t]	1 Tbsp	7	1	5%	0.5	1.5	0	0%
Mayonnaise[tt] (Soybean Oil)	1 Tbsp	11	1.5	8%	0	1.5	5	2%
Shortening[a]	1 Tbsp	13	3.5	18%	4	7.5	0	0%
Potato Chips[a]	Small bag (42.5 g)	11	2	10%	3	5	0	0%
Milk, whole[a]	1 cup	7	4.5	23%	0	4.5	35	12%
Milk, skim[t]	1 cup	0	0	0%	0	0	5	2%
Doughnut[a]	1	18	4.5	23%	5	9.5	25	8%
Cookies[a] (Cream Filled)	3 (30 g)	6	1	5%	2	3	0	0%
Candy Bar[a]	1 (40 g)	10	4	20%	3	7	<5	1%
Cake, pound[a]	1 slice (80 g)	16	3.5	18%	4.5	8	0	0%

*Nutrient values rounded based on FDA's nutrition labeling regulations.
** Butter values from FDA "Table of *Trans* Values," 1/30/95.
[t] Values derived from 2002 USDA "National Nutrient Database for Standard Reference, Release 15."
[tt] Prerelease values derived from 2003 USDA "National Nutrient Database for Standard Reference, Release 16."
[a] 1995 USDA Composition Data.

While scientific reports have confirmed the relationship between *trans* fat and an increased risk of CHD, none has provided a reference value for *trans* fat or any other information that the FDA believes is sufficient to establish a Daily Reference Value or a %DV.

There is, however, a %DV shown for saturated fat and cholesterol. To choose foods low in saturated fat and cholesterol, use the general rule of thumb that 5 percent of the Daily Value or less is low and 20 percent or more is high.

You can also use the %DV to make dietary trade-offs with other foods throughout the day. You don't have to give up a favorite food to eat a healthy diet. When a food you like is high in saturated fat or cholesterol, balance it with foods that are low in saturated fat and cholesterol at other times of the day.

Do Dietary Supplements Contain Trans Fat?

Some dietary supplements contain *trans* fat from partially hydrogenated vegetable oil as well as saturated fat or cholesterol. As a result of the FDA's label requirements, if a dietary supplement contains a reportable amount of *trans* or saturated fat, which is 0.5 gram or more, dietary supplement manufacturers must list the amounts on the Supplement Facts panel. Energy and nutrition bars are dietary supplements that may contain saturated fat, *trans* fat, and cholesterol.

Tips to Limit Fat Consumption

Here are some practical tips you can use every day to keep your consumption of saturated fat, *trans* fat, and cholesterol low while consuming a nutritionally adequate diet.

- Check the Nutrition Facts panel to compare foods because the serving sizes are generally consistent in similar types of foods. Choose foods lower in saturated fat, *trans* fat, and cholesterol. For saturated fat and cholesterol, keep in mind that 5 percent of the daily value (%DV) or less is low and 20 percent or more is high. (There is no %DV for *trans* fat.)

- Choose alternative fats. Replace saturated and *trans* fats in your diet with monounsaturated and polyunsaturated fats. These fats do not raise LDL cholesterol levels and have health benefits when eaten in moderation.

- Sources of monounsaturated fats include olive and canola oils. Sources of polyunsaturated fats include soybean oil, corn oil, sunflower oil, and foods like nuts and fish.

- Choose vegetable oils (except coconut and palm kernel oils) and soft margarines (liquid, tub, or spray) more often because the amounts of saturated fat, *trans* fat, and cholesterol are lower than the amounts in solid shortenings, hard margarines, and animal fats, including butter.

- Consider fish. Most fish are lower in saturated fat than meat. Some fish, such as mackerel, sardines, and salmon, contain omega-3 fatty acids that are being studied to determine if they offer protection against heart disease.

- Choose lean meats, such as poultry without the skin and not fried; lean beef; and pork, not fried, with visible fat trimmed.

- Ask before you order when eating out. Remember to ask which fats are being used in the preparation of your food when eating or ordering out.

- Watch calories. Don't be fooled! Fats are high in calories. All sources of fat contain 9 calories per gram, making fat the most concentrated source of calories. By comparison, carbohydrates and protein have only 4 calories per gram.

The following tips can help you keep your intake of saturated fat, *trans* fat, and cholesterol low:

- Look at the Nutrition Facts panel when comparing products. Choose foods low in the combined amount of saturated fat and *trans* fat and low in cholesterol as part of a nutritionally adequate diet.

- Substitute alternative fats that are higher in mono- and polyunsaturated fats like olive oil, canola oil, soybean oil, corn oil, and sunflower oil.

- Be aware of major food sources of *trans* fat for American adults. (Average daily *trans* fat intake is 5.8 grams or 2.6 percent of calories.)

How Fat Relates to Health

What are the relationships between total fat intake and health?

At low intakes of fat (less than 20 percent of energy) and high intakes of carbohydrates (greater than 65 percent of energy), risk increases for inadequate intakes of vitamin E, a-linolenic acid, and linoleic acid, and for adverse changes in HDL cholesterol and triglycerides. At high intakes of fat (greater than 35 percent of energy), the risk increases for obesity and CHD. This is because fat intakes that exceed 35 percent of energy are associated with both increased calorie and saturated fat intakes. Total fat intake of 20 to 35 percent of calories is recommended for adults and 25 to 35 percent for children age 4 to 18 years. A fat intake of 30 to 35 percent of calories is recommended for children age 2 to 3 years.

What are the relationships between saturated fat intake and health?

The relationship between saturated fat intake and LDL cholesterol is direct and progressive, increasing the risk of cardiovascular disease (CVD). Thus, saturated fat consumption by adults should be as low as possible while consuming a diet that provides 20 to 35 percent calories from fat and meets recommendations for a-linolenic acid and linoleic acid. In particular,

- For adults with LDL cholesterol below 130 mg/dL, less than 10 percent of calories from saturated fatty acids is recommended.
- For adults with an elevated LDL cholesterol (over 130 mg/dL), less than 7 percent of calories from saturated fatty acids is recommended.

What is the relationship between **trans** *fat intake and health?*

The relationship between *trans* fatty acid intake and LDL cholesterol is direct and progressive, increasing the risk of CHD. *Trans* fatty acid consumption by all population groups should be kept as low as possible, which is about 1 percent of energy intake or less.

What is the relationship between cholesterol intake and cardiovascular disease?

The relationship between cholesterol intake and LDL cholesterol concentrations is direct and progressive, increasing the risk of CHD. Thus, cholesterol intake should be kept as low as possible within a nutritionally adequate diet. In particular,

- for adults with an LDL cholesterol less than 130 mg/dL, less than 300 mg of dietary cholesterol per day is recommended.

- for adults with an elevated LDL cholesterol (over 130 mg/dL), less than 200 mg of dietary cholesterol/day is recommended.

Chapter 10

Vitamins: Dietary Insurance

Dietary Insurance: A Daily Multivitamin

If you eat a healthy diet, do you need to take vitamins? Not long ago, the answer from most experts would have been a resounding *no*. Today, though, there is good evidence that taking a daily multivitamin makes sense for most adults.

What has changed? Not only have scientists determined why we need pyridoxine (vitamin B$_6$), but they are also accumulating evidence that this vitamin and others do much more than ward off the so-called diseases of deficiency, things like scurvy and rickets. Intake of several vitamins above the minimum daily requirement may prevent heart disease, cancer, osteoporosis, and other chronic diseases.

This chapter will focus on vitamins with newly recognized or suspected roles in health and disease. It will present some of the evidence about vitamins' possible new roles, point out how to get more of these in your diet, and assess the value of taking a daily multivitamin.

What Are Vitamins?

Nutrition textbooks dryly define vitamins as organic compounds that the body needs in small quantities for normal functioning. Here's the translation: Vitamins are nutrients you must get from food because your body cannot make them from scratch. You need only small amounts (that's why they are often referred to as micronutrients) because the body uses them without breaking them down, as happens to carbohydrates and other macronutrients.

So far, 13 compounds have been classified as vitamins. Vitamins A, D, E, and K, the four fat-soluble vitamins, tend to accumulate in the body. Vitamin C and the eight B vitamins—biotin, folate, niacin, pantothenic acid, riboflavin, thiamin, vitamin B_6, and vitamin B_{12}—dissolve in water, so excess amounts are excreted.

The "letter" vitamins sometimes go by different names. These include the following:

- Vitamin A: retinol, retinaldehyde, retinoic acid
- Vitamin B_1: thiamin
- Vitamin B_2: riboflavin
- Vitamin B_6: pyridoxine, pyridoxal, pyridoxamine
- Vitamin B_{12}: cobalamin
- Vitamin C: ascorbic acid
- Vitamin D: calciferol
- Vitamin E: tocopherol, tocotrienol
- Vitamin K: phylloquinone

Vitamin A

Vitamin A does much more than help you see in the dark. It stimulates the production and activity of white blood cells, takes part in remodeling bone, helps maintain the health of endothelial cells (those lining the body's interior surfaces), and regulates cell growth and division. This latter role had researchers exploring for years whether insufficient vitamin A caused cancer. Several studies have dashed this hypothesis,[1] as have randomized trials of supplements containing beta carotene, a precursor of vitamin A.

Although it is relatively easy to get too little vitamin A, it is also easy to get too much. Intake of up to 10,000 International Units (IU), twice the current recommended daily level, is thought to be safe. However, there is some evidence that this much preformed vitamin A might increase the risk of hip fracture[2] or some birth defects.[3]

Optimal intake: The current recommended intake of vitamin A is 5,000 IU for men and 4,000 IU for women. Many breakfast cereals, juices, dairy products, and other foods are fortified with vitamin A. Many fruits and vegetables, and some supplements, also contain beta-carotene and other vitamin A precursors, which the body can turn into vitamin A.

The 3 Bs: Vitamin B_6, Vitamin B_{12}, and Folic Acid

One of the advances that changed the way we look at vitamins is the discovery that too little folic acid, one of the eight B vitamins, is linked to birth defects such as spina bifida and anencephaly. Fifty years ago, no one knew what caused these birth defects, which occur when the early development of tissues—that eventually become the spinal cord, surrounding tissues, or the brain—goes awry. Twenty-five years ago, British researchers found that mothers of children with spina bifida had low vitamin levels.[4] Eventually, two large trials in which women were randomly assigned to take folic acid or a placebo showed that getting too little folic acid increased a woman's chances of having a baby with spina bifida or anencephaly and that getting enough folic acid could prevent these birth defects.[5, 6]

Enough folic acid, at least 400 micrograms a day, is not always easy to get from food. That is why women of childbearing age are urged to take extra folic acid. It is also why the U.S. Food and Drug Administration (FDA) now requires that folic acid be added to most enriched breads, flour, cornmeal, pastas, rice, and other grain products, along with the iron and other micronutrients that have been added for years.[7]

The other exciting discovery about folic acid and two other B vitamins is that they may help fight heart disease and some types of cancer. It is too early to tell if there is merely an association between increased intake of folic acid and other B vitamins and heart disease or cancer, or if high intakes prevent these chronic diseases.

B Vitamins and Heart Disease

In 1968, a Boston pathologist investigating the deaths of two children from massive strokes wondered if the high levels of a protein breakdown product called homocysteine in their systems could have been the reason their arteries were as clogged with cholesterol as those of a 65-year-old fast food addict.[8] Since then, some—but not all—studies have linked high levels of this breakdown product, called homocysteine, with increased risks of heart disease and stroke.[9, 10]

Folic acid, vitamin B_6, and vitamin B_{12} play key roles in recycling homocysteine into methionine, one of the 20 or so building blocks from which the body builds new proteins. Without enough folic acid, vitamin B_6, and vitamin B_{12}, this recycling process becomes inefficient and homocysteine levels increase. Several observational studies show that high levels of homocysteine are associated with increased risks of heart disease and stroke. Increasing an individual's intake of folic acid, vitamin B_6, and vitamin B_{12}, decreases their homocysteine levels. Also, some observational studies show lower risks of cardiovascular disease among people with higher intakes of folic acid, those who use multivitamin supplements, or those with higher levels of serum folate (the form of folic acid found in the body). However, other prospective studies show little or no association between homocysteine and cardiovascular disease. Ongoing randomized trials, such as the *Women's Antioxidant Cardiovascular Study*[11] and the *Vitamin Intervention in Stroke Prevention Study*[12] should yield more definitive answers regarding homocysteine, B vitamins, and cardiovascular risk.

Folic Acid and Cancer

In addition to recycling homocysteine, folate plays a key role in building deoxyribonucleic acid (DNA), the complex compound that forms our genetic blueprint. Observational studies show that people who get higher than average amounts of folic acid from their diets or supplements have lower risks of colon cancer[13] and breast cancer.[14] This could be especially important for those who drink alcohol, since alcohol blocks the absorption of folic acid and inactivates circulating folate. An interesting observation from the *Nurses' Health Study* is that high intake of folic acid blunts the increased risk of breast cancer seen among women who have more than one alcoholic drink a day.[14]

Optimal intake: The definition of a healthy daily intake of B vitamins is not set in stone, and is likely to change over the next few years as data from ongoing randomized trials are evaluated. Because only a fraction of U.S. adults currently get the recommended daily intake of B vitamins by diet alone, use of a multivitamin supplement will become increasingly important.

Folic Acid: The current recommended intake for folic acid is 400 micrograms per day. There are many excellent sources of folic acid including prepared breakfast cereals, beans, and fortified grains.

Vitamin B_6: A healthy diet should include 1.3 to 1.7 milligrams of vitamin B_6. Higher doses have been tested as a treatment for conditions ranging from premenstrual syndrome to attention deficit disorder and carpal tunnel syndrome. To date, there is little evidence that it works.

Vitamin B$_{12}$: The current recommended intake for vitamin B$_{12}$ is 6 micrograms per day. Barely 100 years ago, a lack of vitamin B$_{12}$ was the cause of a common and deadly disease called pernicious anemia. Its symptoms include memory loss, disorientation, hallucinations, and tingling in the arms and legs. Although full-blown pernicious anemia is less common today, it is still often diagnosed in older people who have difficulty absorbing vitamin B$_{12}$ from food. It is also possible that some people diagnosed with dementia or Alzheimer's disease are actually suffering from the more reversible vitamin B$_{12}$ deficiency.

Vitamin C

Vitamin C has been in the public eye for a long time. Even before its discovery in 1932, nutrition experts recognized that something in citrus fruits could prevent scurvy, a disease that killed as many as 2 million sailors between 1500 and 1800.[15] More recently, Nobel laureate Linus Pauling promoted daily megadoses of vitamin C (the amount in 12 to 24 oranges) as a way to prevent colds and protect the body from other chronic diseases.

There is no question that vitamin C plays a role in controlling infections. It is also a powerful antioxidant that can neutralize harmful free radicals, and it helps make collagen—a tissue needed for healthy bones, teeth, gums, and blood vessels.[16]

The question is: Do you need lots of vitamin C to keep you healthy? No. Vitamin C's cold-fighting potential certainly has not panned out. Small trials suggest that the amount of vitamin C in a typical multivitamin taken at the start of a cold might ease symptoms, but there is no evidence that megadoses make a difference, or that they prevent colds.[17] Studies of vitamin C and heart disease, cancer, and eye diseases, such as cataract and macular degeneration, also show no clear patterns.

Optimal intake: The current recommended dietary intake for vitamin C is 90 milligrams (mg) for men and 75 mg for women (add an extra 35 mg for smokers). There is no good evidence that megadoses of vitamin C improve health. As the evidence continues to unfold, 200 to 300 mg of vitamin C a day appears to be a good target. This is easy to attain with a good diet and a standard multivitamin. Excellent food sources of vitamin C are citrus fruits or citrus juices, berries, green and red peppers, tomatoes, broccoli, and spinach. Many breakfast cereals are also fortified with vitamin C.

Vitamin D

If you live north of the line connecting San Francisco to Philadelphia, you probably do not get enough vitamin D. The same holds true if you do not, or cannot, get outside for at least a 15 minute daily walk in the sun. For example, a study of people admitted to a Boston hospital showed that 57% were deficient in vitamin D.[18]

Vitamin D helps ensure that the body absorbs and retains calcium and phosphorus, both critical for building bone. Laboratory studies also show that vitamin D keeps cancer cells from growing and dividing.

Some preliminary studies indicate that insufficient intake of vitamin D is associated with an increased risk of fractures, and that vitamin D supplementation may prevent them.[19] Other early studies suggest an association between low vitamin D intake and increased risks of prostate, breast, colon, and other cancers.

Optimal intake: The current recommended intake of vitamin D is 5 micrograms up to age 50, 10 micrograms between the ages of 51 and 70, and 15 micrograms after age 70. Very few foods naturally contain vitamin D. Good sources include dairy products and breakfast cereals (which are fortified with vitamin D), and fatty fish such as salmon and tuna. For most people, the best way to get the recommended daily intake is by taking a multivitamin.

Vitamin E

For a time, vitamin E supplements looked like an easy way to prevent heart disease. Promising observational studies, including the *Nurses' Health Study*[20] and *Health Professionals Follow-up Study*,[21] suggested 20% to 40% reductions in coronary heart disease risk among individuals who took vitamin E supplements (usually containing 400 IU or more) for least two years.[22]

The results of several randomized trials have dampened enthusiasm for vitamin E's ability to prevent heart attacks or deaths from heart disease among individuals with heart disease or those at high risk for it. In the *Gruppo Italiano per lo Studio della Sopravvivenza nell'Infarto miocardio* (known as the *GISSI Prevention Trial*), more than three years of treatment with vitamin E had no effect on the rate of heart attacks, strokes, or deaths from any cause among 11,000 heart attack survivors, although it did appear to reduce sudden deaths and deaths due to cardiovascular disease.[23] Results from the *Heart Outcomes Prevention Evaluation (HOPE)* trial also showed no benefit of four years worth of vitamin E supplementation among more than 9,500 men and women already diagnosed with heart disease or at high risk for it.[24]

It is entirely possible that in secondary prevention trials, the use of drugs such as aspirin, beta blockers, and angiotensin-converting enzyme (ACE) inhibitors mask a modest effect of vitamin E, and that it may have benefits among healthier people. Ongoing randomized trials of vitamin E, such as the *Women's Health Study*[25] will tell us more about its possible benefits in the coming years.

Optimal intake: The recommended daily intake of vitamin E from food now stands at 15 milligrams from food. That's the equivalent of 22 IU from natural-source vitamin E or 33 IU of the synthetic form. Researchers are still writing the book on vitamin E. Evidence from observational studies suggests that at least 400 IU of vitamin E per day, and possibly more, are needed for optimal health. Since standard multivitamins usually contain around 30 IU, a separate vitamin E supplement is needed to achieve this level.

Vitamin K

Vitamin K helps make six of the 13 proteins needed for blood clotting. Its role in maintaining the clotting cascade is so important that people who take anticoagulants such as warfarin (Coumadin) must be careful to keep their vitamin K intake stable.

Lately, researchers have demonstrated that vitamin K is also involved in building bone. Low levels of circulating vitamin K have been linked with low bone density, and supplementation with vitamin K shows improvements in biochemical measures of bone health.[26] A report from the *Nurses' Health Study* suggests that women who get at least 110 micrograms of vitamin K a day are 30% less likely to break a hip as women who get less than that.[27] Among the nurses, eating a serving of lettuce or other green leafy vegetable a day cut the risk of hip fracture in half when compared with eating one serving a week. Data from the *Framingham Heart Study* also shows an association between high vitamin K intake and reduced risk of hip fracture.[28]

Optimal intake: The recommended daily intake for vitamin K is 80 micrograms for men and 65 for women. Because this vitamin is found in so many foods, especially green leafy vegetables and commonly used cooking oils, most adults get enough of it. According to a 1996 survey, though, a substantial number of Americans, particularly children and young adults, are not getting the vitamin K they need.[29]

Antioxidants

Our cells must constantly contend with nasty substances called free radicals. They can damage DNA, the inside or artery walls, proteins in the eye, or just about any substance or tissue imaginable. Some are made inside the body, inevitable byproducts of turning food into energy. Others come from the air we breathe and the food we eat.

We are not defenseless against free radicals. We extract free-radical fighters, called antioxidants, from food. Fruits, vegetables, and other plant-based foods deliver dozens, if not hundreds, of antioxidants. The most common are vitamin C, vitamin E, beta-carotene, and related carotenoids. Food also supplies minerals such as selenium and manganese, which are needed by enzymes that destroy free radicals.

During the 1990s, the term antioxidants became a huge nutritional buzz word. They were promoted as wonder agents that could prevent heart disease, cancer, cataracts, memory loss, and a host of other conditions.

It is true that the package of antioxidants, minerals, fiber, and other substances found in fruits, vegetables, and whole grains help prevent a variety of chronic diseases. Whether high doses of vitamin C, vitamin E, or other antioxidants can accomplish the same feat is an open question.

The evidence accumulated so far is not promising. Randomized trials of vitamin C, vitamin E, and beta-carotene have not revealed much in the way of protection from heart disease, cancer, or age-related eye diseases. Ongoing trials of other antioxidants, such as lutein and zeaxanthin for macular degeneration and lycopene for prostate cancer, are underway.

The Bottom Line

A standard multivitamin supplement does not come close to making up for an unhealthy diet. It provides a dozen or so of the vitamins known to maintain health, a mere shadow of what is available from eating plenty of fruits, vegetables, and whole grains. Instead, a daily multivitamin provides a sort of nutritional safety net.

While most people get enough vitamins to avoid the classic deficiency diseases, relatively few get enough of five key vitamins that may be important in preventing several chronic diseases. These include the following:

- Folic acid
- Vitamin B_6
- Vitamin B_{12}
- Vitamin D
- Vitamin E

A standard, store-brand, recommended daily allowance (RDA) multivitamin can supply you with enough of these vitamins for under $40 a year. It is about the least expensive insurance you can buy.

References

1. World Cancer Research Fund. *Food, Nutrition and Cancer.* Washington, DC: American Institute for Cancer Research, 1997.

2. Feskanich D, Singh V, Willett WC, Colditz GA. Vitamin A intake and hip fractures among postmenopausal women. *JAMA* 2002; 287:47-54.

3. Rothman KJ, Moore LL, Singer MR, Nguyen US, Mannino S, Milunsky A. Teratogenicity of high vitamin A intake. *N Engl J Med* 1995; 333:1369-73.

4. Smithells RW, Sheppard S, Schorah CJ. Vitamin deficiencies and neural tube defects. *Arch Dis Child* 1976; 51:944-50.

5. Czeizel AE, Dudas I. Prevention of the first occurrence of neural-tube defects by periconceptional vitamin supplementation. *N Engl J Med* 1992; 327:1832-5.

6. MRC Vitamin Study Research Group. Prevention of neural tube defects: results of the Medical Research Council Vitamin Study. *Lancet* 1991; 338:131-7.

7. Federal Register. *Food Standards: Amendment of Standards of Identity for Enriched Grain Products to Require Addition of Folic Acid.* Final rule, 5 March 1996. Food and Drug Administration: Washington, DC, 1996.

8. McCully KS. Vascular pathology of homocystinemia: implications for the pathogenesis of arteriosclerosis. *Am J Pathol* 1969; 56:111-28.

9. Christen WG, Ajani UA, Glynn RJ, Hennekens CH. Blood levels of homocysteine and increased risks of cardiovascular disease: causal or casual? *Arch Intern Med* 2000; 160:422-34.

10. Welch GN, Loscalzo J. Homocysteine and atherothrombosis. *N Engl J Med* 1998; 338:1042-50.

11. Manson JE, Gaziano JM, Spelsberg A, et al. A secondary prevention trial of antioxidant vitamins and cardiovascular disease in women. Rationale, design, and methods. The WACS Research Group. *Ann Epidemiol* 1995; 5:261-9.

12. Spence JD, Howard VJ, Chambless LE, et al. Vitamin Intervention for Stroke Prevention (VISP) trial: rationale and design. *Neuroepidemiology* 2001; 20:16-25.

13. Giovannucci E, Rimm EB, Ascherio A, Stampfer MJ, Colditz GA, Willett WC. Alcohol, low-methionine—low-folate diets, and risk of colon cancer in men. *J Natl Cancer Inst* 1995; 87:265-73.

14. Zhang S, Hunter DJ, Hankinson SE, et al. A prospective study of folate intake and the risk of breast cancer. *JAMA* 1999; 281:1632-1637.

15. Carpenter KJ. *The history of scurvy and vitamin C.* Cambridge: Cambridge University Press, 1986.

16. Carr AC, Frei B. Toward a new recommended dietary allowance for vitamin C based on antioxidant and health effects in humans. *Am J Clin Nutr* 1999; 69:1086-1097.

17. Douglas RM, Chalker EB, Treacy B. Vitamin C for preventing and treating the common cold. *Cochrane Database Syst Rev* 2000:CD000980.

18. Thomas MK, Lloyd-Jones DM, Thadhani RI, et al. Hypovitaminosis D in medical inpatients. *N Engl J Med* 1998; 338: 777-83.

19. *Osteoporosis Prevention, Diagnosis, and Therapy.* http://consensus.nih.gov/cons/111/111_statement.htm accessed on 10 April 2002.

20. Stampfer MJ, Hennekens CH, Manson JE, Colditz GA, Rosner B, Willett WC. Vitamin E consumption and the risk of coronary disease in women. *N Engl J Med* 1993; 328:1444-9.

21. Rimm EB, Stampfer MJ, Ascherio A, Giovannucci E, Colditz GA, Willett WC. Vitamin E consumption and the risk of coronary heart disease in men. *N Engl J Med* 1993; 328:1450-6.

22. Rimm EB, Stampfer MJ. Antioxidants for vascular disease. *Med Clin North Am* 2000; 84:239-49.

23. Dietary supplementation with n-3 polyunsaturated fatty acids and vitamin E after myocardial infarction: results of the GISSI-Prevenzione trial. Gruppo Italiano per lo Studio della Sopravvivenza nell'Infarto miocardico. *Lancet* 1999; 354:447-55.

24. Yusuf S, Dagenais G, Pogue J, Bosch J, Sleight P. Vitamin E supplementation and cardiovascular events in high-risk patients. The Heart Outcomes Prevention Evaluation Study Investigators. *N Engl J Med* 2000; 342:154-60.

25. Buring JE, Hennekens CH, for the Women's Health Study Research Group. The Women's Health Study: Rationale, background and summary of the study design. *J Myocardial Ischemia* 1992; 4:27-29 and 30-40.

26. Weber P. Vitamin K and bone health. *Nutrition* 2001; 17:880-7.

27. Feskanich D, Weber P, Willett WC, Rockett H, Booth SL, Colditz GA. Vitamin K intake and hip fractures in women: a prospective study. *Am J Clin Nutr* 1999; 69:74-9.

28. Booth SL, Tucker KL, Chen H, et al. Dietary vitamin K intakes are associated with hip fracture but not with bone mineral density in elderly men and women. *Am J Clin Nutr* 2000; 71:1201-8.

29. Booth SL, Pennington JA, Sadowski JA. Food sources and dietary intakes of vitamin K-1 (phylloquinone) in the American diet: data from the FDA Total Diet Study. *J Am Diet Assoc* 1996; 96:149-54.

Chapter 11

Sodium and Potassium

On average, higher salt (sodium chloride) intake directly relates to higher blood pressure. Nearly all Americans consume substantially more salt than they need. Decreasing salt intake is advisable to reduce the risk of elevated blood pressure. Keeping blood pressure in the normal range reduces an individual's risk of coronary heart disease, stroke, congestive heart failure, and kidney disease. Many American adults will develop hypertension (high blood pressure) during their lifetime. Lifestyle changes can prevent or delay the onset of high blood pressure and can lower elevated blood pressure. These changes include reducing salt intake, increasing potassium intake, losing excess body weight, increasing physical activity, and eating a healthy diet.

Key Recommendations

- Consume less than 2,300 milligrams (mg) of sodium per day, approximately 1 tsp of salt.

- Choose and prepare foods with little salt. At the same time, consume potassium-rich foods, such as fruits and vegetables.

This chapter includes excerpts from "Sodium and Potassium," from *Dietary Guidelines for Americans, 2005*, U.S. Department of Health and Human Services (HHS) and U.S. Department of Agriculture (USDA). And, an excerpt titled, "Effects of Salt and Potassium on Health," from *Report of the Dietary Guidelines Advisory Committee on the Dietary Guidelines for Americans 2005*, HHS and USDA.

Key Recommendations for Specific Population Groups

- *Individuals with hypertension, blacks, and middle-aged and older adults.* Aim to consume no more than 1,500 mg of sodium per day, and meet the potassium recommendation (4,700 mg/day) with food.

Salt is sodium chloride. Food labels list sodium rather than salt content. When reading a Nutrition Facts Panel on a food product, look for the sodium content. Foods that are low in sodium (less than 140 mg or 5 percent of the daily value [%DV]) are low in salt.

On average, the natural salt content of food accounts for only about 10 percent of total intake, while discretionary salt use (i.e., salt added at the table or while cooking) provides another 5 to 10 percent of total intake. Approximately 75 percent is derived from salt added by manufacturers. In addition, foods served by food establishments may be high in sodium. It is important to read the food label and determine the sodium content of food, which can vary by several hundreds of milligrams in similar foods. For example, the sodium content in regular tomato soup may be 700 mg per cup in one brand and 1,100 mg per cup in another brand. Reading labels, comparing sodium content of foods, and purchasing the lower sodium brand may be one strategy to lower total sodium intake.

An individual's preference for salt is not fixed. After consuming foods lower in salt for a period of time, taste for salt tends to decrease. Use of other flavorings may satisfy an individual's taste. While salt substitutes containing potassium chloride may be useful for some individuals, they can be harmful to people with certain medical conditions. These individuals should consult a healthcare provider before trying salt substitutes.

Discretionary salt use is fairly stable, even when foods offered are lower in sodium than typical foods consumed. When consumers are offered a lower sodium product, they typically do not add table salt to compensate for the lower sodium content, even when available. Therefore, any program for reducing the salt consumption of a population should concentrate primarily on reducing the salt used during food processing and on changes in food selection (e.g., more fresh, less processed items, less sodium-dense foods) and preparation.

Reducing salt intake is one of several ways that people may lower their blood pressure. The relationship between salt intake and blood pressure is direct and progressive without an apparent threshold. On average, the higher individuals' salt intake, the higher their blood pressure. Reducing blood pressure, ideally to the normal range, reduces the risk of stroke, heart disease, heart failure, and kidney disease.

Another dietary measure to lower blood pressure is to consume a diet rich in potassium. A potassium-rich diet also blunts the effects of salt on blood pressure, may reduce the risk of developing kidney stones, and possibly decrease bone loss with age. The recommended intake of potassium for adolescents and adults is 4,700 mg/day. Recommended intakes for potassium for children 1 to 3 years of age is 3,000 mg/day, 4 to 8 years of age is 3,800 mg/day, and 9 to 13 years of age is 4,500 mg/day. Potassium should come from food sources. Fruits and vegetables which are rich in potassium with its bicarbonate precursors favorably affect acid-base metabolism, which may reduce risk of kidney stones and bone loss. Potassium-rich fruits and vegetables include leafy green vegetables, fruit from vines, and root vegetables. Meat, milk, and cereal products also contain potassium, but may not have the same effect on acid-base metabolism.

Individuals with Hypertension, Blacks, and Middle-Aged and Older Adults

Some individuals tend to be more salt sensitive than others, including people with hypertension, blacks, and middle-aged and older adults. Because blacks commonly have a relatively low intake of potassium and a high prevalence of elevated blood pressure and salt sensitivity, this population subgroup may especially benefit from an increased dietary intake of potassium. Dietary potassium can lower blood pressure and blunt the effects of salt on blood pressure in some individuals. While salt substitutes containing potassium chloride may be useful for some individuals, they can be harmful to people with certain medical conditions. These individuals should consult a health-care provider before using salt substitutes.

Sodium Content Ranges in Food

Table 11.1 exemplifies the importance of reading the food label to determine the sodium content of food which can vary by several hundreds of milligrams in similar foods.

Effects of Salt and Potassium on Health

What are the effects of salt (sodium chloride) intake on health?

The relationship between salt (sodium chloride) intake and blood pressure is direct and progressive without an apparent threshold.

Hence, individuals should reduce their salt intake as much as possible. In view of the currently high levels of salt intake, a daily sodium intake of less than 2,300 mg is recommended. Many persons will benefit from further reductions in salt intake, including hypertensive individuals, blacks, and middle- and older-aged adults. Individuals should concurrently increase their consumption of potassium because a diet rich in potassium blunts the effects of salt on blood pressure.

A recent report from the Institute of Medicine (IOM, 2004) provides the basis for a recommended daily sodium intake or adequate intake (AI) of 1,500 mg and a tolerable upper intake level (UL) of 2,300 mg for adults. These recommendations are based on an extensive examination of the scientific literature by an expert IOM panel. The primary basis for setting the AI was to ensure overall nutrient adequacy, not to prevent chronic disease. In contrast, the UL was set because of the direct relationship of salt intake with blood pressure.

Recommendations for salt (sodium chloride) intake. The IOM set the AI for sodium for adults at 1,500 mg per day to ensure

Table 11.1. Range of Sodium Content for Selected Foods

Food Group	Serving Size	Range (mg)
Breads, all types	1 oz	95 – 210
Frozen pizza, plain, cheese	4 oz	450 – 1200
Frozen vegetables, all types	½ cup	2 – 160
Salad dressing, regular fat, all types	2 Tbsp	110 – 505
Salsa	2 Tbsp	150 – 240
Soup (tomato), reconstituted	8 oz	700 – 1260
Tomato juice	8 oz (~1 cup)	340 – 1040
Potato chips[a]	1 oz (28.4 g)	120 – 180
Tortilla chips[a]	1 oz (28.4 g)	105 – 160
Pretzels[a]	1 oz (28.4 g)	290 – 560

[a] All snack foods are regular flavor, salted.

Source: Agricultural Research Service *Nutrient Database for Standard Reference, Release 17* and recent manufacturers label data from retail market surveys. Serving sizes were standardized to be comparable among brands within a food. Pizza and bread slices vary in size and weight across brands.

Note: None of the examples provided were labeled low-sodium products.

that the overall diet provides sufficient amounts of other nutrients and to cover sodium sweat losses in unacclimatized individuals who are exposed to high temperatures or who are moderately physically active (IOM, 2004). This amount of sodium does not apply to highly active individuals, such as endurance athletes and certain workers (e.g., foundry workers) who lose large amounts of sweat on a daily basis and thus require a higher sodium intake. The IOM set the UL at 2,300 mg of sodium per day (IOM, 2004). In dose-response trials, this level of sodium intake commonly was the next tested level above the AI. The UL of 2,300 mg of sodium daily is not a recommended intake. There is no benefit to consuming sodium in an amount that exceeds the AI.

Sodium intakes. According to data from *National Health and Nutrition Examination Survey 1988-1994 (NHANES III)* (IOM, 2004), the median intakes of sodium among adult men and women age 31 to 50 are 4,300 mg and 2,900 mg of sodium per day, respectively. One-fourth of adult men exceed 5,200 mg of sodium per day, and one-fourth of women exceed 3,500 mg per day. Approximately 95 percent of adult men and 75 percent of adult women exceed the UL of 2,300 mg of sodium per day, and 100 percent exceed the AI of 1,500 mg of sodium per day. On average, blacks and non-blacks consume similar amounts of sodium. The reported sodium intakes probably are underestimates of total sodium intake because the NHANES III did not ask about discretionary salt intake.

What are the effects of potassium intake on health?

Diets rich in potassium can lower blood pressure and lessen the adverse effects of salt on blood pressure, may reduce the risk of developing kidney stones, and possibly decrease bone loss. In view of the health benefits of potassium and its relatively low intake by the general population, a daily potassium intake of at least 4,700 mg is recommended. Blacks are especially likely to benefit from an increased intake of potassium.

In the generally healthy population with normal kidney function, a potassium intake from foods that exceeds 4.7 g per day poses no potential for increased risk because excess potassium is readily excreted in the urine. Hence, the IOM did not set a UL for potassium (IOM, 2004). However, a potassium intake below 4.7 g per day is indicated for individuals whose urinary potassium excretion is impaired. Adverse cardiac effects (arrhythmias) can result from hyperkalemia, which is a markedly elevated serum level of potassium. Common drugs that can substantially impair potassium excretion are angiotensin converting enzyme (ACE) inhibitors, angiotensin receptor blockers (ARB), and potassium-sparing diuretics. Medical conditions associated with impaired potassium excretion include diabetes, chronic kidney disease, end stage renal disease, severe heart failure, and adrenal insufficiency. As a group, elderly individuals are at increased risk of hyperkalemia because they often have one or more of these conditions or take one or more of the above medications.

Chapter 12

Fluids and Nutrition

Water

Physiological Functions

Water is considered an essential nutrient because it must be consumed from outside sources to satisfy metabolic demand. Water constitutes approximately 60% of adult body weight. It is a catalyst for a majority of enzymatic reactions including those involved in nutrient digestion, absorption, transport, and metabolism. It is also required for facilitating excretion of metabolic waste by the kidneys. Inadequate intake of water compromises cell functions by contributing to electrolyte imbalances, contraction of plasma volume, and inability to regulate body temperature.

Factors Affecting Availability

Water is not consumed in sufficient amounts by most individuals since thirst does not develop until body fluids are depleted well below

This chapter includes: "Nutrition Fact Sheet: Water," reprinted with permission from the Department of Preventative Medicine, Northwestern University Feinberg School of Medicine. © 2002 Northwestern University. Also, an excerpt titled, "Fluid Recommendations," from *Report of the Dietary Guidelines Advisory Committee on the Dietary Guidelines for Americans, 2005*, U.S. Department of Health and Human Services (HHS) and U.S. Department of Agriculture (USDA); and excerpts from "Alcoholic Beverages," from *Dietary Guidelines for Americans 2005*, HHS and USDA.

levels required for optimal functioning. Mechanisms that trigger thirst sensations are stimulated by increased osmolality or decreased extracellular volume which are not detected until significant contraction of plasma volume has occurred. Groups most vulnerable to dehydration—infants, elderly adults, and athletes—are either not able to adequately express thirst sensations or to detect them. With extreme heat and excessive perspiration, thirst may lag behind actual water requirements. To prevent dehydration, a minimum of eight cups of fluid is required daily from beverages and foods.

Table 12.1. Water Balance

Water Intake (milliliters)

Beverages	1400
Solid Food	700
Cellular Oxidation	200
Total	2300

Water Output (millimeters)

	Normal Ambient Temperature	High Ambient Temperature	Prolonged Exercise
Urine	1400	1200	500
Feces	100	100	100
Perspiration	100	1400	5000
Skin	350	350	350
Respiratory Tract	350	250	650
Total	2300	3300	6600

Source: Mahan, L.K. and Escott-Stump, S. Krause's *Food, Nutrition & Diet Therapy, 10th Ed.*, 2000.

Deficiency

Loss of body water amounting to 10% of the body weight impairs work performance and is associated with nausea, weakness, delirium, and hyperthermia. Signs of dehydration include poor skin turgor, skin tenting on the forehead, decreased urine output, concentrated urine, sunken eyes, dry mucous membranes in the mouth and nose, orthostatic blood pressure changes, and tachycardia (rapid heart beat). Water losses exceeding 20% of body weight are life-threatening.

Toxicity

Water intoxication may develop if large amounts of water are provided to patients to replenish fluids lost with surgery, trauma, or other conditions associated with fluid and electrolyte losses, especially if compromised renal function or hormonal imbalances are also present. The ensuing increase in intracellular fluid volume can cause swelling of brain tissue accompanied by headaches, nausea, vomiting, muscle twitching, convulsions, and even death.

Requirements

Consumption of approximately 2.5 to 3 liters (10.4–12.5 cups daily) of water is recommended to maintain optimal hydration. Both foods and beverages can satisfy this requirement. The equivalent of 8 cups of water (64 fluid ounces or 2 liters) is the minimum amount of fluid recommended daily to replace water losses under conditions of moderate activity, ambient temperature, and altitude. More specific guidelines are provided in table 12.2.

Dietary Sources

Water requirements are most effectively met by consumption of plain water or beverages which are greater than 90% water by volume. Water may also be obtained from solid foods such as fruits and vegetables which have a high water content. Low moisture foods such as grains and meat products do not contribute significantly to water intake.

Water Content of Selected Foods *

Foods with 91–100% water

- Water, any type
- Milk
- Coffee
- Soup
- Sports drink

- Watermelon
- Strawberries
- Broccoli
- Lettuce
- Tomato

Foods with 80–90% water

- Soda and fruit juices
- Non-carbonated fruit drinks
- Cantaloupe
- Orange
- Apple

- Pear
- Grapes
- Peach
- Gelatin

Foods with 70–79% water

- Peas
- Frozen yogurt
- Banana

- Some fish
- Eggs
- Casseroles

Foods with less than 69% water

- Potatoes
- Bread
- Pasta
- Rice
- Beef

- Poultry
- Nuts
- Baked goods
- Crackers
- Chips

* Source: Nutrient Data System 2.93 software program.

Fluid Recommendations

What amount of fluid is recommended for health?

The combination of thirst and usual drinking behavior, especially the consumption of fluids with meals, is sufficient to maintain normal hydration. Healthy individuals who have routine access to fluids and who are not exposed to heat stress consume adequate water to meet their needs. Purposeful drinking is warranted for individuals who are exposed to heat stress or who perform sustained vigorous activity.

Recommendations from the *Dietary Guidelines for Americans* for water are made to prevent the deleterious, primarily acute, effects of dehydration. These effects include impaired cognitive function and motor control. Although a low intake of water has been associated with some chronic diseases, this evidence is insufficient to establish recommendations for water consumption. The primary indicator of hydration status is plasma or serum osmolality.

Total water intake includes drinking water, water in beverages, and water contained in food. Because normal hydration can be maintained over a wide range of water intakes, the Adequate Intake (AI) for total water was set based on the median total water intake from U.S. survey data (Institute of Medicine [IOM], 2004). The AI should not be interpreted as a specific requirement or recommended intake. Individual water requirements can vary greatly, even on a day-to-day basis, primarily because of differences in physical activity and environmental conditions, but also because of differences in diet. A total water intake above the AI often is required by those individuals who are physically active or who are exposed to heat stress. In individuals who are neither physically active nor exposed to heat stress, daily consumption below the AI can be sufficient to maintain normal hydration. Dietary factors also influence water requirements because total water consumption must be sufficient to excrete metabolites of protein and organic compounds, as well as excess electrolytes. Because healthy individuals have considerable ability to excrete excess water and thereby maintain water balance, the IOM did not set a Tolerable Upper Intake Level (UL) for water. However, acute water toxicity can occur following the rapid consumption of large quantities of fluids that

Table 12.2. Guidelines to Replenish Water Losses during **Moderate Activity**

Life Stage	Fluid per *pound* body weight	Fluid per *kilogram* body weight
Infants	68 milliliters or 2.3 ounces	150 milliliters or 5 ounces
Children	22.7–22.3 milliliters or 0.75–0.91 ounces	50–60 milliliters or 1.7–2.0 ounces
Adults	5.6 milliliters or 0.2 ounces	35 milliliters or 1.2 ounces

Hydration Guidelines during **Strenuous Activity**

Before Exercise	During Exercise	After Exercise
One hour prior: 16 ounces	5–10 ounces every 15–20 minutes or 20–40 ounces every hour	24 ounces per pound weight loss experienced during exercise

greatly exceed the kidney's maximal excretion rate of approximately 0.7 to 1.0 L per hour.

Information about Alcoholic Beverages from the Dietary Guidelines for Americans

The consumption of alcohol can have beneficial or harmful effects depending on the amount consumed, age and other characteristics of the person consuming the alcohol, and specifics of the situation. According to the Behavioral Risk Factor Surveillance System, in 2002, 55 percent of U.S. adults were current drinkers, and forty-five percent of U.S. adults did not drink any alcohol at all. Abstention is an important option. Fewer Americans consume alcohol today as compared to 50 to 100 years ago.

Key Recommendations

- Those who choose to drink alcoholic beverages should do so sensibly and in moderation—defined as the consumption of up to one drink per day for women and up to two drinks per day for men.

- Alcoholic beverages should not be consumed by some individuals, including those who cannot restrict their alcohol intake, women of childbearing age who may become pregnant, pregnant and lactating women, children, adolescents, individuals taking medications that can interact with alcohol, and those with specific medical conditions.

- Alcoholic beverages should be avoided by individuals engaging in activities that require attention, skill, or coordination, such as driving or operating machinery.

Alcoholic beverages supply calories but few essential nutrients. As a result, excessive alcohol consumption makes it difficult to ingest sufficient nutrients within an individual's daily calorie allotment and to maintain a healthy weight. Although the consumption of one to two alcoholic beverages per day is not associated with macronutrient or micronutrient deficiencies or with overall dietary quality, heavy drinkers may be at risk of malnutrition if the calories derived from alcohol are substituted for those in nutritious foods.

American adults who consume alcohol should drink alcoholic beverages in moderation. Moderation is defined as the consumption of up to one drink per day for women and up to two drinks per day for men. Twelve fluid ounces of regular beer, 5 fluid ounces of wine, or 1.5 fluid ounces of 80-proof distilled spirits count as one drink for purposes of explaining moderation. This definition of moderation is not intended as an average over several days, but rather as the amount consumed on any single day.

The effect of alcohol consumption varies depending on the amount consumed and an individual's characteristics and circumstances. Alcoholic beverages are harmful when consumed in excess. Excess alcohol consumption alters judgment and can lead to dependency or addiction and other serious health problems such as cirrhosis of the liver, inflammation of the pancreas, and damage to the heart and brain. Even less than heavy consumption of alcohol is associated with significant risks. Consuming more than one drink per day for women and two drinks per day for men increases the risk for motor vehicle accidents, other injuries, high blood pressure, stroke, violence, some types of cancer, and suicide. Compared with women who do not drink, women who consume one drink per day appear to have a slightly higher risk of breast cancer.

Studies suggest adverse effects even at moderate alcohol consumption levels in specific situations and individuals. Individuals in some situations should avoid alcohol—those who plan to drive, operate machinery, or take part in other activities that require attention, skill, or coordination. Some people, including children, adolescents, women of childbearing age who may become pregnant, pregnant and lactating women, individuals who cannot restrict alcohol intake, individuals taking medications that can interact with alcohol, and individuals with specific medical conditions should not drink at all. Even moderate drinking during pregnancy may have behavioral or developmental consequences for the baby. Heavy drinking during pregnancy can produce a range of behavioral and psychosocial problems, malformation, and mental retardation in the baby.

Moderate alcohol consumption may have beneficial health effects in some individuals. In middle-aged and older adults, a daily intake of one to two alcoholic beverages per day is associated with the lowest all-cause mortality. More specifically, compared to non-drinkers, adults who consume one to two alcoholic beverages a day appear to have a lower risk of coronary heart disease. In contrast, among younger adults alcohol consumption appears to provide little, if any, health benefit, and alcohol use among young adults is associated with a higher risk of traumatic injury and death. A number of strategies reduce the risk of chronic disease, including a healthful diet, physical activity, avoidance of smoking, and maintenance of a healthy weight.

It is not recommended that anyone begin drinking or drink more frequently on the basis of health considerations.

Caloric Intake from Various Alcoholic Beverages

Table 12.3 is a guide to estimate the caloric intake from various alcoholic beverages. An example serving volume and the calories in that drink are shown for beer, wine, and distilled spirits. Higher alcohol content (higher percent alcohol or higher proof) and mixing alcohol with other beverages, such as calorically sweetened soft drinks, tonic water, fruit juice, or cream, increases the amount of calories in the beverage. Alcoholic beverages supply calories, but provide few essential nutrients.

Table 12.3. Calories in Selected Alcoholic Beverages

Beverage	Approximate Calories Per 1 Fluid Oz[a]	Example Serving Volume	Approximate Total Calories[b]
Beer (regular)	12	12 oz	144
Beer (light)	9	12 oz	108
White wine	20	5 oz	100
Red wine	21	5 oz	105
Sweet dessert wine	47	3 oz	141
80 proof distilled spirits (gin, rum, vodka, whiskey)	64	1.5 oz	96

[a] Source: Agricultural Research Service (ARS) *Nutrient Database for Standard Reference (SR),* Release 17 (http://www.nal.usda.gov/fnic/foodcomp/index.html). Calories are calculated to the nearest whole number per 1 fluid oz.

[b] The total calories and alcohol content vary depending on the brand. Moreover, adding mixers to an alcoholic beverage can contribute calories in addition to the calories from the alcohol itself.

Chapter 13

Sweeteners:
With and Without Calories

Sweeteners

Definition

There are two types of sweeteners: caloric (nutritive) and noncaloric (non nutritive). The caloric sweeteners provide 4 calories per gram; and the noncaloric varieties provide zero.

Function

Caloric sweeteners provide sweet flavor and bulk when added to food. They also maintain freshness and contribute to product quality. Caloric sweeteners act as a preservative in jams and jellies, and a flavor enhancer in processed meats. They provide fermentation for breads and pickles, bulk to ice cream, and body to carbonated beverages. Some caloric sweeteners are made by processing sugar compounds and some occur naturally.

Noncaloric sweeteners are used in place of caloric sweeteners in some cases. They do not provide calories, but they do provide the sweet taste. All noncaloric sweeteners are chemically processed.

Food Sources of Caloric Sweeteners

Processed

- Confectioner's sugar (also known as powdered sugar) is finely ground sucrose.

- Corn sweeteners are sugars obtained from corn (for example, corn syrup). Corn syrup is used frequently in carbonated beverages, baked goods, and some canned products. It is a liquid that is a combination of maltose, glucose, and dextrose.

- Dextrose is glucose combined with water.

- Invert sugar is a sugar that is made by dividing sucrose into its two parts: glucose and fructose. Sweeter than sucrose and used in a liquid form, invert sugar helps in maintaining the sweetness of confections and baked items.

- Sucrose includes raw sugar, granulated sugar, brown sugar, confectioner's sugar, and turbinado sugar. It is made up of glucose and fructose. It is made by concentrating sugar beet juice and/or sugar cane.

- Turbinado sugar is made by refining sugar and making it more pure.

Non-processed

- Raw sugar is granulated, solid, or coarse, and is brown in color. It is obtained by the evaporation of the moisture from the juice of the sugar cane.

- Brown sugar is made from the sugar crystals obtained from molasses syrup.

- Fructose is the naturally occurring sugar in all fruits. It is also called levulose or fruit sugar.

- Glucose is found in fruits but in limited amounts; it is also a syrup made from corn starch.

- Honey is a combination of fructose, glucose, and water, produced by bees.

- Lactose (milk sugar) is the carbohydrate that is in milk. It is made up of glucose and galactose.

- Maltose (malt sugar) is produced during the process of fermentation. It is found in beer and in breads.

- Mannitol is a by-product of alcohol production but does not contain any alcohol. It does have a laxative effect when consumed in large quantities. It is used in dietetic food products.

- Maple sugar is obtained from the sap of maple trees. It is made up of sucrose, fructose, and glucose.

- Molasses is obtained from the residue of sugar cane processing.

- Sorbitol is used in many dietetic food products. It is produced from glucose, and it is also found naturally in certain berries and fruits. It is absorbed by the body at a much slower rate than sugar.

Noncaloric Sweeteners

- Aspartame is a combination of phenylalanine and aspartic acid, which are two amino acids. It is also known by its commercial names of Equal, which is available as a packaged sweetener, and as NutraSweet when it is used in food or beverage products. It is 180 to 220 times sweeter than sugar.

- Acesulfame K is an artificial sweetener, also known as Sunett. It is heat stable and can be used in cooking and baking. It is also available as a tabletop sweetener, marketed under the name Sweet One. It is FDA-approved and is used in combination with other sweeteners such as saccharin in carbonated low-calorie beverages and other products.

- Saccharin is 300 times sweeter than sugar. It is the first artificial sweetener. It is used in several dietetic food and beverage products.

- Cyclamates are 30 times sweeter than sugar. They are banned in the United States because in 1970 they were shown to have caused bladder cancer in animals.

References: U.S. Department of Health and Human Services (HHS), National Toxicology Program (NTP) 9th Report on Carcinogens, May 2000.

Side Effects

Sugar provides calories and no other nutrients. There is a concern that sugar or caloric sweeteners can cause tooth decay. A high intake of sugar does not cause diabetes, but if a person is diagnosed with diabetes the amount of simple sugar eaten daily often needs to be reduced.

People have reported side effects from ingesting aspartame, but this has not been proved through scientific studies.

Recommendations

Sugar is on the Food and Drug Administration's (FDA's) list of safe foods. It contains 16 calories per teaspoon and can be used in moderation. All of the various types of sugars described can be used in moderation.

Aspartame has been FDA approved. Recommended safe daily levels are 18 packets of Equal or three 12-ounce diet sodas per day for a 130-pound person. For people with the genetic disorder phenylketonuria (PKU), aspartame is not recommended as they are unable to metabolize it.

In the National Toxicology Program (NTP) 9th Report on Carcinogens, May 2000, saccharin was removed from the list of carcinogenic substances.

Acesulfame K is also FDA approved.

Polyols: Sweet Benefits

According to a 2004 Calorie Control Council survey, 84 percent of consumers (or 180 million) use low-calorie, reduced-sugar, and sugar-free foods and beverages. A number of these products contain polyols or sugar alcohols, especially sugar-free gum, candy, ice cream, frozen desserts, and baked goods.

What Are Polyols?

Polyols, also called sugar alcohols, are a group of low-calorie, carbohydrate-based sweeteners. Polyols deliver the taste and texture of sugar with about half the calories. They are used as a food ingredient, often to replace sugar, cup for cup, in many sugar-free and low-calorie foods. Polyols vary in sweetness from about half as sweet as sugar to equally as sweet. Polyols add sweetness and texture to many sugar-free foods. They are frequently combined with low-calorie sweeteners such as aspartame, acesulfame-K, neotame, saccharin, or sucralose, which are intensely sweet and thus are used in small amounts. For example, polyols are used in foods such as sugar-free chewing gums, ice cream, candies, frozen desserts, and baked goods. In addition to mild sweetness, polyols provide the bulk and texture of sugar in food products.

How to Spot Polyols

Common polyols listed on food labels are:

- erythritol;
- hydrogenated starch hydrolysates (polyglycitol, polyglucitol);
- isomalt;
- lactitol;
- maltitol (including maltitol syrups);
- mannitol;
- sorbitol;
- xylitol.

Polyol content may be included voluntarily on the Nutrition Facts Panel. If a claim such as "sugar-free" is made on the label, the polyol content must be listed. According to U.S. Food and Drug Administration (FDA) guidelines, the specific polyol may be listed in the Nutrition Facts Panel if only one polyol is in the food. If more than one, the term "sugar alcohols" must be used. Don't be confused, the term sugar alcohols refers to the chemical structure. Polyols are neither sugar nor alcohol. FDA is currently evaluating whether the term "polyol" would be less confusing to consumers than "sugar alcohol."

Benefits of Polyols

Low-calorie, sugar-free foods that are sweetened with polyols offer many benefits:

- Polyols taste like sugar, but have fewer calories than sugar.
- Polyols do not promote tooth decay.
- Polyols produce a low glycemic response that benefits all consumers, including those with diabetes.

Promote Dental Health

The FDA approved the use of the health claim "does not promote tooth decay" for sugar-free products containing polyols. And, the American Dental Association issued a position statement that sugar-free foods do not promote tooth decay.

111

Low in Calories

Since polyols are only partially absorbed by the body, they have fewer calories than sugar. Polyols range from 0.2 to 3 calories per gram, compared to sugar with 4 calories per gram. That's why foods made with polyols provide sweetness with fewer calories.

Recognizing the Dietary Impact

According to diabetes management guidelines, if all the carbohydrate in a food is from polyols and the total carbohydrate is less than 10 grams, it is considered a "free food." To calculate the grams of available carbohydrate in foods with more than 10 grams, subtract half the grams of polyols from total carbohydrate grams.

Glycemic Effect

Polyols can be used to replace sugar, glucose, and certain types of starch in a variety of foods such as dairy products, baked goods, sweets, and candy. Polyols have a lower rate of digestion and absorption than sugars. This results in a lower rise in blood glucose and insulin levels than sugars and other carbohydrates. Food manufacturers are introducing many new food products using polyols to reduce the calories and the blood glucose response of foods.

Consume in Moderation

As with any food, consume foods with high amounts of low-digestible carbohydrates, like polyols, in moderate amounts. For some individuals, overconsumption of polyol-containing foods (about 50 grams of polyols or more per day) may cause laxative effects similar to prunes, beans, or certain high-fiber foods.

The Future Is Sweet

The future for products using polyols is a "sweet one." With current consumer preferences for low-calorie, sugar-free products, as well as the increased availability of polyols and innovations in food technology, consumers can enjoy additional good tasting, sugar-free, and reduced-calorie products. These products may assist in maintaining good oral health and managing weight and blood glucose levels.

Chapter 14

Food and Color Additives

For centuries, ingredients have served useful functions in a variety of foods. Our ancestors used salt to preserve meats and fish, added herbs and spices to improve the flavor of foods, preserved fruit with sugar, and pickled cucumbers in a vinegar solution. Today, consumers demand and enjoy a food supply that is flavorful, nutritious, safe, convenient, colorful, and affordable. Food additives and advances in technology help make that possible.

There are thousands of ingredients used to make foods. The Food and Drug Administration (FDA) maintains a list of over 3000 ingredients in its data base "Everything Added to Food in the United States," many of which we use at home every day (e.g., sugar, baking soda, salt, vanilla, yeast, spices, and colors).

Still, some consumers have concerns about additives because they may see the long, unfamiliar names and think of them as complex chemical compounds. In fact, every food we eat—whether a just-picked strawberry or a homemade cookie—is made up of chemical compounds that determine flavor, color, texture, and nutrient value. All food additives are carefully regulated by federal authorities and various international organizations to ensure that foods are safe to eat and are accurately labeled.

Excerpts from "Food Ingredients and Colors," reprinted from the International Food Information Council Foundation and the United States Food and Drug Administration, 2004.

Why Are Food and Color Ingredients Added to Food?

Additives perform a variety of useful functions in foods that consumers often take for granted. Some additives could be eliminated if we were willing to grow our own food, harvest and grind it, spend many hours cooking and canning, or accept increased risks of food spoilage. But most consumers today rely on the many technological, aesthetic, and convenient benefits that additives provide.

Ingredients are added to foods for the following reasons:

1. **To maintain or improve safety and freshness:** Preservatives slow product spoilage caused by mold, air, bacteria, fungi, or yeast. In addition to maintaining the quality of the food, they help control contamination that can cause foodborne illness, including life-threatening botulism. One group of preservatives—antioxidants—prevents fats and oils, and the foods containing them, from becoming rancid or developing an off-flavor. They also prevent cut, fresh fruits, such as apples, from turning brown when exposed to air.

2. **To improve or maintain nutritional value:** Vitamins and minerals (and fiber) are added to many foods to make up for those lacking in a person's diet, lost in processing, or to enhance the nutritional quality of a food. Such fortification and enrichment has helped reduce malnutrition in the U.S. and worldwide. All products containing added nutrients must be appropriately labeled.

3. **To improve taste, texture, and appearance:** Spices, natural and artificial flavors, and sweeteners are added to enhance the taste of food. Food colors maintain or improve appearance. Emulsifiers, stabilizers, and thickeners give foods the texture and consistency consumers expect. Leavening agents allow baked goods to rise during baking. Some additives help control the acidity and alkalinity of foods, while other ingredients help maintain the taste and appeal of foods with reduced fat content.

What Is a Food Additive?

In its broadest sense, a food additive is any substance added to food. Legally, the term refers to "any substance the intended use of which results or may reasonably be expected to result—directly or indirectly—in its becoming a component or otherwise affecting the characteristics of any food." This definition includes any substance used in the production, processing, treatment, packaging, transportation, or storage of food. The purpose of the legal definition, however, is to impose a pre-market approval requirement. Therefore, this definition excludes ingredients whose use is generally recognized as safe (where government approval is not needed), those ingredients approved for use by FDA or the U.S. Department of Agriculture prior to the food additives provisions of law, and color additives and pesticides where other legal pre-market approval requirements apply.

Direct food additives are those that are added to a food for a specific purpose in that food. For example, xanthan gum—used in salad dressings, chocolate milk, bakery fillings, puddings, and other foods to add texture—is a direct additive. Most direct additives are identified on the ingredient label of foods.

Indirect food additives are those that become part of the food in trace amounts due to its packaging, storage, or other handling. For instance, minute amounts of packaging substances may find their way into foods during storage. Food packaging manufacturers must prove to the U.S. Food and Drug Administration (FDA) that all materials coming in contact with food are safe before they are permitted for use in such a manner.

What Is a Color Additive?

A color additive is any dye, pigment, or substance which when added or applied to a food, drug, cosmetic, or to the human body, is capable (alone or through reactions with other substances) of imparting color. FDA is responsible for regulating all color additives to ensure that foods containing color additives are safe to eat, contain only approved ingredients, and are accurately labeled.

Color additives are used in foods for many reasons: 1) to offset color loss due to exposure to light, air, temperature extremes, moisture, and storage conditions; 2) to correct natural variations in color; 3) to enhance colors that occur naturally; and 4) to provide color to colorless and fun foods. Without color additives, colas wouldn't be brown, margarine wouldn't be yellow, and mint ice cream wouldn't be green. Color additives are now recognized as an important part of practically all processed foods.

FDA's permitted colors are classified as subject to certification or exempt from certification, both of which are subject to rigorous safety standards prior to their approval and listing for use in foods.

- **Certified colors** are synthetically produced (or human made) and used widely because they impart an intense, uniform color, are less expensive, and blend more easily to create a variety of hues. There are nine certified color additives approved for use in the United States. Certified food colors generally do not add undesirable flavors to foods.

- **Colors that are exempt from certification** include pigments derived from natural sources such as vegetables, minerals, or animals. Nature derived color additives are typically more expensive than certified colors and may add unintended flavors to foods. Examples of exempt colors include annatto extract (yellow), dehydrated beets (bluish-red to brown), caramel (yellow to tan), beta-carotene (yellow to orange), and grape skin extract (red, green).

How Are Additives Approved for Use in Foods?

Today, food and color additives are more strictly studied, regulated, and monitored than at any other time in history. FDA has the primary legal responsibility for determining their safe use. To market a new food or color additive (or before using an additive already approved for one use in another manner not yet approved), a manufacturer or other sponsor must first petition FDA for its approval. These petitions must provide evidence that the substance is safe for the ways in which it will be used. As a result of recent legislation, since 1999, indirect additives have been approved via a pre-market notification process requiring the same data as was previously required by petition.

When evaluating the safety of a substance and whether it should be approved, FDA considers: 1) the composition and properties of the substance, 2) the amount that would typically be consumed, 3) immediate and long-term health effects, and 4) various safety factors. The evaluation determines an appropriate level of use that includes a built-in safety margin—a factor that allows for uncertainty about the levels of consumption that are expected to be harmless. In other words, the levels of use that gain approval are much lower than what would be expected to have any adverse effect.

Because of inherent limitations of science, FDA can never be absolutely certain of the absence of any risk from the use of any substance. Therefore, FDA must determine—based on the best science available—if there is a reasonable certainty of no harm to consumers when an additive is used as proposed.

If an additive is approved, FDA issues regulations that may include the types of foods in which it can be used, the maximum amounts to be used, and how it should be identified on food labels. In 1999, procedures changed so that FDA now consults with USDA during the review process for ingredients that are proposed for use in meat and poultry products. Federal officials then monitor the extent of Americans' consumption of the new additive and results of any new research on its safety to ensure its use continues to be within safe limits.

If new evidence suggests that a product already in use may be unsafe, or if consumption levels have changed enough to require another look, federal authorities may prohibit its use or conduct further studies to determine if the use can still be considered safe.

Regulations known as Good Manufacturing Practices (GMP) limit the amount of food ingredients used in foods to the amount necessary to achieve the desired effect.

Questions and Answers about Food and Color Additives

How are ingredients listed on a product label?

Food manufacturers are required to list all ingredients in the food on the label. On a product label, the ingredients are listed in order of predominance, with the ingredients used in the greatest amount first, followed in descending order by those in smaller amounts. The label must list the names of any FDA-certified color additives. But some ingredients can be listed collectively as flavors, spices, artificial flavoring, or in the case of color additives exempt from certification, artificial colors, without naming each one. Declaration of an allergenic ingredient in a collective or single color, flavor, or spice could be accomplished by simply naming the allergenic ingredient in the ingredient list.

What are dyes and lakes in color additives?

Certified color additives are categorized as either dyes or lakes. Dyes dissolve in water and are manufactured as powders, granules, liquids, or other special-purpose forms. They can be used in beverages, dry mixes, baked goods, confections, dairy products, pet foods, and a variety of other products. Lakes are the water insoluble form of the dye. Lakes are more stable than dyes and are ideal for coloring products containing fats and oils or items lacking sufficient moisture to dissolve dyes. Typical uses include coated tablets, cake and donut mixes, hard candies, and chewing gums.

Do additives cause childhood hyperactivity?

No. Although this hypothesis was popularized in the 1970's, well-controlled studies conducted since then have produced no evidence that food additives cause hyperactivity or learning disabilities in children. A Consensus Development Panel of the National Institutes of Health concluded in 1982 that there was no scientific evidence to support the claim that additives or colorings cause hyperactivity. However, for some children with attention deficit hyperactivity disorder (ADHD) and confirmed food allergy, dietary modification has produced some improvement in behavior.

What is the difference between natural and artificial ingredients? Is a naturally produced ingredient safer than an artificially manufactured ingredient?

Natural ingredients are derived from natural sources (e.g., soybeans and corn provide lecithin to maintain product consistency; beets provide beet powder used as food coloring). Other ingredients are not found in nature, and therefore, must be synthetically produced as artificial ingredients. Also, some ingredients found in nature can be manufactured artificially and produced more economically, with greater purity and more consistent quality, than their natural counterparts. For example, vitamin C or ascorbic acid may be derived from an orange or produced in a laboratory. Food ingredients are subject to the same strict safety standards regardless of whether they are naturally or artificially derived.

Are certain people sensitive to Food, Drug, and Cosmetic (FDC) Yellow No. 5 in foods?

Yellow No. 5, is used to color beverages, dessert powders, candy, ice cream, custards, and other foods. FDA's Committee on Hypersensitivity to Food Constituents concluded in 1986 that Yellow No. 5 might cause hives in fewer than one out of 10,000 people. It also concluded that there was no evidence the color additive in food provokes asthma attacks. The law now requires Yellow No. 5 to be identified on the ingredient line. This allows the few who may be sensitive to the color to avoid it.

Do low-calorie sweeteners cause adverse reactions?

No. Food safety experts generally agree there is no convincing evidence of a cause and effect relationship between these sweeteners and negative health effects in humans. The FDA has monitored consumer complaints of possible adverse reactions for more than 15 years. However, persons with a rare hereditary disease known as phenylketonuria (PKU) must control their intake of phenylalanine from all sources, including aspartame. Although aspartame contains only a small amount of phenylalanine, labels of aspartame-containing foods and beverages must include a statement advising phenylketonurics of the presence of phenylalanine.

Individuals who have concerns about possible adverse effects from food additives or other substances should contact their physicians.

How do they add vitamins and minerals to fortified cereals?

Adding nutrients to a cereal can cause taste and color changes in the product. This is especially true with added minerals. Since no one wants cereal that tastes like a vitamin supplement, a variety of techniques are employed in the fortification process. In general, those nutrients that are heat stable (such as vitamins A and E and various minerals) are incorporated into the cereal itself (they're baked right in). Nutrients that are not stable to heat (such as B-vitamins) are applied directly to the cereal after all heating steps are completed. Each cereal is unique—some can handle more nutrients than others can.

What is the role of modern technology in producing food additives?

Many new techniques are being researched that will allow the production of additives in ways not previously possible. One approach is the use of biotechnology, which can use simple organisms to produce food additives. These additives are the same as food components found in nature. In 1990, FDA approved the first bioengineered enzyme, rennin, which traditionally had been extracted from calves' stomachs for use in making cheese.

Types of Food Ingredients

Table 14.1. lists the types of common food ingredients, why they are used, and some examples of the names that can be found on product labels. Some additives are used for more than one purpose.

Table 14.1. Food Ingredients: Uses, Examples, and Names

Preservatives

What They Do: Prevent food spoilage from bacteria, molds, fungi, or yeast (antimicrobials); slow or prevent changes in color, flavor, or texture and delay rancidity (antioxidants); maintain freshness

Examples of Uses: Fruit sauces and jellies, beverages, baked goods, cured meats, oils and margarines, cereals, dressings, snack foods, fruits, and vegetables

Names Found on Product Labels: Ascorbic acid, citric acid, sodium benzoate, calcium propionate, sodium erythorbate, sodium nitrite, calcium sorbate, potassium sorbate, butylated hydroxyanisole (BHA), butylated hydroxytoluene (BHT), ethylenediaminetetraacetic acid (EDTA), tocopherols (Vitamin E)

Sweeteners

What They Do: Add sweetness with or without the extra calories

Examples of Uses: Beverages, baked goods, confections, table-top sugar, substitutes, many processed foods

Names Found on Product Labels: Sucrose (sugar), glucose, fructose, sorbitol, mannitol, corn syrup, high fructose corn syrup, saccharin, aspartame, sucralose, acesulfame potassium (acesulfame-K), neotame

Color Additives

What They Do: Offset color loss due to exposure to light, air, temperature extremes, moisture, and storage conditions; correct natural variations in color; enhance colors that occur naturally; provide color to colorless and fun foods

Examples of Uses: Many processed foods, (candies, snack foods margarine, cheese, soft drinks, jams/jellies, gelatins, pudding, and pie fillings)

Names Found on Product Labels: FDC Blue Nos. 1 and 2, FDC Green No. 3, FDC Red Nos. 3 and 40, FDC Yellow Nos. 5 and 6, Orange B, Citrus Red No. 2, annatto extract, beta-carotene, grape skin extract, cochineal extract or carmine, paprika oleoresin, caramel color, fruit and vegetable juices, saffron (Note: Exempt color additives are not required to be declared by name on labels, but may be declared simply as colorings or color added)

Table 14.1. (*continued*) Food Ingredients: Uses, Examples, and Names

Flavors and Spices

What They Do: Add specific flavors (natural and synthetic)

Examples of Uses: Pudding and pie fillings, gelatin dessert mixes, cake mixes, salad dressings, candies, soft drinks, ice cream, BBQ sauce

Names Found on Product Labels: Natural flavoring, artificial flavor, and spices

Flavor Enhancers

What They Do: Enhance flavors already present in foods (without providing their own separate flavor)

Examples of Uses: Many processed foods

Names Found on Product Labels: Monosodium glutamate (MSG), hydrolyzed soy protein, autolyzed yeast extract, disodium guanylate, or inosinate

Fat Replacers (and components of formulations used to replace fats)

What They Do: Provide expected texture and a creamy texture in reduced-fat foods

Examples of Uses: Baked goods, dressings, frozen desserts, confections, cake and dessert mixes, dairy products

Names Found on Product Labels: Olestra, cellulose gel, carrageenan, polydextrose, modified food starch, microparticulated egg white protein, guar gum, xanthan gum, whey protein concentrate

Nutrients

What They Do: Replace vitamins and minerals lost in processing (enrichment); add nutrients that may be lacking in the diet (fortification)

Examples of Uses: Flour, breads, cereals, rice, macaroni, margarine, salt, milk, fruit beverages, energy bars, instant breakfast drinks

Names Found on Product Labels: Thiamine hydrochloride, riboflavin (Vitamin B_2), niacin, niacinamide, folate or folic acid, beta carotene, potassium iodide, iron or ferrous sulfate, alpha tocopherols, ascorbic acid, Vitamin D, amino acids (L-tryptophan, L-lysine, L-leucine, L-methionine)

Table 14.1. (*continued*) Food Ingredients: Uses, Examples, and Names

Emulsifiers

What They Do: Allow smooth mixing of ingredients, prevent separation. Keep emulsified products stable, reduce stickiness, control crystallization, keep ingredients dispersed, and to help products dissolve more easily

Examples of Uses: Salad dressings, peanut butter, chocolate, margarine, frozen desserts

Names Found on Product Labels: Soy lecithin, mono- and diglycerides, egg yolks, polysorbates, sorbitan monostearate

Stabilizers, Thickeners, Binders, Texturizers

What They Do: Produce uniform texture

Examples of Uses: Frozen desserts, dairy products, cakes, pudding and gelatin mixes, dressings, jams and jellies, sauces

Names Found on Product Labels: Gelatin, pectin, guar gum, carrageenan, xanthan gum, whey

pH Control Agents and Acidulants

What They Do: Control acidity and alkalinity, prevent spoilage

Examples of Uses: Beverages, frozen desserts, chocolate, low acid canned foods, baking powder

Names Found on Product Labels: Lactic acid, citric acid, ammonium hydroxide, sodium carbonate

Leavening Agents

What They Do: Promote rising of baked goods

Examples of Uses: Breads and other baked goods

Names Found on Product Labels: Baking soda, monocalcium phosphate, calcium carbonate

Anti-Caking Agents

What They Do: Keep powdered foods free-flowing, prevent moisture absorption

Examples of Uses: Salt, baking powder, confectioner's sugar

Names Found on Product Labels: Calcium silicate, iron ammonium citrate, silicon dioxide

Table 14.1. (*continued*) Food Ingredients: Uses, Examples, and Names

Humectants

What They Do: Retain moisture

Examples of Uses: Shredded coconut, marshmallows, soft candies, confections

Names Found on Product Labels: Glycerin, sorbitol

Yeast Nutrients

What They Do: Promote growth of yeast

Examples of Uses: Breads and other baked goods

Names Found on Product Labels: Calcium sulfate, ammonium phosphate

Dough Strengtheners and Conditioners

What They Do: Produce more stable dough

Examples of Uses: Breads and other baked goods

Names Found on Product Labels: Ammonium sulfate, azodicarbonamide, L-cysteine

Firming Agents

What They Do: Maintain crispness and firmness

Examples of Uses: Processed fruits and vegetables

Names Found on Product Labels: Calcium chloride, calcium lactate

Enzyme Preparations

What They Do: Modify proteins, polysaccharides and fats

Examples of Uses: Cheese, dairy products, meat

Names Found on Product Labels: Enzymes, lactase, papain, rennet, chymosin

Gases

What They Do: Serve as propellant, aerate, or create carbonation

Examples of Uses: Oil cooking spray, whipped cream, carbonated beverages

Names Found on Product Labels: Carbon dioxide, nitrous oxide

Additional Information

Center for Food Safety and Applied Nutrition (CFSAN)
5100 Paint Branch Parkway
College Park, MD 20740-3835
Toll-Free: 888-723-3366
Website: http://www.cfsan.fda.gov

Food Allergy and Anaphylaxis Network (FAAN)
11781 Lee Jackson Hwy.
Suite 160
Fairfax, VA 22033
Toll-Free: 800-929-4040
Fax: 703-691-2713
Website: http://
www.foodallergy.org
E-mail: faan@foodallergy.org

Food Safety and Inspection Service
1400 Independence Ave., S.W.
Room 2932-S
Washington, DC 20250-3700
Toll-Free Meat and Poultry
Hotline: 800-535-4555
Toll-Free TTY: 800-256-7072
Website: http://www.fsis.usda.gov
Food Additives Website: http://
www.fsis.usda.gov/OA/pubs/
additive.htm
E-mail: fsis@usda.gov

Institute of Food Technologists
525 W. Van Buren
Suite 1000
Chicago, IL 60607
Toll-Free: 800-IFT-FOOD (438-3663)
Phone: 312-782-8424
Fax: 312-782-8348
Website: http://www.ift.org
E-mail: info@ift.org

International Food Information Council Foundation
1100 Connecticut Ave., N.W.
Suite 430
Washington, DC 20036
Phone: 202-296-6540
Fax: 202-296-6547
Website: http://www.ific.org
E-mail: foodinfo@ific.org

U.S. Food and Drug Administration
5600 Fishers Lane
Rockville, MD 20857
Toll-Free: 888-463-6335
Website: http://www.fda.gov

Chapter 15

Food and Nutrition Misinformation

Types of Nutrition Misinformation

The public is bombarded with an overwhelming amount of food and nutrition information. Unfortunately, it is not always clear how to distinguish nutrition facts from nutrition misinformation. Nutrition facts result from application of the scientific method and can withstand replication and peer review.

Nutrition misinformation, on the other hand, consists of erroneous information, formulated with or without malicious intent, or misinterprets food and nutrition science. The danger of nutrition misinformation is that it may be harmful to health, or be used to fuel food faddism, quackery, or health fraud.

Food fads involve unreasonable or exaggerated beliefs that foods, supplements, or their components, may cure disease, convey special health benefits, or offer quick weight loss. Food fads may also involve combining or eliminating certain foods from the diet. The U.S. Surgeon General's Report on Nutrition and Health defines food quackery as "the promotion for profit of special foods, products, processes, or appliances with false or misleading health or therapeutic claims." Food quackery is exploitative and entrepreneurial. Nevertheless, many people who promote quackery schemes may themselves be victims of misinformation or incomplete information and may sincerely

Excerpted with permission from "Position of the American Dietetic Association: Food and Nutrition Misinformation," *Journal of the American Dietetic Association* 102:260–266. © 2002 American Dietetic Association.

believe that they are promoting accurate information. Health fraud shares many of the characteristics of food faddism and food quackery, yet it is always deliberate and done for gain. According to the American Dietetic Association (ADA)'s *Complete Food and Nutrition Guide*, "Health fraud means promoting for financial gain, a health remedy that doesn't work—or hasn't yet been proven to work."

The Harmful Effects on the Health and Economic Status of Consumers

The public has seen a shift in the health and nutrition environment that recognizes the link between diet, disease prevention, and optimal health. New science has revealed a place for functional foods and the assimilation of some forms of complementary medicine into mainstream healthcare. Consumers are taking greater responsibility for self-care, perhaps as a byproduct of an evolving healthcare system, and are hungry for food and nutrition information. With these changes have also come increased opportunities for food and nutrition misinformation to impact the health and economic status of consumers, leaving them perhaps more vulnerable to fraud than ever before. Indeed, nutrition products have been found to be among the most commonly misused. This issue becomes even more critical as the population ages, as there is evidence that the majority of victims of healthcare fraud—up to 60%—are older people. The population is also becoming more overweight and is spending billions of dollars annually to combat obesity. Americans have spent $33 billion annually on weight loss foods, products, and services. Yet fewer than half of obese patients have reported receiving any advice from healthcare professionals to lose weight, suggesting that qualified professionals need to be more proactive in providing sound information about appropriate weight loss methods and referrals to qualified dietetics professionals. The true cost of health fraud is difficult to calculate, but is likely in the tens of billions of dollars, especially when considering the cost of purchasing products that may do no harm, but also provide no benefit, whether purported or not.

Dietary supplements are a particular area of concern because of the rapid expansion of the market and changing federal regulations. No longer limited to vitamins and minerals, a plethora of herbal, botanical, sports supplements, and other products now comprises over half the dietary supplement industry and have helped sales increase by over 60% to $13.9 billion. Consumer spending on dietary supplements, natural/organic food, natural personal care products, and functional foods totaled $128 billion in 2000. Herbs and botanicals, sports and meal supplements, and other specialty products account for slightly more than half of these sales yet only 12% use herbal supplements. Many supplements, such as herbs, remain largely uncontrolled and unregulated so long as their labels contain no health claims. The Dietary Supplement Health Education Act of 1994 established specific guidelines for health claims and the labeling of dietary supplements, but also shifted the burden of proving the accuracy of claims, safety, and quality from the manufacturer to the Food and Drug Administration (FDA). This shift towards having to prove harm rather than safety can potentially impact consumers by lending an air of credibility to misinformation or fraud simply because the federal government has not yet discovered or taken action against it. Over 1,000 new dietary supplements are added annually to the already 29,000 already available. Monitoring the claims made by marketers of those products creates an overwhelming task for the FDA, further delaying the time when information can be retracted or products removed from the marketplace.

The health consequences of food quackery, faddism, misinformation, or the misuse or misinterpretation of emerging science, may include: delay or failure to seek legitimate medical care or continue essential treatment, undesirable drug/nutrient interactions, the effects of nutrient toxicities or toxic components of products, and interference with sound nutrition education and practices. Economic harm occurs when purported remedies, treatments, and cures fail to work, and when products are purchased needlessly. With the burden of proof now on the federal government, there are fewer roadblocks to developing costly but useless products. Indirect impact on health and economic status can occur when the media report conflicting stories or stories that contain information that may be accurate but incomplete.

Sources of Nutrition Misinformation

Consumers receive nutrition information from a variety of sources. According to the ADA's *Nutrition and You: Trends* 2000 survey, the media are consumers' leading source of nutrition information, with television (48%), magazines (47%), and newspapers (18%) cited as the top three information sources. Other sources cited include books (12%), doctors (11%), and family and friends (11%). Dietitians (1%) and nutritionists (1%) were not frequently cited.

The Internet is a burgeoning source of health and nutrition information. According to a Harris Interactive poll, an estimated 100 million consumers sought health information on the Internet in the year 2000, up from 70 million in 1999 (*Wall Street Journal*, 12/29/00).

Consumer interest in health and nutrition information is high, and more than four in 10 (43%) consumers say they like to hear about new studies. However, one in five consumers (22%) report being confused by reports giving dietary advice. The sheer volume and varying quality of the information received, as well as perceptions that the information is always changing, fuels consumer confusion about who or what to believe. Specific sources of nutrition misinformation include the following areas.

Misinterpretation of Scientific Studies in the Media

Scientific progress alone does not prevent or eliminate nutrition misinformation. Too often the popular media capitalize on preliminary research data in an effort to enhance audience and readership ratings. Promoters quickly turn legitimate research findings into sales pitches, products, and services. Therefore, universities, research groups, and commercial enterprises that fund a study and release the results to the media must use caution in presenting their findings.

In addition, news reports on food and nutrition rarely provide enough context for consumers to interpret the advice given. Frequently absent are details about how much more or less of a food to eat, how often to eat a food, and to whom the advice applies. Both the news media and researchers must share responsibility for reporting accurate, balanced, and complete information to the public.

The *New England Journal of Medicine*, concerned about the way scientific articles in their journal are sensationalized by the media, has responded by developing the following four caveats for the media to use when assessing research findings:

- An association between two events is not the same as a cause and effect.

- Demonstrating one link in a postulated chain of events does not mean that the whole chain is proved.

- Probabilities are not the same as certainties.

- The way a scientific result is framed can greatly affect its impact.

The evaluation of nutrition information through the media is best done through proper interpretation of scientific studies by qualified dietetics professionals and other credentialed experts. Initiatives such as the ADA's national media spokesperson program have made great strides nationally and locally in relaying accurate food and nutrition information to the public and positioning registered dietitians as the experts. Yet, a competitive field of celebrities, fitness experts, psychologists, and others without nutrition credentials are frequent sources for nutrition-related interviews.

For their part, researchers must put their own findings into context by explaining the connection with other studies that show different outcomes. Researchers can also lay the groundwork for ensuring that their findings are presented accurately by critically evaluating the supporting documentation used in their research. One model to follow is the rigorous criteria used by the National Research Council in determining what studies to cite in the report *Diet and Health: Implications for Reducing Chronic Disease Risk*. The Council first assessed the strengths and weaknesses of each kind of study and then evaluated the total evidence against six criteria: strength of association, dose-response relationship, temporally correct association, consistency of association, specificity of association, and biological plausibility. To properly evaluate reports of scientific studies, such criteria are needed, as well as knowledge of whether the studies were conducted by experienced investigators.

Dietetics professionals must be trained in critical research skills, including how to interpret research findings and communicate them to the public. They must recognize and communicate the fact that studies done on small, select groups are not applicable to the general population and that a single study should not form the basis for clinical practice. Dietetics professionals also must recognize that scientific studies will always be open to differences of interpretation; a clear scientific consensus on an issue may not emerge for many years.

Challenges from the Internet

The emergence of the Internet as a major source of health and nutrition information reflects the fact that consumers are taking more responsibility for researching and participating in their own health-care decisions. However, consumers must be reminded that the accuracy of information appearing on Web sites is not governed by any regulatory agency. Therefore, sites featuring sound science-based content coexist with sites containing questionable, inaccurate, or alarming information promoted by individuals and groups espousing unscientific views. Chat rooms, listservs, and electronic bulletin boards that are not supervised by qualified health professionals can provide a forum for the exchange of inaccurate advice about nutrition and health.

In addition, the popularization of electronic mail has resulted in rapid and widespread dissemination of false nutrition and health-related stories via the Internet. Examples of these unfounded "urban health myths" are that bananas from Costa Rica carry flesh-eating bacteria, and that the sweetener aspartame causes numerous ills such as multiple sclerosis and lupus.

Several health organizations are addressing the proliferation of misinformation on the Internet. For example, the American Medical Association has issued guidelines for medical and health information sites on the Internet. The Health On the Net Foundation sets ethical standards for Web site developers and strives to guide medical practitioners and consumers to useful and reliable online medical and health information.

Influence of Culture and Food Beliefs

Nutrition misinformation and mistaken beliefs flourish to some degree because they often are deeply rooted in our cultural milieu. Throughout history, many cultures have ascribed health promoting powers to certain foods, and many religions have followed specific dietary practices. The Chinese "herbs of immortality" that were a popular fad among the ancient Egyptians have their modern manifestation in Chinese herbs promoted to bodybuilders in health food stores.

An example of a cultural belief is the concept of "hot" and "cold" foods rooted in Hispanic culture. This belief refers to food's influence on health and well-being, not to the temperature or spiciness of foods. "Cold" foods include most vegetables, tropical fruits, dairy products, and inexpensive cuts of meat. "Hot" foods include chili peppers, garlic, onion, most grains, expensive cuts of meat, oils, and alcohol. Pregnancy is considered a "hot" condition during which many Latinos typically avoid "hot" foods, believing this will prevent the infant from contracting a "hot" illness, such as a skin rash.

In contrast to the Hispanic "hot/cold" beliefs, the Chinese believe that pregnancy is a "cold" condition during which the expectant mother should consume "hot" foods to keep herself in balance for good health.

Fundamental to mistaken beliefs about nutrition is the statement "you are what you eat," which implies that everything from mood and behavior to intellectual capacity is determined by diet. "Bee pollen boosts energy," "Fish is brain food," and "Eating grapefruit burns body fat," are some common mistaken beliefs about food.

Although some food beliefs that are rooted in traditional cultures and religions are unsupported by scientific evidence, they can be respected as long as they do not result in possible harm and economic exploitation to adherents.

Other Sources of Misinformation

Nutrition misinformation is often disseminated by multilevel marketing companies that promote unproven health products such as dietary supplements, weight loss products, and herbs. These companies claim that their products can prevent or cure disease. Product literature may contain illegal therapeutic claims or product distributors may supply such information through anecdotes and independently published literature.

Testimonials also may spread misinformation. People tend to believe information that is reinforced by sports figures, celebrities, health food store personnel, teachers, coaches, ministers, legislators, health-care workers, media commentators, health professionals, and other persons they respect. When such public role models give scientifically unfounded testimonials about the benefits of specific nutritional practices, the effects can be far-reaching and potentially harmful to the public. Thus, these role models should carefully examine the accuracy and reliability of any nutrition information they disseminate and sharpen their skills at making appropriate inferences from scientific reports. When they are uncertain about the scientific merit of nutrition products they are asked to endorse, or do not have the scientific expertise to identify nutrition misinformation, role models should seek the advice of dietetics professionals. Dietetics professionals must be aware of the various sources and forms of nutrition misinformation and be prepared to counter them with science-based information.

The Role of Consumers in Reviewing Science-Based Food and Nutrition Information

Self-care is a consumer trend; today's consumers are more proactive in gathering nutrition and health information. To take responsibility for their personal health behaviors, consumers need to meet the communication process halfway. Consumers need to recognize qualified dietetics professionals as credible resources for nutrition information and for helping consumers make sound decisions that match their personal needs. Knowing how to access credible information is one important skill. Consumers need to learn how to recognize science-based nutrition and health advice, to critically examine what they read or hear, and to distinguish fact from fiction.

Many consumers may not even be aware that misinformation exits. To avoid being lured by misinformation, consumers need to:

- question the qualifications of authors, presenters, and other nutrition advocates, as well as the evidence for any claims or advice;

- take steps to evaluate nutrition reports or promotions before they become victims of the ploys, by becoming more aware of the many ways misinformation, food fraud, and quackery are conveyed;

- think critically about food and nutrition messages used to promote the sale of a products or services;

- ask a qualified nutrition expert for help in evaluating a statement, product, or service;

- inquire at the medical or nutrition department of a nearby university or college, or at the food and nutrition department of a local hospital/medical center, to obtain current and accurate information and to find nutrition services for the public.

Additional Information

American Dietetic Association (ADA)
120 S. Riverside Plaza, Suite 2000
Chicago, IL 60606-6995
Toll-Free: 800-877-1600
Fax: 312-899-4899
Website: http://www.eatright.org/Public
E-mail: hotline@eatright.org

Chapter 16

Ten Nutrition Myths That Won't Quit

Myths may be the wrong word. It's not that these beliefs are dead wrong. More often, they're promising theories that are backed by too little evidence. Or they're outdated ideas that have crumpled under the weight of recent research. In this chapter, the evidence is clarified on 10 assumptions that people rarely question.

1. Soy Foods Prevent Breast Cancer

Most women will do whatever they can to reduce the risk of breast cancer. Maybe that's why they're so willing to believe that the plant estrogens (phytoestrogens) in soy can keep the disease at bay. Yet so far, the evidence is weak.

Researchers in the Netherlands reviewed 13 studies—largely from China and Japan—that looked at soy and the risk of breast cancer.[1] "Overall, results do not show protective effects, with the exception maybe for women who consume phytoestrogens at adolescence or at very high doses," concludes Petra Peeters of the University Medical Center in Utrecht.

What's more, if you exclude studies that asked women who already have breast cancer what they used to eat, that leaves only four studies that asked healthy women about soy and then waited to see who got cancer, she adds. "And none of them found statistically significant breast cancer reductions." The bottom line: it's still too early to say whether soy—or other phytoestrogens —might protect the breast. What else might soy do?

Prostate cancer. Soy's impact on the risk of prostate cancer is still muddy, in part because most Americans eat too little soy for studies to detect any lower risk. However, researchers have tested soy's impact on PSA (prostate-specific antigen) levels, with mixed results. In a recent study, soy grits (about two ounces a day) lowered PSA by 13 percent in eight men with prostate cancer.[2] In studies on healthy men, though, PSA didn't budge.[3] And experts are now questioning whether small changes in PSA levels matter.

Hot flashes. So far, well-designed studies have found that soy (or plant estrogens from supplements like red clover) has little impact on hot flashes and other symptoms of menopause. Researchers at the University of Minnesota examined 20 trials on menopause and soy foods, beverages, powders, or extracts. Nearly all came up empty.[4] "The available evidence suggests that phytoestrogens available as soy foods, soy extracts, and red clover extracts do not improve hot flushes or other menopausal symptoms," conclude Minnesota's Erin Krebs and colleagues.

The bottom line: soy foods do seem to lower cholesterol, so they may help protect your heart. But whether they do more is a question mark.

2. Olive Is the Healthiest Oil

Fish oil is probably the healthiest, but you can't pour it on your salad or cook with it. Olive is certainly one of the good oils. Whether it's the best is unclear.

"The data suggest that any oil that's high in unsaturated fats— whether it's polyunsaturated or monounsaturated—is associated with a decreased risk of cardiovascular disease," says Alice Lichtenstein of the U.S. Department of Agriculture Jean Mayer Human Nutrition Research Center on Aging at Tufts University in Boston. "Canola is probably better than olive oil because it's lower in saturated fat," Lichtenstein explains. What's more, canola has more polyunsaturated fat than olive oil, "and polys lower LDL [bad cholesterol] more than monos."

So why not stick with soy and canola? Both have more of a polyunsaturated fat called alpha-linolenic acid (ALA) than olive. ALA is an omega-3 fat that may help lower the risk of heart disease. But if preliminary studies hold up, ALA may also raise (slightly) the risk of prostate cancer. Right now that's a big if. "I don't think the data is strong enough for recommendations," says Lichtenstein.

And there are other ways to cut back on ALA. "Red meat and dairy fat are also sources of ALA, and they have been more consistently related to higher prostate cancer risk," says Ed Giovannucci of the Harvard School of Public Health.

Our advice: at home, switch off between canola and olive. Since roughly 80 percent of the oil used in the U.S. is soy, odds are you already get plenty from salad dressings, mayonnaise, and restaurant foods. You wouldn't want olive oil in your blueberry muffin recipe anyway.

3. Vitamin C Prevents Colds

Ever since Linus Pauling, people have rushed for a bottle of vitamin C at the first sniffle. And some take extra vitamin C all winter in hopes of keeping germs at bay.

Researchers recently looked carefully at 30 trials that tested the vitamin and colds. Their conclusion: taking high doses (up to 1,000 mg—or one gram—a day) for several winter months didn't ward off those pesky cold germs.[5] However, vitamin C did appear to shorten colds slightly—by a little less than half a day per cold. On average, the vitamin reduced days of misery by about eight percent, but the results varied widely. It doesn't hurt to try vitamin C—about 1,000 mg a day—once you feel that sore throat or reach for the tissues. Just don't expect miracles.

4. If Your Blood Sugar, Triglycerides, Cholesterol, and Blood Pressure Aren't High, Don't Worry

Even before you hit high, you hit trouble. Your risk of a heart attack, stroke, or diabetes doesn't jump from low to high when your number crosses a sharp cutoff. It's gradual. That's why experts keep ratcheting down what's normal. For example:

Blood sugar. In April 2004, the National Institute of Diabetes and Digestive and Kidney Diseases (NIDDK) announced that 40 percent of U.S. adults have pre-diabetes, which means their fasting blood sugar is between 100 and 125. (Over 125 is diabetes.) Using the old cutoff (110), only 20 percent of adults had pre-diabetes.

135

Blood pressure. In May 2003, the National Heart, Lung, and Blood Institute (NHLBI) declared that an estimated 22 million Americans have pre-hypertension—that is, blood pressure over 120 (systolic) or over 80 (diastolic). Another 25 percent have hypertension, or high blood pressure, which starts at 140 over 90.

Triglycerides. Triglycerides under 200 used to be normal. Now normal ends at 150, and borderline high ranges from 150 to 200, says the NHLBI.

HDL (good) cholesterol. The lower your HDL, the higher your risk of heart disease. Low used to be 35 or below. Now it's 40 or below (for men) and 50 or below (for women).

LDL (bad) cholesterol. A borderline high LDL is 130 to 160. But 129 isn't ideal. So NHLBI now makes it clear that only LDLs under 100 are optimal. An LDL between 100 and 129 is above optimal.

Why do the numbers keep dropping (or rising for HDL)? Studies show that people in that gray area between low and high are at risk. Take blood sugar. "Many people with pre-diabetes go on to develop type 2 diabetes within 10 years," says the NIDDK. But not if they do something about it.

"Research has clearly shown that losing five to seven percent of body weight through diet and increased physical activity can prevent or delay pre-diabetes from progressing to type 2 diabetes," explains NIDDK director Allen Spiegel.

"The emphasis has shifted from treatment to prevention," says Tufts's Alice Lichtenstein. And most people can prevent illness with diet, exercise, or other lifestyle changes. "We're trying to minimize disease progression without putting everyone on medication," she says.

5. People Gain a Lot of Weight over the Holidays.

Office parties, neighborhood gatherings, family celebrations—from Thanksgiving to New Year's Day, most Americans are surrounded by luscious, tempting, irresistible food. So the conventional wisdom—that most of us start the new year about five pounds heavier—seems reasonable. Reasonable but not necessarily true.

In 2000, researchers tracked 200 people from late September to early March, and, in some cases, into June.[6] On average, they gained only about a pound during the holidays. But that doesn't mean you can live it up from turkey to eggnog.

You might not lose what you gained. In the study, most people lost little weight after the holidays, whether they tried to or not. And one pound is half of what the average person gains in a year. Those two pounds may not seem like much, but after 10 years, they could easily move you from trim to chubby.

You may not be average. Among the overweight or obese participants in the study, 14 percent gained more than five pounds. What's more, the participants may not be typical. "The study followed employees of the National Institutes of Health, an upscale, professional, health-conscious bunch if ever there was one," notes Susan Roberts of the Human Nutrition Research Center on Aging at Tufts University. "Weight gain is a likely consequence of overindulgence," she cautions. "It's always easier to overeat than to lose weight, because our bodies don't seem to count a few thousand extra calories, but start screaming hunger if we cut a few thousand."

6. Antioxidants Prevent Cancer and Heart Disease

It sounded so convincing. Damage caused by renegade oxygen could trigger cancer, injure arteries, hamper vision, and accelerate aging, said enthusiasts. And antioxidants—like beta-carotene and vitamins C and E—could neutralize the damage before it took hold. But so far, the best studies—trials that randomly assigned people to take antioxidants or a placebo—have flopped.

Cancer. In two trials, high doses of beta-carotene raised the risk of lung cancer in smokers. In other studies, the antioxidant had no impact on skin, mouth, or throat cancer. And when European researchers pooled the results of 14 studies on more than 170,000 people, they found that vitamins A, C, E, and beta-carotene—separately or together—failed to cut the risk of cancers of the colon, pancreas, stomach, or esophagus.[7] "We could not find evidence that antioxidant supplements can prevent gastrointestinal cancers," the authors concluded.

Heart disease. "With vitamin E and heart disease, the evidence looked rosy a few years ago," says Meir Stampfer, chairman of the department of epidemiology at the Harvard School of Public Health.

Since then, researchers examined evidence from three trials testing beta-carotene supplements on 70,000 people and five trials testing vitamin E on 29,000 patients at high risk of cardiovascular disease.[8]

"The results of these trials have been disappointing and failed to confirm any protective effect of these vitamins for either cancer or for cardiovascular disease," wrote Robert Clarke of the Radcliffe Infirmary in Oxford, England.

That's not to say that all antioxidants are useless. "The door isn't closed," says Stampfer. For example, a large trial is still testing whether vitamin E and selenium can prevent prostate cancer. The mistake, he explains, is to assume that if antioxidants work, it's because they're antioxidants. "It's a myth that antioxidants are a meaningful category," says Stampfer. "Some, like vitamin C, are antioxidants in one setting and pro-oxidants in others. You have to look at the specifics." If vitamin E and selenium protect the prostate, it may not be because they're antioxidants. "They may work through different pathways," says Stampfer. "To say that a food is rich in antioxidants is meaningless."

7. A High-Fiber Diet Prevents Colon Cancer

"The National Cancer Institute believes eating the right foods may reduce your risk of some kinds of cancer," said the All-Bran label in 1984. "That's why a healthy diet includes high-fiber foods like bran cereals." Within months, President Reagan underwent surgery for colon cancer. The media advised people to eat more fiber to lower their risk. But the evidence wasn't as airtight as it sounded.

In 2000, two trials testing fiber-rich diets on precancerous colon polyps came up empty. One found no fewer polyps in roughly 1,000 people who ate a diet rich in fiber (33 grams a day) and fruits and vegetables (6½ servings a day), than in 1,000 people who ate their usual diet (with about 19 grams of fiber) for four years.[9] A second trial found no fewer polyps in 700 people who ate 14 grams a day of wheat bran fiber than in nearly 600 people who ate only two grams a day of fiber for three years.[10]

It's always possible that the trials didn't last long enough, but many experts have thrown in the towel. "The theory is close to disproved," says Stampfer. But don't throw out your All-Bran yet, he adds. "People should still eat fiber because we have strong evidence that it has other benefits." Among them: "Fiber—especially grain fiber—has been consistently linked to a lower risk of cardiovascular disease," Stampfer explains. Researchers aren't sure how fiber may protect the heart, but the link shows up in study after study.[11] "And there's no question that fiber decreases the risk of constipation and diverticulitis," he adds. "They're not marquee diseases, but they make people uncomfortable and kill some."

8. Don't Drink Milk If You Have a Cold

"Milk makes mucus," goes the conventional wisdom. Yet few studies have tested milk's effect on cold sufferers. (Okay, so it's not a life-or-death issue that's crying out for research funds.) However, Australian researchers took up the challenge in 1990.[12] They infected 50 volunteers with a cold virus and asked them to keep track of how much milk or other dairy foods they consumed for 10 days. Meanwhile, all used tissues were weighed to measure nasal secretions. The results: mucus ranged from zero to one ounce a day, and milk ranged from zero to 11 glasses a day, but one had nothing to do with the other.

It's hard to know how to sort out the good and bad things you hear about dairy these days. Here's a brief rundown:

Weight loss. "Burn more fat, lose weight," promise the milk ads. "3 servings of dairy a day in a reduced calorie diet supports weight loss." In fact, the evidence comes largely from research by Michael Zemel, a University of Tennessee professor. His only published study in humans showed more weight loss in 11 people who had three servings of dairy a day.[13] But Zemel has a stake in finding that dairy aids weight loss because he has a patent on the claim. (He's already licensed it to Yoplait, the American Dairy Association, and the National Dairy Council.) Until other researchers get into the act, stay skeptical.

Cancer. It's not so much dairy, but calcium that's under scrutiny. So far, it looks like too much calcium—more than 1,500 mg a day—may slightly raise the risk of prostate cancer.[14] That's how much you'd get in a typical diet plus four servings of milk (or yogurt or cheese). However, other studies show that roughly 1,000 mg of calcium, or at least one glass of milk a day, may cut the risk of colon cancer.[15]

Where does that leave consumers? Women can simply go for the recommended levels (from food and supplements). That's 1,000 mg a day if you're 50 or younger, and 1,200 mg a day if you're over 50. Women have a higher risk of osteoporosis than men anyway.

Men, on the other hand, should try not to exceed the recommended levels. "We know of no benefits at intakes that exceed 1,500 milligrams a day," says Ed Giovannucci of the Harvard School of Public Health.

"So it may be advisable for men to not exceed about 1,000 milligrams of calcium a day." If that seems scary, remember that if calcium raises the risk of prostate cancer, it's not by much.

9. Hamburgers Are Safe to Eat when the Meat Is No Longer Pink

Chicken is safe when the pink is gone, the juices run clear, the leg moves easily in its socket, or the thigh reaches an internal temperature of 180° F (170° F for a breast). That's enough to kill Salmonella and Campylobacter, the usual poultry contaminants.

But ground beef is a different story. *Escherichia coli* (*E coli*) O157:H7 can survive even when the pink is gone and the juices are clear. And you don't want to mess around with O157:H7. In some people, it can cause severe bloody diarrhea and stomach cramps. They're the lucky ones. Roughly two to seven percent of infections—often those in the elderly and children under five—lead to hemolytic uremic syndrome. Red blood cells are destroyed, the kidneys fail, and even with intensive care, three to five percent die. (Antibiotics don't help and may even hurt.) About a third of the survivors have abnormal kidney function many years later, and a few require long-term dialysis. Another eight percent have lifelong complications like high blood pressure, seizures, blindness, or paralysis, or lose part of their bowel.

How can you tell when your burger is done? Use a thermometer to make sure the internal temperature reaches 160° F. (Chain restaurants typically cook burgers enough to kill *E. coli*.)

Beyond burgers, make sure your milk, juice, or apple cider has been pasteurized. Pasteurizing heats beverages enough to kill the *E. coli*. If you're elderly, under age five, have a weak immune system, or simply want to play it safe, skip raw bean or alfalfa sprouts. You can wash other fruits and vegetables, but there's no way (yet) to make sure that sprouts are clean.

10. Being Overweight Is Largely a Threat to Your Heart and Risk of Diabetes

Extra pounds can make your heart pound when you exercise. Maybe that's why people remember that being overweight puts a strain on the heart. And many know that the risk of diabetes shoots up with weight gain. But they tend to forget that obesity can wreak havoc elsewhere. For example, after tobacco smoking, obesity is the principal cause of cancer in the U.S.

"Being heavy or gaining weight as an adult increases the risk for a number of cancers," says Rachel Ballard-Barbash of the National Cancer Institute. "The list includes postmenopausal breast cancer, colorectal cancer, endometrial cancer, esophageal cancer, and kidney cancer." And it's not just cancer.

"Many people aren't aware that obesity also increases the risk of stroke, hypertension, gastroesophageal reflux disease, gallstones, osteoarthritis, and venous thrombosis—that's when blood clots form in the legs and sometimes travel to the lungs," says JoAnn Manson of Harvard Medical School and Brigham and Women's Hospital in Boston.

What's more, some risks start to climb with just a small spare tire. "Even a weight gain of 15 to 20 pounds during adulthood increases the risk of diabetes, high blood pressure, and coronary heart disease," she adds. On the flip side, losing 10 to 20 pounds can cut those risks. "If you're overweight, losing even five to 10 percent of your starting weight can significantly improve blood pressure, cholesterol levels, and blood sugar levels," says Manson.

References

1. *Breast Cancer Res. Treat.* 77: 171, 2003.

2. *Urology* 64: 510, 2004.

3. *Cancer Epidemiol. Biomarkers Prev.* 13: 644, 2004.

4. *Obstet. Gynecol.* 104: 824, 2004.

5. *Cochrane Database Syst. Rev. 2*: CD000980, 2000.

6. *New Eng. J. Med.* 342: 861, 2000.

7. *Lancet* 364: 1219, 2004.

8. *Cardiovasc. Drugs Ther.* 16: 411, 2002.

9. *New Eng. J. Med.* 342: 1149, 2000.

10. *New Eng. J. Med.* 342: 1156, 2000.

11. *Arch. Intern. Med.* 164: 370, 2004.

12. *Amer. Rev. Respir. Dis.* 141: 352, 1990.

13. *Obes. Res.* 12: 582, 2004.

14. *Cancer Epidemiol. Biomarkers Prev.* 12: 597, 2003.

15. *J. Nat. Cancer Inst.* 96: 1015, 2004.

Part Two

Nutrition Intake and Proportions

Chapter 17

Adequate Nutrients within Calorie Needs

Many Americans consume more calories than they need without meeting recommended intakes for a number of nutrients. This circumstance means that most people need to choose meals and snacks that are high in nutrients but low to moderate in energy content; that is, meeting nutrient recommendations must go hand in hand with keeping calories under control. Doing so offers important benefits—normal growth and development of children, health promotion for people of all ages, and reduction of risk for a number of chronic diseases that are major public health problems.

Based on dietary intake data or evidence of public health problems, intake levels of the following nutrients may be of concern for:

- **Adults:** calcium, potassium, fiber, magnesium, and vitamins A (as carotenoids), C, and E.

- **Children and adolescents:** calcium, potassium, fiber, magnesium, and vitamin E.

This chapter includes: Excerpts from "Adequate Nutrients within Calorie Needs," from *Dietary Guidelines for Americans 2005*, U.S. Department of Health and Human Services (HHS) and U.S. Department of Agriculture (USDA); excerpts titled, "Aiming to Meet Nutrient Intake Recommendations," and "Nutrient Contributions of Each Food Group," from *Report of the Dietary Guidelines Advisory Committee on the Dietary Guidelines for Americans, 2005*, HHS and USDA; and "Food Intake Patterns," MyPyramid, USDA, 2005.

- **Specific population groups** (pregnant women, dark-skinned people, and people over age 50): vitamin B_{12}, iron, folic acid, and vitamins E and D.

At the same time, in general, Americans consume too many calories and too much saturated and *trans* fats, cholesterol, added sugars, and salt.

Meeting Recommended Intakes within Energy Needs

A basic premise of the Dietary Guidelines is that food guidance should recommend diets that will provide all the nutrients needed for growth and health. To this end, food guidance should encourage individuals to achieve the most recent nutrient intake recommendations of the Institute of Medicine, referred to collectively as the Dietary Reference Intakes (DRI).

An additional premise of the Dietary Guidelines is that the nutrients consumed should come primarily from foods. Foods contain not only the vitamins and minerals that are often found in supplements, but also hundreds of naturally occurring substances, including carotenoids, flavonoids and isoflavones, and protease inhibitors that may protect against chronic health conditions. There are instances when fortified foods may be advantageous. These include providing additional sources of certain nutrients that might otherwise be present only in low amounts in some food sources, providing nutrients in highly bioavailable forms, and where the fortification addresses a documented public health need.

Two examples of eating patterns that exemplify the Dietary Guidelines are the DASH (Dietary Approaches to Stop Hypertension) Eating Plan and the U.S. Department of Agriculture (USDA) Food Guide. These two similar eating patterns are designed to integrate dietary recommendations into a healthy way to eat and are used in the Dietary Guidelines to provide examples of how nutrient-focused recommendations can be expressed in terms of food choices. Both the USDA Food Guide and the DASH Eating Plan differ in important ways from common food consumption patterns in the United States. In general, they include:

- more dark green vegetables, orange vegetables, legumes, fruits, whole grains, and low-fat milk and milk products.

- less refined grains, total fats (especially cholesterol, and saturated and *trans* fats), added sugars, and calories.

Variety among and within Food Groups

Each basic food group is the major contributor of at least one nutrient while making substantial contributions of many other nutrients. The food groups in the USDA Food Guide are: grains; vegetables; fruits; milk, yogurt, and cheese; and meat, poultry, fish, dry beans, eggs, and nuts. Food groups in the DASH Eating Plan are: grains and grain products; vegetables; fruits; low-fat or fat-free dairy; meat, poultry, and fish; and nuts, seeds, and dry beans. Because each food group provides a wide array of nutrients in substantial amounts, it is important to include all food groups in the daily diet.

Both illustrative eating patterns include a variety of nutrient-dense foods within the major food groups. Selecting a variety of foods within the grain, vegetable, fruit, and meat groups may help to ensure that an adequate amount of nutrients and other potentially beneficial substances are consumed. For example, fish contains varying amounts of fatty acids that may be beneficial in reducing cardiovascular disease risk.

Nutrient-Dense Foods

Nutrient-dense foods are those foods that provide substantial amounts of vitamins and minerals (micronutrients) and relatively few calories. Foods that are low in nutrient density are foods that supply calories but relatively small amounts of micronutrients, sometimes none at all. The greater the consumption of foods or beverages that are low in nutrient density, the more difficult it is to consume enough nutrients without gaining weight, especially for sedentary individuals. The consumption of added sugars, saturated and *trans* fats, and alcohol provides calories while providing little, if any, of the essential nutrients.

Selecting low-fat forms of foods in each group and forms free of added sugars—in other words nutrient-dense versions of foods—provides individuals a way to meet their nutrient needs while avoiding the overconsumption of calories and of food components such as saturated fats. However, Americans generally do not eat nutrient-dense forms of foods. Most people will exceed calorie recommendations if they consistently choose higher fat foods within the food groups—even if they do not have dessert, sweetened beverages, or alcoholic beverages.

If only nutrient-dense foods are selected from each food group in the amounts proposed, a small amount of calories can be consumed as added fats or sugars, alcohol, or other foods—the discretionary calorie allowance.

Nutrients of Concern

The actual prevalence of inadequacy for a nutrient can be determined only if an Estimated Average Requirement (EAR) has been established and the distribution of usual dietary intake can be obtained. If such data are not available for a nutrient, but there is evidence for a public health problem associated with low intakes, a nutrient might still be considered to be of concern.

Efforts may be warranted to promote increased dietary intakes of:

- potassium, fiber, and possibly vitamin E, regardless of age;
- calcium and possibly vitamins A (as carotenoids) and C and magnesium by adults;
- calcium and possibly magnesium by children age 9 years or older;
- adolescent females in general.

Low intakes of fiber tend to reflect low intakes of whole grains, fruits, and vegetables. Low intakes of calcium tend to reflect low intakes of milk and milk products. Low intakes of vitamins A (as carotenoids) and C and magnesium tend to reflect low intakes of fruits and vegetables. Selecting fruits, vegetables, whole grains, and low-fat and fat-free milk and milk products in the amounts suggested by the USDA Food Guide and the DASH Eating Plan will provide adequate amounts of these nutrients.

Most Americans of all ages also need to increase their potassium intake. To meet the recommended potassium intake levels, potassium-rich foods from the fruit, vegetable, and dairy groups must be selected in both the USDA Food Guide and the DASH Eating Plan.

Most Americans may need to increase their consumption of foods rich in vitamin E while decreasing their intake of foods high in energy but low in nutrients. The vitamin E content in both the USDA Food Guide and the DASH Eating Plan is greater than current consumption, and specific vitamin E-rich foods need to be included in the eating patterns to meet the recommended intake of vitamin E. Breakfast cereal that is fortified with vitamin E is an option for individuals seeking to increase their vitamin E intake while consuming a low-fat diet.

In addition, most Americans need to decrease sodium intake. The DASH Eating Plan provides guidance on how to keep sodium intakes within recommendations. When using the USDA Food Guide, selecting foods that are lower in sodium than others is especially necessary to meet the recommended intake level at calorie levels of 2,600/day and above.

Considerations for Specific Population Groups

People over 50 and Vitamin B$_{12}$: Although a substantial proportion of individuals over age 50 have reduced ability to absorb naturally occurring vitamin B$_{12}$, they are able to absorb the crystalline form. Thus, all individuals over the age of 50 should be encouraged to meet their Recommended Dietary Allowance (RDA) (2.4 micrograms [µg]/day) for vitamin B$_{12}$ by eating foods fortified with vitamin B$_{12}$ such as fortified cereals, or by taking the crystalline form of vitamin B$_{12}$ supplements.

Women and Iron: Based on blood values, substantial numbers of adolescent females and women of childbearing age are iron deficient. Thus, these groups should eat foods high in heme-iron (e.g., meats), and/or consume iron-rich plant foods (e.g., spinach), or iron-fortified foods with an enhancer of iron absorption such as foods rich in vitamin C (e.g., orange juice).

Women and Folic Acid: Since folic acid reduces the risk of the neural tube defects, spina bifida, and anencephaly, a daily intake of 400 µg/day of synthetic folic acid (from fortified foods or supplements in addition to food forms of folate from a varied diet) is recommended for women of childbearing age who may become pregnant. Pregnant women should consume 600 µg/day of synthetic folic acid (from fortified foods or supplements) in addition to food forms of folate from a varied diet. It is not known whether the same level of protection could be achieved by using food that is naturally rich in folate.

Special Groups and Vitamin D: Adequate vitamin D status, which depends on dietary intake and cutaneous synthesis, is important for optimal calcium absorption, and it can reduce the risk for bone loss. The elderly and individuals with dark skin (because the ability to synthesize vitamin D from exposure to sunlight varies with degree of skin pigmentation) are at a greater risk of low serum 25-hydroxyvitamin D concentrations. Also at risk are those exposed to insufficient ultraviolet radiation (i.e., sunlight) for the cutaneous production of vitamin D (e.g., housebound individuals).

For individuals within the high-risk groups, substantially higher daily intakes of vitamin D (i.e., 25 µg or 1,000 International Units (IU) of vitamin D per day) have been recommended. Three cups of vitamin D-fortified milk (7.5 µg or 300 IU), 1 cup of vitamin D-fortified orange juice (2.5 µg or 100 IU), and 15 µg (600 IU) of supplemental vitamin D would provide 25 µg (1,000 IU) of vitamin D daily.

Fluid

The combination of thirst and normal drinking behavior, especially the consumption of fluids with meals, is usually sufficient to maintain normal hydration. Healthy individuals who have routine access to fluids and who are not exposed to heat stress consume adequate water to meet their needs. Purposeful drinking is warranted for individuals who are exposed to heat stress or perform sustained vigorous activity.

Flexibility of Food Patterns for Varied Food Preferences

The USDA Food Guide and the DASH Eating Plan are flexible to permit food choices based on individual and cultural food preferences, cost, and availability. Both can also accommodate varied types of cuisines and special needs due to common food allergies. Two adaptations of the USDA Food Guide and the DASH Eating Plan are vegetarian and milk substitutions.

Vegetarian Choices: Vegetarians of all types can achieve recommended nutrient intakes through careful selection of foods. These individuals should give special attention to their intakes of protein, iron, and vitamin B_{12}, as well as calcium and vitamin D if avoiding milk products. In addition, vegetarians could select only nuts, seeds, and legumes from the meat and beans group, or they could include eggs if so desired. At the 2,000-calorie level, they could choose about 1.5 ounces of nuts and ²/₃ cup legumes instead of 5.5 ounces of meat, poultry, and/ or fish. One egg, ½ ounce of nuts, or ¼ cup of legumes is considered equivalent to 1 ounce of meat, poultry, or fish in the USDA Food Guide.

Substitutions for Milk and Milk Products: Since milk and milk products provide more than 70 percent of the calcium consumed by Americans, guidance on other choices of dietary calcium is needed for those who do not consume the recommended amount of milk products. Milk product consumption has been associated with overall diet quality and adequacy of intake of many nutrients, including calcium, potassium, magnesium, zinc, iron, riboflavin, vitamin A, folate, and vitamin D. People may avoid milk products because of allergies, cultural practices, taste, or other reasons. Those who avoid all milk products need to choose rich sources of the nutrients provided by milk, including potassium, vitamin A, and magnesium in addition to calcium and vitamin D. Some non-dairy sources of calcium are shown in Table 17.2. The bioavailability of the calcium in these foods varies.

Those who avoid milk because of its lactose content may obtain all the nutrients provided by the milk group by using lactose-reduced or low-lactose milk products, taking small servings of milk several times a day, taking the enzyme lactase before consuming milk products, or eating other calcium-rich foods.

Calorie Requirements by Age, Gender, and Activity Level

Estimated amounts of calories needed to maintain energy balance for various gender and age groups at three different levels of physical activity. The estimates are rounded to the nearest 200 calories. These levels are based on Estimated Energy Requirements (EER) from the Institute of Medicine (IOM) *Dietary Reference Intakes Macronutrients Report, 2002*, calculated by gender, age, and activity level for reference-sized individuals. "Reference size," as determined by IOM, is based on median height and weight for ages up to age 18 years of age and median height and weight for that height to give a BMI of 21.5 for adult females and 22.5 for adult males.

Aiming to Meet Nutrient Intake Recommendations

What dietary pattern is associated with achieving recommended nutrient intakes?

Two major aspects of the USDA dietary pattern contribute to meeting nutrient intake recommendations:

1. Consumption of foods from each of the basic food groups:
    - fruits
    - vegetables
    - grain
    - milk, yogurt, and cheese
    - meat, poultry, fish, dry beans, eggs, and nuts

2. Consumption of a variety of food commodities within each of those food groups—since higher energy intake is strongly associated with greater variety and higher nutrient intake,

attention also should be given to food group choices that maintain appropriate energy balance.

What factors related to diet or physical activity may help or hinder achieving recommended nutrient intakes?

A sedentary lifestyle limits the amount of calories needed to maintain one's weight. Careful food selection is needed to meet recommended

Table 17.1. Estimated Calorie Requirements (in Kilocalories) for Each Gender and Age Group at Three Levels of Physical Activity

		Activity Level [a,b,c,]		
Gender	Age (years)	Sedentary[a]	Moderately Active[b]	Active[c]
Child	2–3	1,000	1,000–1,400[d]	1,000–1,400[d]
Female	4–8	1,200	1,400–1,600	1,400–1,800
	9–13	1,600	1,600–2,000	1,800–2,200
	14–18	1,800	2,000	2,400
	19–30	2,000	2,000–2,200	2,400
	31–50	1,800	2,000	2,200
	51+	1,600	1,800	2,000–2,200
Male	4–8	1,400	1,400–1,600	1,600–2,000
	9–13	1,800	1,800–2,200	2,000–2,600
	14–18	2,200	2,400–2,800	2,800–3,200
	19–30	2,400	2,600–2,800	3,000
	31–50	2,200	2,400–2,600	2,800–3,000
	51+	2,000	2,200–2,400	2,400–2,800

[a] Sedentary means a lifestyle that includes only the light physical activity associated with typical day-to-day life.

[b] Moderately active means a lifestyle that includes physical activity equivalent to walking about 1.5 to 3 miles per day at 3 to 4 miles per hour, in addition to the light physical activity associated with typical day-to-day life.

[c] Active means a lifestyle that includes physical activity equivalent to walking more than 3 miles per day at 3 to 4 miles per hour, in addition to the light physical activity associated with typical day-to-day life.

[d] The calorie ranges shown are to accommodate needs of different ages within the group. For children and adolescents, more calories are needed at older ages. For adults, fewer calories are needed at older ages.

nutrient intakes within this calorie limit. Diets that include foods with a high nutrient content relative to calories are helpful in achieving recommended nutrient intakes without excess calories. Diets that include a large proportion of foods or beverages that are high in calories but low in nutrients are unlikely to meet recommended intakes for micronutrients and fiber, especially for sedentary individuals.

Table 17.2. Summary of the Nutrient Contributions of Each Food Group, Averaged Over Food Patterns at All Energy Levels (*continued on next page*)

Food Group	Major contribution(s)[1]	Substantial contribution(s) (greater than 10% of total)[2]
Fruit Group	Vitamin C	Thiamin Vitamin B$_6$ Folate Magnesium Copper Potassium Carbohydrate Fiber
Vegetable Group	Vitamin A Potassium	Vitamin E Vitamin C Thiamin Niacin Vitamin B$_6$ Folate Calcium Phosphorus Magnesium Iron Zinc Copper Carbohydrate Fiber Alpha-linolenic acid
Vegetable Subgroups		
Dark green vegetables	Vitamin C	Vitamin A
Orange vegetables	Vitamin A	
Legumes		Folate Copper Fiber

153

Table 17.2. (*continued*) Summary of the Nutrient Contributions of Each Food Group, Averaged Over Food Patterns at All Energy Levels

Food Group	Major contribution(s)[1]	Substantial contribution(s) (greater than 10% of total)[2]
Vegetable Subgroups (*continued*)		
Starchy vegetables		Vitamin B_6 Copper
Other vegetables		Vitamin C
Grain Group	Thiamin Folate Magnesium Iron Copper Carbohydrate Fiber	Vitamin A Riboflavin Niacin Vitamin B_6 Vitamin B_12 Calcium Phosphorus Zinc Potassium Protein Linoleic acid Alpha-linolenic acid
Grain Subgroups		
Whole grains	Folate(tie)[1] Magnesium Iron Copper Carbohydrate(tie)[1] Fiber Zinc Protein	Thiamin Riboflavin Niacin Vitamin B_6 Vitamin B_12 Phosphorus
Enriched grains	Folate(tie)[1] Thiamin Carbohydrate(tie)[1] Copper	Riboflavin Niacin Iron
Meat, poultry, fish, eggs, and nuts group	Niacin Vitamin B_6 Zinc Protein	Vitamin E Thiamin Riboflavin Vitamin B_12 Phosphorus Magnesium Iron Copper Potassium Linoleic acid

Table 17.2. (*continued*) Summary of the Nutrient Contributions of Each Food Group, Averaged Over Food Patterns at All Energy Levels

Food Group	Major contribution(s)[1]	Substantial contribution(s) (greater than 10% of total)[2]
Milk group	Riboflavin Vitamin B_{12} Calcium Phosphorus	Vitamin A Thiamin Vitamin B_6 Magnesium Zinc Potassium Carbohydrate Protein
Milk group	Vitamin E Linoleic acid Alpha-linolenic acid	
Oils and soft margarines	Vitamin E Linoleic acid Alpha-linolenic acid	

[1] Major contribution means that the food group or subgroup provides more of the nutrient than any other single food group, averaged over all calorie levels. When two food groups or subgroups provide equal amounts, it is noted as a tie.

[2] A substantial contribution means that the food group or subgroup provides 10% or more of the total amount of the nutrient in the food patterns, averaged over all calorie levels.

MyPyramid Food Intake Patterns

Table 17.3. lists the suggested amounts of food to consume from the basic food groups, subgroups, and oils to meet recommended nutrient intakes at 12 different calorie levels. Nutrient and energy contributions from each group are calculated according to the nutrient-dense forms of foods in each group (e.g., lean meats and fat-free milk). The table also gives the discretionary calorie allowance that can be accommodated within each calorie level, in addition to the suggested amounts of nutrient-dense forms of foods in each group.

155

Table 17.3. Daily Amount of Food from Each Group

Calorie Level[1]	1,000	1,200	1,400	1,600	1,800	2,000	2,200	2,400	2,600	2,800	3,000	3,200
Fruits[2]	1 cup	1 cup	1.5 cups	1.5 cups	1.5 cups	2 cups	2 cups	2 cups	2 cups	2.5 cups	2.5 cups	2.5 cups
Vegetables[3]	1 cup	1.5 cups	1.5 cups	2 cups	2.5 cups	2.5 cups	3 cups	3 cups	3.5 cups	3.5 cups	4 cups	4 cups
Grains[4]	3 oz-eq*	4 oz-eq	5 oz-eq	5 oz-eq	6 oz-eq	6 oz-eq	7 oz-eq	8 oz-eq	9 oz-eq	10 oz-eq	10 oz-eq	10 oz-eq
Meat and Beans[5]	2 oz-eq	3 oz-eq	4 oz-eq	5 oz-eq	5 oz-eq	5.5 oz-eq	6 oz-eq	6.5 oz-eq	6.5 oz-eq	7 oz-eq	7 oz-eq	7 oz-eq
Milk[6]	2 cups	2 cups	2 cups	3 cups	3 cups	3 cups	3 cups	3 cups	3 cups	3 cups	3 cups	3 cups
Oils[7]	3 tsp	4 tsp	4 tsp	5 tsp	5 tsp	6 tsp	6 tsp	7 tsp	8 tsp	8 tsp	10 tsp	11 tsp
Discretionary calorie allowance[8]	165	171	171	132	195	267	290	362	410	426	512	648

* eq = equivalent

[1] **Calorie Levels** are set across a wide range to accommodate the needs of different individuals.

[2] **Fruit Group** includes all fresh, frozen, canned, and dried fruits and fruit juices. In general, 1 cup of fruit or 100% fruit juice, or ½ cup of dried fruit can be considered as 1 cup from the fruit group.

[3] **Vegetable Group** includes all fresh, frozen, canned, and dried vegetables and vegetable juices. In general, 1 cup of raw or cooked vegetables or vegetable juice, or 2 cups of raw leafy greens can be considered as 1 cup from the vegetable group.

[4] **Grains Group** includes all foods made from wheat, rice, oats, cornmeal, barley, such as bread, pasta, oatmeal, breakfast cereals, tortillas, and grits. In general, 1 slice of bread, 1 cup of ready-to-eat cereal, or ½ cup of cooked rice, pasta, or cooked cereal can be considered as 1 ounce equivalent (eq) from the grains group. At least half of all grains consumed should be whole grains.

[5] **Meat and Beans Group** in general, 1 ounce of lean meat, poultry, or fish, 1 egg, 1 Tbsp. peanut butter, ¼ cup cooked dry beans, or ½ ounce of nuts or seeds can be considered as 1 ounce equivalent from the meat and beans group.

[6] **Milk Group** includes all fluid milk products and foods made from milk that retain their calcium content, such as yogurt and cheese. Foods made from milk that have little to no calcium, such as cream cheese, cream, and butter, are not part of the group. Most milk group choices should be fat-free or low-fat. In general, 1 cup of milk or yogurt, 1½ ounces of natural cheese, or 2 ounces of processed cheese can be considered as 1 cup from the milk group.

[7] **Oils** include fats from many different plants and from fish that are liquid at room temperature, such as canola, corn, olive, soybean, and sunflower oil. Some foods are naturally high in oils, like nuts, olives, some fish, and avocados. Foods that are mainly oil include mayonnaise, certain salad dressings, and soft margarine.

[8] **Discretionary Calorie Allowance** is the remaining amount of calories in a food intake pattern after accounting for the calories needed for all food groups—using forms of foods that are fat-free or low-fat and with no added sugars.

Table 17.4. Vegetable Subgroup Amounts Per Week

c/wk= cup/week

Calorie Level[1]	1,000	1,200	1,400	1,600	1,800	2,000	2,200	2,400	2,600	2,800	3,000	3,200
Dark green veg	1 c/wk	1.5 c/wk	1.5 c/wk	2 c/wk	3 c/wk	3 c/wk	3 c/wk	3 c/wk	3 c/wk	3 c/wk	3 c/wk	3 c/wk
Orange veg.	.5 c/wk	1 c/wk	1 c/wk	1.5 c/wk	2 c/wk	2 c/wk	2 c/wk	2 c/wk	2.5 c/wk	2.5 c/wk	2.5 c/wk	2.5 c/wk
Legumes	.5 c/wk	1 c/wk	1 c/wk	2.5 c/wk	3 c/wk	3 c/wk	3 c/wk	3 c/wk	3.5 c/wk	3.5 c/wk	3.5 c/wk	3.5 c/wk
Starchy veg.	1.5 c/wk	2.5 c/wk	2.5 c/wk	2.5 c/wk	3 c/wk	3 c/wk	6 c/wk	6 c/wk	7 c/wk	7 c/wk	9 c/wk	9 c/wk
Other veg.	3.5 c/wk	4.5 c/wk	4.5 c/wk	5.5 c/wk	6.5 c/wk	6.5 c/wk	7 c/wk	7 c/wk	8.5 c/wk	8.5 c/wk	10 c/wk	10 c/wk

Chapter 18

How Much Are You Eating: Servings and Food Groups

"Make that mega-sized."

"I'll have the gigantic-gulp."

"I don't believe I ate the whole thing!"

Many people feel that the bigger the portion, the better. But is that so? Not if you're trying to manage your weight. One key to getting or keeping your weight in a healthy range is to eat sensible portions. That's easy to say—but not always so easy to do! This chapter gives tips to help you decide what sensible portions are for you, and to help you stick to those reasonable portion sizes.

How Much Do You Eat?

Suppose you had dinner at an Italian restaurant last night. You ordered spaghetti with meatballs. While you were waiting for your order, you ate 2 slices of garlic bread. How can you tell if this dinner is too much food for you? You need to estimate how much you ate, and then compare that to Food Guide Pyramid recommendations.

Think about your plateful of spaghetti and meatballs. Estimate the amounts of spaghetti, sauce, and meat. You may decide, for example, that the spaghetti portion was about 2 cups, the tomato sauce looked like about 1 cup, and the meatballs were about 6 ounces. With the 2

Excerpted from "How Much Are You Eating," Center for Nutrition Policy and Promotion, U.S. Department of Agriculture (USDA), March 2002.

slices of garlic bread, you now have an idea about how much you ate for dinner. But how do your portions translate into standard servings? According to the Pyramid, your portions equal the number of servings in Table 18.1.

Pyramid Recommendations

To figure out if your spaghetti dinner was the right amount of food for you, review the number of servings recommended for each Pyramid food group, based on your calorie needs. Over a day, you should plan on eating the number of servings recommended from each group.

The number of servings from each food group recommended by the Pyramid depends on your calorie needs.

- Children ages 2 to 6 years, many inactive women, and some older adults may need about 1,600 calories per day.

- Most children over 6, teen girls, active women, and many inactive men may need about 2,200 calories per day.

- Teen boys and active men may need about 2,800 calories per day.

For example, if you need about 1,600 calories a day, the Pyramid recommends 6 daily servings from the Grains (Bread, Cereal, Rice, and Pasta) group. How does this compare to your spaghetti dinner? Your dinner had 6 servings—the total daily recommendation for someone with your calorie needs. If you had counted your portions of spaghetti and bread as only 1 serving each, you might think you had only eaten 2 servings from the Grains group. But, you actually ate 6. By comparing the portion you ate with a standard Pyramid serving, you can judge whether your daily intake is right for you.

Table 18.1. Spaghetti Dinner

Food	Your portion	One Pyramid serving	Pyramid Food Group	Number of Pyramid Servings you ate
Spaghetti	2 cups	½ cup	Grains	4
Garlic bread	2 slices	1 slice	Grains	2
Tomato Sauce	1 cup	½ cup	Vegetables	2
Meatballs	6 oz.	2–3 oz.	Meat and beans	2–3

Pyramid serving sizes and the recommended number of servings from each group are guides to help determine your daily intake. Your portions do not have to match the standard serving size—they can be larger or smaller. But, the amount you eat over the day should match the total amount of a food that is recommended. Often, the food portions of grains and meats that people choose are larger than the Pyramid serving size. Be especially careful when counting servings from these groups to figure out how many Pyramid servings are in your portions.

Portions and Servings—What's the Difference?

A portion is the amount of food you choose to eat. There is no standard portion size and no single right or wrong portion size.

A serving is a standard amount used to help give advice about how much to eat, or to identify how many calories and nutrients are in a food. For example: You eat a sandwich with 2 slices of bread. The Food Guide Pyramid serving size for bread is 1 slice. Your portion is 2 slices, which equals 2 servings from the Pyramid Grains group. Your 2 servings are one-third of the Pyramid recommendation of 6 servings for people needing 1,600 calories per day.

Table 18.2. shows the size of a portion you may choose or be served. They are not recommendations. This table compares these portions to Pyramid servings, so that you can judge how they might fit into your overall daily eating plan.

How Can You Follow Pyramid Recommendations?

One key to making wise food choices is knowing how much you are eating, as well as how much you should eat. This is especially important if you are trying to lose weight or manage your weight. Note that an active man may need about 2,800 calories each day. This man's Grains group recommendation would be 11 servings per day. The full spaghetti dinner might fit easily within his recommended food choices for the day.

Tips to Help You Choose Sensible Portions

When Eating Out

- Choose a small or medium portion. This includes main dishes, side dishes, and beverages as well. Remember that water is always a good option for quenching your thirst.

Table 18.2. Sample Food Portions Larger than 1 Pyramid Serving

Food	Sample portion you receive	Compare to Pyramid serving size	Approximate Pyramid servings in this portion
Grains Group			
Bagel	1 bagel 4 ½" in diameter (4 ounces)	½ bagel 3" in diameter (1 ounce)	4
Muffin	1 muffin 3 ½" in diameter (4 ounces)	1 muffin 2 ½" in diameter (1½ ounces)	3
English muffin	1 whole muffin	½ muffin	2
Sweet roll or cinnamon bun	1 large from bakery (6 ounces)	1 small (1 ½ ounces)	4
Pancakes	4 pancakes 5" in diameter (10 ounces)	1 pancake 4" in diameter (1 ½ ounces)	6
Burrito-sized flour tortilla	1 tortilla 9" in diameter (2 ounces)	1 tortilla 7" in diameter (1 ounce)	2
Individual bag of tortilla chips	1¾ ounces	12 tortilla chips (¾ ounce)	2
Popcorn	16 cups (movie theatre, medium)	2 cups	8
Hamburger bun	1 bun	½ bun	2
Spaghetti	2 cups (cooked)	½ cup (cooked)	4
Rice	1 cup (cooked)	½ cup (cooked)	2
Vegetable Group			
Baked potato	1 large (7 ounces)	1 small (2¼ ounces)	3
French fries	1 medium order (4 ounces)	½ cup, 10 French fries (1 ounce)	4
Meat and Beans Group			
Broiled chicken breast	6 ounces	2 to 3 ounces	2
Fried chicken	3 pieces (7 to 8 ounces)	2 to 3 ounces	3
Broiled fish	6 to 9 ounces	2 to 3 ounces	3
Sirloin steak	8 ounces (cooked, trimmed)	2 to 3 ounces	3
Porterhouse steak or prime rib	13 ounces (cooked, trimmed)	2 to 3 ounces	5
Ham or roast beef (in deli sandwich)	5 ounces	2 to 3 ounces	2
Tuna salad (in deli sandwich)	6 ounces	2 to 3 ounces	2

- If main dish portions are larger than you want, order an appetizer or side dish instead, or share a main dish with a friend. Resign from the "clean your plate club"—when you've eaten enough, leave the rest. If you can chill the extra food right away, take it home in a doggie bag.

- Ask for salad dressing to be served on the side so you can add only as much as you want.

- Order an item from the menu instead of the all-you-can-eat buffet.

At Home

- Once or twice, measure your typical portion of foods you eat often. Use standard measuring cups. This will help you estimate the portion size of these foods and similar foods.

- Be especially careful to limit portions of foods high in calories, such as cookies, cakes, other sweets, fats, oils, and spreads.

- Try using a smaller plate for your meal.

- Put sensible portions on your plate at the beginning of the meal, and don't take second helpings.

Don't Be Fooled by Large Portions

Many items sold as single portions actually provide 2 or more Pyramid servings. For example, a large bagel may actually be equal to 3 or 4 servings from the Grains group. A restaurant portion of steak may be more than the recommended amount for the whole day. Table 18.2 lists other common examples of foods that are often sold or prepared in portions larger than one Pyramid serving.

Nutrition Facts Label Serving Sizes

The serving sizes listed on the Nutrition Facts label may be different from Food Guide Pyramid serving sizes. Many Pyramid serving sizes are smaller than those on the Nutrition Facts label. For example, 1 serving of cooked cereal, rice, or pasta is 1 cup for the label, but only ½ cup for the Pyramid.

Use the Nutrition Facts label to make nutritional comparisons of similar products. The label serving size is not meant to tell you how much to eat, but to help identify nutrients in a food and to make product comparisons easier. To compare the calories and nutrients in two foods, first check the serving size and the number of servings in the package. Serving sizes are provided in familiar units, such as cups or pieces.

The Bottom Line

Choosing sensible portions is a key to controlling calorie intake and getting or keeping your weight in a healthy range. What is sensible for you?

- Each day, choose the recommended amount from the five Pyramid food groups—depending on your calorie needs.

- A Pyramid serving may not be the same as the portion you choose to eat—compare to find out how many servings are in your portion.

- Keep sensible portions in mind at restaurants as well as at home.

Chapter 19

Portion Size: The Forgotten Factor

It began slowly, beneath the notice of most Americans. Decades ago, fast food chains started competing for consumer dollars by offering larger portions. Soon, value meals and super sizes became commonplace. In the meantime, modestly-sized bagels and muffins disappeared from American cafes, replaced by creations three or four times their size. Even table-service restaurants started using larger plates laden with more food to assure customers they were getting their money's worth. At the same time, portion sizes began expanding in the home.

Central to the New American Plate is a recognition that it is not just what we eat that matters, but also how much we eat of each food. According to statistics from the Centers for Disease Control and Prevention, the average number of calories Americans eat each day has risen from 1,996 to 2,247 over the last 20 years. That significant increase—251 calories per day—theoretically works out to an extra 26 pounds every year.

Learning about Servings

A good way to figure out the actual amount of food on your plate is by becoming familiar with the standard serving sizes established

Excerpted from *The New American Plate: Meals for a healthy weight and a healthy life, Revised Edition.* © 2004 American Institute for Cancer Research. Also, Table 19.2 is from "Table E-4," *Report of the Dietary Guidelines Advisory Committee on the Dietary Guidelines for Americans, 2005,* U.S. Department of Health and Human Services (HHS) and U.S. Department of Agriculture (USDA).

by the U.S. Department of Agriculture (USDA). Standard serving sizes provide accepted measurements for calories, fat, cholesterol, carbohydrates, protein, vitamins, and minerals. Referring to serving sizes allows us to speak the same language as health professionals and food manufacturers.

Table 19.1 lists standard serving sizes for a variety of foods. One look makes it clear that these servings are smaller than most people usually eat. For example, the American Institute for Cancer Research (AICR) recommends seven or more servings of whole grains, beans, and other starches per day. If this sounds like a great deal of food to you, consider the following:

- The two cups of spaghetti covering your dinner plate equals not one, but four grain servings.

Table 19.1. Standard Serving Sizes

Food	Serving	Looks Like
Chopped Vegetables	½ cup	½ baseball or rounded handful for average adult
Raw Leafy Vegetables (such as lettuce)	1 cup	1 baseball or fist of an average adult
Fresh Fruit	1 medium piece or ½ cup chopped	1 baseball, ½ baseball, or rounded handful for average adult
Dried Fruit	¼ cup	1 golf ball or scant handful for average adult
Pasta, Rice, Cooked Cereal	½ cup	½ baseball or rounded handful for average adult
Ready-to-Eat Cereal	1 oz., which varies from ½ cup to 1¼ cups (check label)	
Meat, Poultry, Seafood	3 oz. (boneless cooked weight from 4 oz. raw)	Deck of Cards
Dried beans	½ cup cooked	1/2 baseball or rounded handful for average adult
Nuts	1/3 cup	Level handful for average adult
Cheese	1½ oz. (2 oz. if processed cheese)	1 oz. looks like 4 dice

Source: U.S. Department of Agriculture (USDA).

- Those small bagels found in grocery store freezer aisles equal about two grain servings. The jumbo bagels commonly served in shops and cafes are closer to four or five.

- The full bowl of whole grain cereal you pour yourself in the morning may amount to two or three grain servings.

"Eyeball" What You Eat

You can use USDA standard serving sizes to develop an important weight management skill. (Often, but not always, the serving sizes listed on Nutrition Facts food labels are equivalent to these standard serving sizes.) It takes only a few minutes to learn, and it is a tool you will use many times.

At your next meal, check the serving size chart for a favorite food. Fill a measuring cup or spoon with that amount and empty the food onto a clean plate. Now take a good look. Make a mental snapshot of how much of the plate is covered by a single serving.

Do the same thing with some of your other favorite foods. You will only have to measure once or twice, and in no time you'll develop a real-world sense for serving sizes. Why is this helpful? Once you know how a standard serving is supposed to look on your plate, you can use this information at future meals. You will also know exactly how many servings of certain foods you have been eating and can consider whether your portion sizes have grown too large. This knowledge can help you make important changes for health.

Fad Diets and the New American Plate

No doubt you have heard a lot about high-protein and low-carb diets. Behind these quick-fix plans lies the notion that certain kinds of foods are bad and should be avoided. Unfortunately, people have had difficulty staying on diets that eliminate whole categories of food. Thus, weight that is lost with great effort is soon gained back.

But perhaps the worst thing about low-carb diets is the confusion they cause. Vegetables, fruits, whole grains, and beans are powerful tools in the fight against chronic disease and overweight. Yet they all contain considerable amounts of carbohydrates. Loose talk about cutting carbs may lead people to reduce consumption of these highly beneficial foods.

There is no need to eliminate any category of food from your diet in order to lose weight. Just form some healthy eating habits and stick to them. Maintain a healthy proportion of plant-based food to animal-based food on your plate, reduce portion size all around, and keep physically active.

Servings Versus Portions

Serving sizes may have been standardized by the government, but each individual has very different caloric needs and weight management goals. That is why it is important to distinguish between a serving, which is simply a standard unit of measure, and a portion, which is the amount of a food you actually eat.

For example, those who sit at a desk all day may need only one cup of cereal (the standard serving size) in the morning. Others who run three miles a day may need two or three cups (servings) for their portion. The size of the portion you eat should depend on your needs. Do you exercise regularly? Is your body experiencing an increased energy demand, as happens during puberty or pregnancy? Are you trying to cut back on calories in order to work toward a healthy weight? Then your plate should feature portions that reflect these needs.

Portions and Weight Loss

Looking to lose weight? Remember that the New American Plate features more food and fewer calories than a traditional meat-based meal. That is why it is possible to feel satisfied eating a meal built around vegetables, fruits, whole grains, and beans and still work toward a healthy weight. Add some regular physical activity, and you have a safe, effective way to manage your weight for the long term.

But what if the problem persists? You make the switch to a healthy diet, but still cannot seem to maintain a healthy weight. There may be many factors at play here, but consider the obvious one first. Are your portion sizes too large?

It may be time to eyeball those standard servings once again. Pour out your usual portion of a favorite food on a plate. Then using the chart, take a moment to measure out a standard serving of the same food on the same size plate. Compare. How many standard servings go into the portions you eat regularly? Are you eating three standard servings of potatoes when you are full after only two? Are you pouring two standard servings of cereal when your activity level requires only one?

Gradually cut back on the number of servings you include in your regular portions. Reducing your portion of mashed potatoes from two cups to one will save you 230 calories. Cutting back that bowl of cereal from two standard servings to one means 100 calories less. Consistently eating smaller portions can make a substantial difference.

Don't forget to watch your portion size when eating away from home as well. Choosing a regular burger instead of a quarter-pounder saves you about 160 calories. Stopping after one cup of pasta on a three-cup platter saves almost 300 calories. In eateries where portions are absurdly large, divide the plate of food in half and ask for a doggie bag for the extra half.

Eating a plant-based diet and reducing your portions are two important strategies in any weight loss plan. The third strategy is, of course, increasing your physical activity.

AICR recommends one hour a day of brisk physical activity and one hour a week of more vigorous exercise. That's the recommendation for reducing cancer risk. But any exercise you do is better than none at all. In working toward this activity level, you will burn more calories, which will help lower your weight. Always check with your doctor before starting or changing your exercise program.

A fad diet that has not stood up to rigorous scientific testing is not the way to go. Obesity became an epidemic at the same time portion sizes grew enormous. It is likely that you can reach a healthy weight on your own by simply increasing the proportion of plant foods on your

Table 19.2. How Portion Sizes Have Changed

Food Item	Calories per Portion 20 Years Ago	Calories per Portion Today
Bagel	140 calories (3 in. diameter)	350 calories (6 in. diameter)
Fast food cheeseburger	333 calories	590 calories
Spaghetti and meatballs	500 calories (1 cup of spaghetti with sauce and 3 small meatballs)	1,025 calories (2 cups of spaghetti and 3 large meatballs)
Bottle of soda	85 calories (6.5 oz.)	250 calories (20 oz.)
Fast food French fries	210 calories (2.4 oz)	610 calories (6.9 oz)
Turkey sandwich	320 calories	820 calories (10 in. sub)

Source: Adapted from the Portion Distortion Quiz on the NHLBI Web site.

plate, reducing the size of the portions you eat, and exercising more. If you still do not see your weight gradually moving in a healthy direction, contact your doctor or a registered dietitian for a more individualized plan.

Final Message

What's new about the New American Plate? It's the idea that eating for a healthy life can also mean eating for a healthy weight. There is no need to follow the latest diet trend. You just need to keep an eye on the proportion of foods on your plate, and the size of the portions you eat.

A diet based mostly on vegetables, fruits, whole grains, and beans can help prevent cancer, heart disease, type 2 diabetes, and stroke. It can also keep your weight in a healthy range. And because eating from the New American Plate is as pleasurable as it is beneficial, you will soon find it becomes a permanent part of your life.

Additional Information

American Institute for Cancer Research
1759 R Street N.W.
Washington, DC 20009
Toll-Free: 800-843-8114
Phone: 202-328-7744
Fax: 202-328-7226
Website: http://www.aicr.org
E-mail: aicrweb@aicr.org

AICR has recipes available on the website and a new cookbook with 200 recipes available in bookstores.

Chapter 20

Calories:
Necessary and Discretionary

Calories and Diet

Definition

The energy stored in food is measured in terms of calories. Technically, one calorie is the amount of energy required to raise the temperature of 1 gram of water 1 degree Centigrade (from 14.5 to 15.5). The calorie measure used commonly to discuss the energy content of food is actually a kilocalorie or 1000 real calories; this is the amount of energy required to raise one kilogram of water (about 2.2 pounds) one degree Centigrade.

Different foods can be used by the body to produce different amounts of energy—which is why a small piece of chocolate can have many more calories than a similarly sized piece of lettuce. However, since calories are a measure of energy, there cannot be, as some diet books claim, different types of calories. A fat calorie has the same amount of energy as a protein calorie by definition.

A person's caloric need is determined using a variety of mathematical equations. Age, height, current weight, desired weight, and height are taken into account.

This chapter includes, "Calories," © 2003 A.D.A.M., Inc. Reprinted with permission. Also, an excerpt titled, "Discretionary Calories," from *Report of the Dietary Guidelines Advisory Committee on the Dietary Guidelines for Americans, 2005*, U.S. Department of Health and Human Services (HHS) and U.S. Department of Agriculture (USDA).

Function

The amount of calories in a diet refers to how much energy the diet can provide for the body. A well-balanced diet is one that delivers an adequate amount of calories while providing the maximum amount of nutrients.

The body breaks down food molecules to release the energy stored within them. This energy is needed for vital functions like movement, thought, growth—anything that you do requires the use of fuel. The body stores energy it does not need in the form of fat cells for future use.

The process of breaking down food for use as energy is called metabolism. Increased activity results in increased metabolism as the body needs more fuel. The opposite is also true. With decreased activity the body continues to store energy in fat cells and does not use it up. Therefore, weight gain is the result of increased intake of food, decreased activity, or both.

The nutrition labels on food packages indicate the number of calories contained in the food.

Food Sources

Naturally, different foods provide different amounts of calories. Some foods, such as ice-cream, have many calories; while others, like leafy vegetables, have few.

Side Effects

- Inappropriate dieting (fad dieting) can lead to rebound weight gain.

- Altered body image can lead to anorexia nervosa or bulimia.

- Diets that are excessively low in calories are considered dangerous and do not result in healthful weight loss. A more desirable method of weight reduction is one that is moderate in calories and that encourages routine exercise.

- Children and young adults should not limit calories below the Recommended Daily Allowance because they require a certain amount of calories for growth and development. Better eating habits for the entire family often accomplish the caloric decrease that is required for a child or young adult to reach a desirable weight.

Recommendations

Recommendations for limiting calories:

- Do not eat meat more than once a day. Fish and poultry are recommended instead of red or processed meats because they are less fattening.

- Avoid frying food because your food absorbs the fats from the cooking oils and this increases your dietary fat intake. Bake or broil food instead. If you do fry, use polyunsaturated oils, such as corn oil.

- Cut down on your salt intake, whether it be table salt, or flavor intensifiers that contain salt such as monosodium glutamate (MSG).

- Include adequate fiber in your diet. Fiber is found in green leafy vegetables, fruit, beans, bran flakes, nuts, root vegetables, and whole grain foods.

- Do not eat more than 4 eggs per week. Although they are a good source of protein and low in saturated fat, eggs are very high in cholesterol, and should be eaten in moderation for that reason.

- Choose fresh fruit for desserts rather than cookies, cake, or pudding.

- Too much of anything has its drawbacks, whether it be calories, or a particular type of food. A well-balanced diet with creativity and variety is best suited to your needs.

Ask a registered dietitian to help you calculate the amount of calories your body needs.

Discretionary Calories

Discretionary calories can be viewed from two different perspectives—in the context of 1) the sedentary lifestyle and typical food consumption of Americans, or 2) diet planning.

The daily amount of food a person needs to consume is driven by two factors: the need to meet recommended nutrient intakes, and the need to consume enough calories to match energy expenditure and therefore maintain a stable weight. By carefully choosing foods with higher-nutrient densities and/or lower-energy densities, people can meet recommended nutrient intakes while still consuming fewer calories than their daily energy needs. In this situation, an individual has a certain amount of calories left in his or her daily caloric allowance—calories that can be used flexibly, since nutrient needs already have been fulfilled. These remaining calories are called discretionary calories—the difference between total energy requirements and the energy consumed to meet recommended nutrient intakes.

Discretionary Calories in the Context of the Sedentary Lifestyle and Typical Food Consumption of Americans

Because of sedentary lifestyles and food choices that frequently are relatively high in added sugars and solid fats, most Americans have used up discretionary calories even before meeting recommendations for nutrient intakes. The maximum amount of discretionary calories is based on the difference between their total daily calorie requirement and the number of calories used to meet nutrient recommendations.

Discretionary calories can be available only when the amount of calories used to meet recommended nutrient intakes is less than the total daily calorie expenditure. The magnitude of this difference, and whether it is positive or negative, depends on two factors: the nutrient content of the foods consumed, and the total energy requirement, which, in turn, is greatly dependent on the level of physical activity.

Consuming more calories than expended appears to be common in the U.S. population. Food intake surveys (e.g., the National Health and Nutrition Examination Survey) show that most adults have used up all or most of their discretionary calories. At present, Americans are consuming calories in excess of calorie needs (as manifested by the high prevalence of overweight and obesity). Many Americans, however, have inadequate intakes of nutrients. This pattern of nutrient inadequacy in the face of calorie excess results because Americans often consume nutrient-poor foods (e.g., sugar-sweetened beverages), because they choose to consume more energy-dense foods (e.g., whole-fat rather than nonfat milk), and because they are sedentary. Hence, persons who follow typical American eating and activity patterns have used up all their discretionary calories, and more likely are consuming diets well in excess of their energy requirements for their age, gender, and physical activity level.

It seems clear that the desirable goal for a person is to have some discretionary calories available. This would allow more flexibility in food choices, and would give extra room to consume additional healthy foods, such as fruits and vegetables. How can a person increase his or her discretionary calories? There are two ways:

1. By increasing physical activity—burning more calories increases total caloric needs, and increases the maximum amount of calories a person can consume daily. The active level is the desirable level of physical activity.

2. By consuming nutrient-dense foods that are relatively lower in energy density (i.e., a healthy diet).

Ways That Discretionary Calories Are Used Up

Most people have no discretionary calories because of their sedentary lifestyle and selection of energy-dense foods. However, if discretionary calories are available, they can be used in a variety of ways. Often, discretionary calories come from intrinsic fats found in foods in one or more of the basic food groups. For example, drinking low-fat milk rather than skim milk uses some discretionary calories, as does eating a medium-fat hamburger patty instead of a lean cut of meat. The U.S. Department of Agriculture (USDA) food modeling method counts most solid fats and all added sugars as discretionary. Alcoholic beverages also count as discretionary calories. Discretionary calories add up quickly. For example, a 12 ounce soft drink counts as about 150 discretionary calories because of the added sugars it provides, the fat in one cup of 2 percent milk counts as about 32 discretionary calories, and a 12 ounce can of beer counts as about 150 discretionary calories. This exceeds the total amount of discretionary calories that could be available for many persons.

Key Points Regarding Discretionary Calories

- The best way to increase the number of discretionary calories is to increase physical activity. The greater the amount of physical activity, the more discretionary calories will be available.

- Another way to increase the number of discretionary calories is to make nutrient-dense selections from the basic food groups, especially of foods that are good sources of vitamin E, potassium, calcium, and fiber.

- For good health, the goal is to be sure to obtain recommended nutrient intakes from the basic food groups and oils/*trans*-free soft margarines before consuming discretionary calories.

- Even if many discretionary calories are available, keeping saturated and *trans* fat intake very low is advisable to help reduce the risk of heart disease.

- Intake of no more than one serving of alcohol per day for women and two servings per day for men is advisable—even if many discretionary calories are available.

- For weight maintenance, the aim is to consume essential calories plus discretionary calories to equal total energy expenditure. For weight loss, the aim is to consume essential calories, but to consume only part of the discretionary calories. In this way, calorie intake will be less than total energy expenditure, but recommended nutrient intakes will be achieved.

Chapter 21

Food Labels

Chapter Contents

Section 21.1

How to Understand and Use the Nutrition Facts Label

U.S. Food and Drug Administration (FDA), November 2004.

The Nutrition Facts Label

People look at food labels for different reasons. Whatever the reason, many consumers would like to know how to use this information more effectively and easily. The information in this chapter will make it easier to use nutrition labels to make quick, informed food choices that contribute to a healthy diet.

The information in the top section of a Nutrition Facts label can vary with each food product. It contains product-specific information (serving size, calories, and nutrient information). The bottom part contains a footnote with Daily Values (DV) for 2,000 and 2,500 calorie diets. This footnote provides recommended dietary information for important nutrients, including fats, sodium, and fiber. The footnote is found only on larger packages and does not change from product to product.

The Serving Size

The serving size is listed as #1 in Figure 21.1. The first place to start when you look at the Nutrition Facts label is the serving size and the number of servings in the package. Serving sizes are standardized to make it easier to compare similar foods; they are provided in familiar units, such as cups or pieces, followed by the metric amount listing the number of grams.

The size of the serving on the food package influences the number of calories and all the nutrient amounts listed on the top part of the label. Pay attention to the serving size, especially how many servings there are in the food package. Then ask yourself, "How many servings am I consuming?" (e.g., 1/2 serving, 1 serving, or more). In the sample label, one serving of macaroni and cheese equals one cup. If you ate the whole package, you would eat two cups. That doubles the calories and other nutrient numbers, including the %Daily Values as shown in Figure 21.1.

Calories (and Calories from Fat)

Calories (#2 in Figure 21.1) provide a measure of how much energy you get from a serving of this food. Many Americans consume more calories than they need without meeting recommended intakes for a number of nutrients. The calorie section of the label can help you manage your weight (i.e., gain, lose, or maintain). Remember: the number of servings you consume determines the number of calories you actually eat (your portion amount).

In Figure 21.1, there are 250 calories in one serving of this macaroni and cheese. How many calories from fat are there in one serving? There are 110 calories, which means almost half the calories in a single serving come from fat. What if you ate the whole package content? Then, you would consume two servings, or 500 calories, and 220 calories would come from fat.

General Guide to Calories

The General Guide to Calories provides a general reference for calories when you look at a Nutrition Facts label. This guide is based on a 2,000 calorie diet. Eating too many calories per day is linked to excessive weight and obesity.

- 40 calories is low
- 100 calories is moderate
- 400 calories or more is high

The Nutrients: How Much?

Look at the top of the nutrient section labeled #3 and 4 in Figure 21.1. It shows you some key nutrients that impact on your health and separates them into two main groups.

Limit These Nutrients

The nutrients listed first are the ones Americans generally eat in adequate amounts, or even too much. The nutrients listed by #3 of Figure 21.1 should be limited. Eating too much fat, saturated fat, *trans* fat, cholesterol, or sodium may increase your risk of certain chronic diseases such as heart disease, some cancers, or high blood pressure. Important: Health experts recommend that you keep your intake of saturated fat, *trans* fat and cholesterol as low as possible as part of a nutritionally balanced diet.

Get Enough of These Nutrients

Most Americans do not get enough dietary fiber, vitamin A, vitamin C, calcium, and iron in their diets. The nutrients listed by #4 of Figure 21.1 may need to be increased. Eating enough of these nutrients can improve your health and help reduce the risk of some diseases and conditions. For example, getting enough calcium may reduce the risk of osteoporosis, a condition that results in brittle bones as

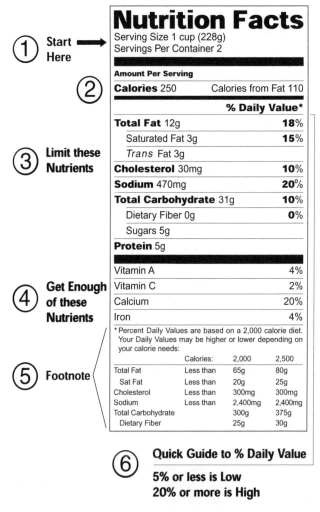

Figure 21.1 Nutrition Facts Label Sample for Macaroni and Cheese

people age. Eating a diet high in dietary fiber promotes healthy bowel function. Additionally, a diet rich in fruits, vegetables, and grain products that contain dietary fiber, particularly soluble fiber, and low in saturated fat and cholesterol may reduce the risk of heart disease.

Remember: You can use the Nutrition Facts label not only to help limit those nutrients you want to cut back on but also to increase those nutrients you need to consume in greater amounts.

Understanding the Footnote on the Bottom of the Nutrition Facts Label

Note the * used after the heading "%Daily Value" on the Nutrition Facts label. It refers to the Footnote (#5 in Figure 21.1) in the lower part of the nutrition label, which states "Percent Daily Value are based on a 2,000 calorie diet." This statement must be on all food labels. But

Table 21.1. Example of Double Serving

	Single Serving	% DV	Double Serving	% DV
Serving Size	1 cup (228 g)		2 cups (456 g)	
Calories	250		500	
Calories from Fat	110		220	
Total Fat	12g	18%	24 g	36%
Trans Fat	1.5 g		3 g	
Saturated Fat	3 g	15%	6 g	30%
Cholesterol	30 mg	10%	60 mg	20%
Sodium	470 mg	20%	940 mg	40%
Total Carbohydrate	31 g	10%	62 g	20%
Dietary Fiber	0 g	0%	0 g	0%
Sugars	5 g		10 g	
Protein	5 g		10 g	
Vitamin A		4%		8%
Vitamin C		2%		4%
Calcium		20%		40%
Iron		4%		8%

the remaining information in the full footnote may not be on the package if the size of the label is too small. When the full footnote does appear, it will always be the same. It does not change from product to product, because it shows recommended dietary advice for all Americans—it is not about a specific food product.

Daily Values (DV) are recommended levels of intakes. DV in the footnote is based on a 2,000 or 2,500 calorie diet. Note how the DV for some nutrients change, while others (for cholesterol and sodium) remain the same for both calorie amounts.

How the Daily Values Relate to the % DV

Upper Limit—Eat Less Than

The nutrients that have upper daily limits are listed first on the footnote of larger labels and in Table 21.2. Upper limits means it is recommended that you stay below—eat less than—the daily value amounts the nutrients listed per day. For example, the DV for saturated fat is 20g. This amount is 100% DV for this nutrient. What is the goal or dietary advice? To eat less than 20g or 100% DV for the day.

Lower Limit—Eat At Least

The DV for dietary fiber is 25g, which is 100% DV. This means it is recommended that you eat at least this amount of dietary fiber per day. The DV for total carbohydrate is 300g or 100% DV. This amount is recommended for a balanced daily diet that is based on 2,000 calories, but can vary, depending on your daily intake of fat and protein.

Table 21.2. Examples of DV Versus % DV Based on a 2,000 Calorie Diet

Nutrient	DV	% DV	Goal
Total Fat	65 g	= 100% DV	Less than
Sat Fat	20 g	= 100% DV	Less than
Cholesterol	300 mg	= 100% DV	Less than
Sodium	2400 mg	= 100% DV	Less than
Total Carbohydrate	300 g	= 100% DV	At least
Dietary Fiber	25 g	= 100% DV	At least

The Percent Daily Value (% DV)

Figure 21.1, #6 shows the % Daily Values (% DV) which are based on the daily value recommendations for key nutrients, but only for a 2,000 calorie daily diet—not 2,500 calories. You, like most people, may not know how many calories you consume in a day. But you can still use the % DV as a frame of reference whether or not you consume more or less than 2,000 calories.

The % DV helps you determine if a serving of food is high or low in a nutrient. A few nutrients, like *trans* fat, do not have a % DV.

Do you need to know how to calculate percentages to use the % DV? No, the label (the % DV) does the math for you. It helps you interpret the numbers (grams and milligrams) by putting them all on the same scale for the day (0–100% DV). The % DV column does not add up vertically to 100%. Instead each nutrient is based on 100% of the daily requirements for that nutrient (for a 2,000 calorie diet). This way you can tell high from low and know which nutrients contribute a lot, or a little, to your daily recommended allowance.

Using the % DV

Comparisons: The % DV makes it easy for you to make comparisons. You can compare one product or brand to a similar product. Just make sure the serving sizes are similar, especially the weight (e.g., gram, milligram, ounces) of each product. It is easy to see which foods are higher or lower in nutrients because the serving sizes are generally consistent for similar types of foods, except in a few cases like cereals.

Nutrient Content Claims: Use the % DV to help you quickly distinguish one claim from another, such as reduced fat vs. light or nonfat. Just compare the % DV for total fat in each food product to see which one is higher or lower in that nutrient—there is no need to memorize definitions. This works when comparing all nutrient content claims, e.g., less, light, low, free, more, high, etc.

Dietary Trade-Offs: You can use the % DV to help you make dietary trade-offs with other foods throughout the day. You do not have to give up a favorite food to eat a healthy diet. When a food you like is high in fat, balance it with foods that are low in fat at other times of the day. Also, pay attention to how much you eat so that the total amount of fat for the day stays below 100% DV.

Calcium: A Nutrient with a % DV but No Listed Weight

Calcium: Look at the % DV for calcium on food packages so you know how much one serving contributes to the total amount you need per day. Remember, a food with 20% DV or more contributes a lot of calcium to your daily total, while one with 5% DV or less contributes a little.

Experts advise adult consumers to consume adequate amounts of calcium, that is, 1,000 mg or 100% DV in a daily 2,000 calorie diet. This advice is often given in milligrams (mg), but the Nutrition Facts label only lists a % DV for calcium.

For certain populations, they advise that adolescents, especially girls, consume 1,300 mg (130% DV), and post-menopausal women consume 1,200 mg (120% DV) of calcium daily. The DV for calcium on food labels is 1,000 mg.

Do not be fooled—always check the label for calcium because you cannot make assumptions about the amount of calcium in specific food categories. Example: the amount of calcium in milk, whether skim or whole, is generally the same per serving, whereas the amount of calcium in the same size yogurt container (8 oz) can vary from 20–45% DV.

Calcium Equivalencies

- 30% DV = 300 mg calcium = one cup of milk
- 100% DV = 1,000 mg calcium
- 130% DV = 1,300 mg calcium

Nutrients without a % DV: Trans *Fats, Protein, and Sugars*

To limit nutrients that have no % DV, like *trans* fat and sugars, compare the labels of similar products and choose the food with the lowest amount.

***Trans* Fat:** Experts could not provide a reference value for *trans* fat nor any other information that FDA believes is sufficient to establish a DV or % DV. Scientific reports link *trans* fat (and saturated fat) with raising blood low density lipoprotein (LDL), or bad, cholesterol levels, both of which increase your risk of coronary heart disease, a leading cause of death in the U.S. Health experts recommend that you keep your intake of saturated fat, *trans* fat and cholesterol as low as possible as part of a nutritionally balanced diet.

Protein: A % DV is required to be listed if a claim is made for protein, such as high in protein. Otherwise, unless the food is meant for use by infants and children under 4 years old, none is needed. Current scientific evidence indicates that protein intake is not a public health concern for adults and children over 4 years of age.

Sugars: No daily reference value has been established for sugars because no recommendations have been made for the total amount to eat in a day. Keep in mind, the sugars listed on the Nutrition Facts label include naturally occurring sugars (like those in fruit and milk) as well as those added to a food or drink. Check the ingredient list for specifics on added sugars.

If you are concerned about your intake of sugars, make sure that added sugars are not listed as one of the first few ingredients. Other names for added sugars include: corn syrup, high-fructose corn syrup, fruit juice concentrate, maltose, dextrose, sucrose, honey, and maple syrup.

Section 21.2

Food Health Claims Permitted by the U.S. Food and Drug Administration (FDA)

This section includes excerpts from "Claims That Can Be Made for Conventional Foods and Dietary Supplements," and excerpts from "Summary of Qualified Health Claims Permitted," U.S. Food and Drug Administration (FDA), September 2003.

Claims That Can Be Made for Conventional Foods and Dietary Supplements

Claims that can be used on food and dietary supplement labels fall into three categories: health claims, nutrient content claims, and structure/function claims. The responsibility for ensuring the validity of these claims rests with the manufacturer, FDA, or in the case of advertising, with the Federal Trade Commission.

Health Claims

Health claims describe a relationship between a food, food component, or dietary supplement ingredient, and reducing risk of a disease or health-related condition. The FDA exercises oversight in determining which health claims may be used on a label or in labeling for a food or dietary supplement.

A health claim by definition has two essential components: (1) a substance (whether a food, food component, or dietary ingredient); and (2) a disease or health-related condition. A statement lacking either one of these components does not meet the regulatory definition of a health claim.

NLEA Authorized Health Claims. The Nutrition Labeling and Education Act (NLEA) of 1990, the Dietary Supplement Act of 1992, and the Dietary Supplement Health and Education Act of 1994 (DSHEA), provide for health claims used on labels that characterize a relationship between a food, a food component, dietary ingredient, or dietary supplement and risk of a disease (for example, diets high in calcium may reduce the risk of osteoporosis), provided the claims meet certain criteria and are authorized by an FDA regulation. FDA authorizes these types of health claims based on an extensive review of the scientific literature, generally as a result of the submission of a health claim petition, using the significant scientific agreement standard to determine that the nutrient/disease relationship is well established.

Health Claims Based on Authoritative Statements. The Food and Drug Administration Modernization Act of 1997 (FDAMA) provides a second way for the use of a health claim on foods to be authorized. FDAMA allows certain health claims to be made as a result of a successful notification to FDA of a health claim based on an authoritative statement from a scientific body of the U.S. Government or the National Academy of Sciences. FDA has prepared a guide on how a firm can make use of authoritative statement-based health claims. FDAMA does not include dietary supplements in the provisions for health claims based on authoritative statements. Consequently, this method of oversight for health claims cannot be used for dietary supplements at this time.

Qualified Health Claims. FDA's 2003 *Consumer Health Information for Better Nutrition Initiative* provides for the use of qualified health claims when there is emerging evidence for a relationship between a food, food component, or dietary supplement, and reduced risk of a disease or health-related condition. In this case, the evidence is not well enough established to meet the significant scientific agreement standard required for FDA to issue an authorizing regulation. Qualifying language is included as part of the claim to indicate that the evidence supporting the claim is limited. Both conventional foods and dietary supplements may use qualified health claims. FDA uses its enforcement discretion for qualified health claims after evaluating and ranking the quality and strength of the totality of the scientific evidence. Although FDA's enforcement discretion letters are issued to the petitioner requesting the qualified health claim, the qualified claims are available for use on any food or dietary supplement product meeting the enforcement discretion conditions specified in the letter.

Nutrient Content Claims

The Nutrition Labeling and Education Act of 1990 (NLEA) permits the use of label claims that characterize the level of a nutrient in a food (i.e., nutrient content claims) made in accordance with FDA's authorizing regulations. Nutrient content claims describe the level of a nutrient or dietary substance in the product, using terms such as free, high, and low, or they compare the level of a nutrient in a food to that of another food, using terms such as more, reduced, and lite.

An accurate quantitative statement (e.g., 200 mg of sodium) that does not characterize the nutrient level may be used to describe any amount of a nutrient present. However, a statement such as "only 200 mg of sodium" characterizes the level of sodium as being low, and would need to conform to the criteria of an appropriate nutrient content claim or carry a disclosure statement that it does not comply with the claim.

Most nutrient content claim regulations apply only to those nutrients or dietary substances that have an established daily value. The requirements that govern the use of nutrient content claims help ensure that descriptive terms, such as high or low, are used consistently for all types of food products and are thus meaningful to consumers. Healthy has been defined by a regulation as an implied nutrient content claim that characterizes a food that has healthy levels of total fat, saturated fat, cholesterol, and sodium.

Percentage claims for dietary supplements are another category of nutrient content claims. These claims are used to describe a percentage level of a dietary ingredient for which there is no established DV. Examples include simple percentage statements such as "40% omega-3 fatty acids, 10 mg per capsule," and comparative percentage claims such as "twice the omega-3 fatty acids per capsule (80 mg) as in 100 mg of menhaden oil (40 mg)."

Structure/Function Claims

Structure/function claims have historically appeared on the labels of conventional foods and dietary supplements as well as drugs. However, the Dietary Supplement Health and Education Act of 1994 (DSHEA) established some special regulatory procedures for such claims for dietary supplement labels. Structure/function claims describe the role of a nutrient or dietary ingredient intended to affect normal structure or function in humans, for example, "calcium builds strong bones." In addition, they may characterize the means by which a nutrient or dietary ingredient acts to maintain such structure or function, for example, "fiber maintains bowel regularity," or "antioxidants maintain cell integrity," or they may describe general well-being from consumption of a nutrient or dietary ingredient.

Structure/function claims may also describe a benefit related to a nutrient deficiency disease (like vitamin C and scurvy), as long as the statement also tells how widespread such a disease is in the U.S. The manufacturer is responsible for ensuring the accuracy and truthfulness of these claims; they are not pre-approved by FDA, but must be truthful and not misleading. If a dietary supplement label includes such a claim, it must state in a disclaimer that FDA has not evaluated the claim. The disclaimer must also state that the dietary supplement product is not intended to diagnose, treat, cure or prevent any disease, because only a drug can legally make such a claim. Manufacturers of dietary supplements that make structure/function claims on labels or in labeling must submit a notification to FDA no later than 30 days after marketing the dietary supplement that includes the text of the structure/function claim.

Qualified Health Claims Permitted by the U.S. Food and Drug Administration

Qualified Claims about Cancer Risk

Selenium and Cancer

Claim Statements:

1. Selenium may reduce the risk of certain cancers. Some scientific evidence suggests that consumption of selenium may reduce the risk of certain forms of cancer. However, FDA has determined that this evidence is limited and not conclusive.

2. Selenium may produce anticarcinogenic effects in the body. Some scientific evidence suggests that consumption of selenium may produce anticarcinogenic effects in the body. However, FDA has determined that this evidence is limited and not conclusive.

Eligible foods: Dietary supplements containing selenium.

Antioxidant Vitamins

Claim Statements:

1. Some scientific evidence suggests that consumption of antioxidant vitamins may reduce the risk of certain forms of cancer. However, FDA has determined that this evidence is limited and not conclusive.

2. Some scientific evidence suggests that consumption of anti-oxidant vitamins may reduce the risk of certain forms of cancer. However, FDA does not endorse this claim because this evidence is limited and not conclusive.

3. FDA has determined that although some scientific evidence suggests that consumption of antioxidant vitamins may reduce the risk of certain forms of cancer, this evidence is limited and not conclusive.

Eligible foods: Dietary supplements containing vitamin E and/or vitamin C.

Qualified Claims about Cardiovascular Disease Risk

Nuts and Heart Disease

Claim Statement: Scientific evidence suggests, but does not prove, that eating 1.5 ounces per day of most nuts such as [name of specific nut] as part of a diet low in saturated fat and cholesterol may reduce the risk of heart disease. [See nutrition information for fat content.]

Notes: The bracketed phrase naming a specific nut is optional. The bracketed fat content disclosure statement is applicable to a claim made for whole or chopped nuts, but not a claim made for nut-containing products.

Eligible Foods: Types of nuts eligible for this claim are restricted to almonds, hazelnuts, peanuts, pecans, some pine nuts, pistachio nuts, and walnuts. Types of nuts on which the health claim may be based are restricted to those nuts that were specifically included in the health claim petition, but that do not exceed 4 g saturated fat per 50 g of nuts. Nuts must be: (1) whole or chopped nuts that are raw, blanched, roasted, salted, and/or lightly coated, and/or flavored; any fat or carbohydrate added in the coating or flavoring must meet the definition of an insignificant amount; and (2) nut-containing products other than whole or chopped nuts that contain at least 11 g of one or more of the nuts.

Walnuts and Heart Disease

Claim Statement: Supportive, but not conclusive, research shows that eating 1.5 ounces per day of walnuts, as part of a low saturated fat and low cholesterol diet, and not resulting in increased caloric intake, may reduce the risk of coronary heart disease. See nutrition information for fat [and calorie] content.

Note: The bracketed phrase [and calorie] is optional in that FDA does not intend for the presence or absence of such phrase to be a factor in whether it considers enforcement discretion for the use of the qualified health claim. FDA considered this additional information might be beneficial to consumers to heighten their awareness of the caloric contribution from walnuts, and encourages companies to include it in product labeling.

Eligible Foods: Whole or chopped walnuts.

Omega-3 Fatty Acids and Coronary Heart Disease

Claim Statement: Consumption of omega-3 fatty acids may reduce the risk of coronary heart disease. FDA evaluated the data and determined that, although there is scientific evidence supporting the claim, the evidence is not conclusive.

Eligible Foods: Dietary supplements containing the omega-3 long chain polyunsaturated fatty acids, eicosapentaenoic acid (EPA) and/or docosahexaenoic acid (DHA).

B Vitamins and Vascular Disease

Claim Statement: As part of a well-balanced diet that is low in saturated fat and cholesterol, folic acid and vitamins B_6 and B_{12} may reduce the risk of vascular disease. FDA evaluated the above claim and found that, while it is known that diets low in saturated fat and cholesterol reduce the risk of heart disease and other vascular diseases, the evidence in support of the above claim is inconclusive.

Eligible Foods: Dietary supplements containing vitamins B_6, B_{12}, and/or folic acid.

Monounsaturated Fatty Acids from Olive Oil and Coronary Heart Disease

Claim Statement: Limited and not conclusive scientific evidence suggests that eating about 2 tablespoons (23 grams) of olive oil daily may reduce the risk of coronary heart disease due to the monounsaturated fat in olive oil. To achieve this possible benefit, olive oil is to replace a similar amount of saturated fat, and not increase the total number of calories you eat in a day. One serving of this product contains [x] grams of olive oil.

Note: The last sentence of the claim "One serving of this product contains [x] grams of olive oil" is optional when the claim is used on the label or in the labeling of olive oil.

Eligible Foods:

- All products that are essentially pure olive oil and are labeled as such.

- Dressings for salads (i.e., salad dressings) that contain 6 g or more olive oil per reference amount customarily consumed per eating occasion (RACC), and are low in cholesterol, and do not contain more than 4 g of saturated fat per RACC.

- Vegetable oil spreads that contain 6 g or more olive oil per RACC, are low in cholesterol, and do not contain more than 4 g of saturated fat per RACC.

- Olive oil-containing foods that contain 6 g or more olive oil per RACC, are low in cholesterol, contain at least 10% of either vitamin A, vitamin C, iron, calcium, protein, or dietary fiber. If the RACC of the olive oil-containing food is greater than 30 g, the food cannot contain more than 4 g of saturated fat per RACC, and if the RACC of the olive oil-containing food is 30 g or less the food cannot contain more than 4 g of saturated fat per 50 g.

- Shortenings that contain 6 g or more olive oil per RACC and are low in cholesterol, and do not contain more than 4 g of saturated fat per RACC.

- Meal products or main dish products are not eligible for the claim.

Qualified Claims about Cognitive Function

Phosphatidylserine and Cognitive Dysfunction and Dementia

Claim Statements:

1. Consumption of phosphatidylserine may reduce the risk of dementia in the elderly. Very limited and preliminary scientific

research suggests that phosphatidylserine may reduce the risk of dementia in the elderly. FDA concludes that there is little scientific evidence supporting this claim.

2. Consumption of phosphatidylserine may reduce the risk of cognitive dysfunction in the elderly. Very limited and preliminary scientific research suggests that phosphatidylserine may reduce the risk of cognitive dysfunction in the elderly. FDA concludes that there is little scientific evidence supporting this claim.

Eligible Foods: Dietary supplements containing soy-derived phosphatidylserine.

Qualified Claims about Neural Tube Birth Defects

Claim Statement: 0.8 mg folic acid in a dietary supplement is more effective in reducing the risk of neural tube defects than a lower amount in foods in common form. FDA does not endorse this claim. Public health authorities recommend that women consume 0.4 mg folic acid daily from fortified foods or dietary supplements or both to reduce the risk of neural tube defects.

Eligible Foods: Dietary supplements containing folic acid.

Section 21.3

Definitions of Nutrient Content

"A Food Labeling Guide: Appendix A,"
U.S. Food and Drug Administration (FDA), November 2004.

Synonyms for Free, Low, Reduced, or Less

- **Free:** Zero, no, without, trivial source of, negligible source of, dietarily insignificant source of, and free for meals and main dishes is the stated value per labeled serving.

- **Low:** Little, (few for calories), contains a small amount of, or a low source of the nutrient.

- **Reduced/Less:** Lower; (fewer, for calories); *modified* may be used in statement of identity; for meals and main dishes reduced/ less are the same as for individual foods on a per 100 g basis.

Note: Free, very low, or low, must indicate if food meets a definition without benefit of special processing, alteration, formulation, or reformulation (e.g., "broccoli, a fat-free food" or "celery, a low calorie food").

Calories

- **Free:** Less than 5 calories per reference amount and per labeled serving. Not defined for meals or main dishes.

- **Low:** 40 cal or less per reference amount (and per 50 g if reference amount is small). Meals and main dishes: 120 cal or less per 100 g.

- **Reduced/Less:** At least 25% fewer calories per reference amount than an appropriate reference food. Reference food may not be low calorie and would use the term fewer, rather than less.

Notes: Light (or Lite)—if 50% or more of the calories are from fat, fat must be reduced by at least 50% per reference amount. If less than

50% of calories are from fat, fat must be reduced at least 50% or calories reduced at least 1/3 per reference amount. Light (or Lite) meal or main dish product meets definition for low calorie, or low fat meal, and is labeled to indicate which definition is met. For dietary supplements: Calorie claims can only be made when the reference product is greater than 40 calories per serving.

Total Fat

- **Free:** Less than 0.5 g per reference amount and per labeled serving (or for meals and main dishes, less than 0.5 g per labeled serving). No ingredient that is fat or understood to contain fat, except when noted (e.g., adds a trivial amount of fat).

- **Low:** 3 g or less per reference amount (and per 50 g if reference amount is small). Meals and main dishes: 3 g or less per 100 g and not more than 30% of calories from fat.

- **Reduced/Less:** At least 25% less fat per reference amount than an appropriate reference food. Reference food may not be low fat.

Notes: "__% Fat Free"—okay if meets the requirements for low fat. If stated, "100% fat free," the food must be fat free. For dietary supplements: calorie claims cannot be made for products that are 40 calories or less per serving.

Saturated Fat

- **Free:** Less than 0.5 g saturated fat and less than 0.5 g *trans* fatty acids per reference amount and per labeled serving (or for meals and main dishes, less than 0.5 g saturated fat and less than 0.5 g *trans* fatty acids per labeled serving). No ingredient that is understood to contain saturated fat except when noted (e.g., adds a trivial amount of saturated fat).

- **Low:** 1 g or less per reference amount and 15% or less of calories from saturated fat. Meals and main dishes: 1 g or less per 100 g and less than 10% of calories from saturated fat.

- **Reduced/Less:** At least 25% less saturated fat per reference amount than an appropriate reference food. Reference food may not be low saturated fat.

Notes: Next to all saturated fat claims, must declare the amount of cholesterol if 2 mg or more per reference amount; and the amount of total fat if more than 3 g per reference amount (or 0.5 g or more of total fat for "saturated fat free"). For dietary supplements: saturated fat claims cannot be made for products that are 40 calories or less per serving.

Cholesterol

- **Free:** Less than 2 mg per reference amount and per labeled serving (or for meals and main dishes, less than 2 mg per labeled serving). No ingredient that contains cholesterol except when noted (e.g., adds a trivial amount of cholesterol). If less than 2 mg per reference amount by special processing and total fat exceeds 13 g per reference amount and labeled serving, the amount of cholesterol must be substantially less (25%) than in a reference food with significant market share (5% of market).

- **Low:** 20 mg or less per reference amount (and per 50 g of food if reference amount is small). If qualifies by special processing and total fat exceeds 13 g per reference and labeled serving, the amount of cholesterol must be substantially less (25%) than in a reference food with significant market share (5% of market). Meals and main dishes: 20 mg or less per 100 g.

- **Reduced/Less:** At least 25% less cholesterol per reference amount than an appropriate reference food. Reference food may not be low cholesterol.

Notes: Cholesterol claims only allowed when food contains 2 g or less saturated fat per reference amount; or for meals and main dish products per labeled serving size for free claims, or per 100 g for low and reduced/less claims. Must declare the amount of total fat next to cholesterol claim when fat exceeds 13 g per reference amount and labeled serving (or per 50 g of food if reference amount is small), or when the fat exceeds 19.5 g per labeled serving for main dishes or 26 g for meal products. For dietary supplements: cholesterol claims cannot be made for products that are 40 calories or less per serving.

Sodium

- **Free:** Less than 5 mg per reference amount and per labeled serving (or for meals and main dishes, less than 5 mg per labeled serving). No ingredient that is sodium chloride or generally understood to contain sodium except when noted (e.g., adds a trivial amount of sodium).

- **Low:** 140 mg or less per reference amount (and per 50 g if reference amount is small). Meals and main dishes: 140 mg or less per 100g.

- **Reduced/Less:** At least 25% less sodium per reference amount than an appropriate reference food. Reference food may not be low sodium.

Notes:

- *Light* (for sodium reduced products): if food is low calorie and low fat and sodium is reduced by at least 50%.

- *Light in Sodium:* if sodium is reduced by at least 50% per reference amount. Entire term *Light in Sodium* must be used in same type, size, color, and prominence. *Light in Sodium* for meals = *Low in Sodium*.

- *Very Low Sodium*: 35 mg or less per reference amount (and per 50 g if reference amount is small). For meals and main dishes: 35 mg or less per 100 g.

- *Salt Free:* must meet criterion for sodium free.

- *No Salt Added, and Unsalted:* must list conditions of use and must declare "This is not a sodium free food" on information panel if food is not sodium free.

- *Lightly Salted:* 50% less sodium than normally added to reference food and if not low sodium, must be so labeled on information panel.

Sugars

- **Free:** Sugar free is less than 0.5 g sugars per reference amount and per labeled serving (or for meals and main dishes, less than 0.5 g per labeled serving). No ingredient that is a sugar or generally understood to contain sugars except when noted (e.g., adds a trivial amount of sugar). Disclose calorie profile (e.g., low calorie).

- **Low:** Not defined. No basis for recommended intake.

- **Reduced/Less:** At least 25% less sugars per reference amount than an appropriate reference food. May not use this claim on dietary supplements of vitamins and minerals.

Notes: "No added sugars" and "without added sugars" are allowed if no sugar or sugar containing ingredient is added during processing.

State if food is not low or reduced calorie. The terms unsweetened, and no added sweeteners remain as factual statements. Claims about reducing dental caries are implied health claims. Does not include sugar alcohols.

Terms

Reference Amount: Reference amount customarily consumed (RACC).

Small Reference Amount: Reference amount of 30 g or less, or 2 tablespoons or less (for dehydrated foods that are typically consumed when rehydrated with water or a diluent containing an insignificant amount, of all nutrients per reference amount, the 50 g criterion refers to the prepared form of the food).

When levels exceed: 13 g fat, 4 g saturated fat, 60 mg cholesterol, and 480 mg sodium per reference amount, per labeled serving, or for foods with small reference amounts, per 50 g, a disclosure statement is required as part of claim (e.g., "See nutrition information for___content" with the blank filled in with nutrient(s) that exceed the prescribed levels).

Additional Information

U.S. Food and Drug Administration (FDA)
5600 Fishers Lane
Rockville, MD 20857
Toll-Free: 888-463-6335
Website: http://www.fda.gov

Part Three

Life Stage Nutrition Issues

Chapter 22

Introducing Food to Infants and Toddlers

Chapter Contents

Section 22.1

Breast-Feeding and Bottle-Feeding

This information was provided by KidsHealth, one of the largest resources online for medically reviewed health information written for parents, kids, and teens. For more articles like this one, visit www.KidsHealth.org, or www.TeensHealth.org. © 2001 The Nemours Center for Children's Health Media, a division of The Nemours Foundation.

One of the first decisions new parents must make is how to feed their baby. We join such medical organizations as the American Academy of Pediatrics and the World Health Organization in recommending breast milk as the ideal form of infant nutrition. For those women who are unable to breast-feed, or who choose not to, today's formulas provide a good alternative in terms of how easy they are for babies to digest and the nutrients they provide.

Making a decision to breast-feed or bottle-feed your baby is a personal one, but there are some points you should consider to help you decide which option is best for you and your baby. Your child's doctor or a lactation consultant can provide excellent guidance.

Feeding your baby, whether by breast or by bottle, is an important time of connection between mother and baby. Breast-feeding mothers seem to particularly value the "skin to skin" warmth of a nursing baby. But no matter the feeding method, it should be a time that is unhurried and quiet.

Following are some issues you might want to consider as you decide which option is best for you and your baby. Once you do make the decision, you'll most likely have a number of questions. How should you get started? How much—and how often—should your baby eat? This chapter addresses these questions as well.

Breast-Feeding

- *Fights infection.* Antibodies passed from mother help protect baby from some conditions, such as ear infections, diarrhea, allergies, pertussis (whooping cough), and coughs due to pneumonia and other respiratory infections. As a group, breast-fed babies tend to have fewer infections than babies fed formula.

- *Promotes digestion.* Enzymes and other substances in breast milk make digestion somewhat easier and aid in the absorption of nutrients. Manufactured formulas do a fairly good job of imitating breast milk, but some of breast milk's more complex substances are too difficult to manufacture, and some have not yet been identified.

- *Cost-free.* Breast milk is free. A nursing mother needs to spend about 500 extra calories per day to produce breast milk. You should talk with your doctor or breast-feeding counselor (lactation consultant) about whether or not this means you need to consume extra calories while you are nursing.

- *Convenient.* There are no bottles to mix and sterilize, no last-minute runs to the store for more formula, and it's always fresh and available.

- *Prevents obesity.* A recent study indicates that breast-feeding may help prevent childhood obesity.

- *Bacteria-free.* Breast milk is free of bacteria (but the bottles used for expressed breast milk may not be).

- *Perfect temperature.* Breast milk is always the right temperature when the infant sucks it directly from the breast.

- *Unsafe with some medical conditions.* Maternal medical conditions, such as HIV or AIDS or some types of hepatitis, or those that involve chemotherapy or treatment with certain medications (such as some antiseizure medicines to treat epilepsy) may make breast-feeding inadvisable because the disease or components of the medicine may be transmitted to the baby through breast milk. (Check with your child's doctor or lactation consultant before taking any medication, though.)

- *Difficult with breast surgery.* Women who have had major breast surgery, such as breast reduction, may have difficulty breast-feeding because their breasts may not produce enough milk or the ducts through which the milk travels in the breast may have been severed. (Women can use a Supplementary Nursing System (SNS) or a nursing trainer—a small tube attached to the nipple that provides additional formula or donor breast milk to the baby.)

- *Limit caffeine.* Caffeine intake should be limited to 300 milligrams (about 3 cups of coffee) per day because this stimulant may cause problems for some babies.

- *Frequent feedings.* Breast-fed babies usually need to eat more often.

- *Personal discomfort.* Some women feel uncomfortable with the idea of breast-feeding, but with adequate education and support, most women can overcome any initial inhibitions or concerns they may have. Some mothers may find it difficult to work, run errands, or travel because of a breast-feeding schedule or a need to express breast milk during the day. Any physical discomfort associated with breast-feeding, such as sore nipples, are usually easily handled by observing proper technique and the advice of doctors, lactation counselors, and other experienced breast-feeders.

Bottle-Feeding

- *Convenient.* Either parent (or another caregiver) can feed the baby at any time (and expressed breast milk also can be given in these circumstances).

- *Flexible.* A mother who bottle-feeds has a bit more flexibility in regard to separation from her baby (to go to work, run errands, or go on a trip) without disrupting the feeding schedule. For those times when baby can't come along, expressed and stored breast milk can also be used.

- *Lacks antibodies.* None of the important antibodies that are found in breast milk are found in manufactured formula.

- *Expensive.* Formula can be expensive (powdered formula is less expensive than premixed, liquid formula, though), and extra care must be taken when mixing formula to ensure your baby gets the right amount of nutrients.

- *Not bacteria-free.* Bottles, nipples, and formula may transmit bacteria if not cleaned properly or stored in sterile containers.

- *Longer preparation time.* Formula must be prepared and bottles must be warmed (but not too hot!) before feeding.

- *May produce gas and constipation.* Bottle-feeding may cause more gas or firmer bowel movements.

- *Can't match complexity.* Manufactured formulas have yet to duplicate the complexity of breast milk, which changes as the baby's needs change.

How to Breast-Feed Your Infant

Arrange for your baby to room with you in the hospital so that you can nurse your baby whenever he's hungry, and let the nurses know that you're going to breast-feed so that they don't give your baby a bottle.

Your milk may take a few days to come in, especially if you have received larger amounts of pain medication or anesthetics for a vaginal birth or a caesarean section (C-section). In the meantime, your baby will benefit from your colostrum (the pre-milk in your breasts during late pregnancy and the first few days following delivery). Colostrum contains many concentrated protective properties, including immune system-boosting and antibacterial substances.

Try to nurse your baby as soon as possible after birth. Let your baby breast-feed at one breast until he no longer seems interested in eating, then switch him to the other side. Before switching, you may want to try burping your baby. Often, the movement alone can be enough to cause a baby to burp, but if this doesn't happen, you can try again when your baby's finished with the second breast.

A lactation consultant or hospital nurse (or perhaps someone from La Leche League) should be available to help you find a comfortable position and help your baby latch on properly. Latching on, which refers to the suction created by your baby's mouth at your nipple, is an important key to successful nursing. It may take a few times before getting it right, but it's important that your baby nurses with a wide-open mouth and takes as much as possible of your areola (the dark-colored area of the breast) in his mouth (not just the tip of the nipple, to help avoid sore nipples).

If your baby is sleepy from a difficult birth, you may have to wake him up to nurse—this will help ensure that your baby's getting enough to eat and that your milk supply is increasing. (This also will lessen the likelihood of uncomfortable engorgement of your breasts.) Follow your baby's cues—many newborns seem to nurse almost constantly during the first few weeks of life.

When feeding your baby, keep the distractions to a minimum. Sit in a quiet room and in a chair that provides you with enough support to keep your baby comfortable and facing your breast. It may take a few days or weeks for you to find the feeding positions that work best for you and your baby. A nursing or feeding pillow (or some cushions) may help. Or if you're recovering from a C-section, consider the football hold (feeding or nursing your baby while he's tucked under your arm and supported by a pillow), rather than lying across your stomach and putting pressure on your incision.

To make nighttime feedings easier, you may want to consider letting your baby sleep in a crib or bassinet in your room for the first few months. The exception: babies should never sleep in the same room with people who are smoking, because of a higher risk of SIDS (sudden infant death syndrome) associated with this sleeping situation.

If your baby sleeps in another room, keep that room dark for nighttime nursing and keep stimulation to a minimum. This will help your baby to realize that nighttime is for sleeping—not playing—and will encourage him to return to sleep.

Avoid supplementing (unless your child's doctor recommends it) your breast milk with formula until your milk supply has had a chance to develop and stabilize; early supplements can lead to nipple confusion for your baby and a reduction in your milk supply. Most lactation professionals recommend that parents wait at least 3 weeks before offering pacifiers or artificial nipples of any kind. Many of the health benefits of breast-feeding come from the first 2 months of feeding.

How to Bottle-Feed Your Infant

The first thing you'll need to do if you decide to bottle-feed your baby is to decide which formula to use. There are many brands on the market, including cow's milk-based formulas, formulas with added iron, soy-based formulas, and specialized formulas for infants born prematurely or those with certain medical conditions. Ask your child's doctor which type would be best for your infant.

Formula comes in ready-to-feed (which is a ready-to-eat liquid), concentrates (which are liquids that require diluting with water), and powders (which require mixing with water). Follow the instructions on the label when preparing your baby's bottles, and always refrigerate any bottles you fill for later feedings to prevent bacteria from growing. Throw away mixed formula after 24 hours.

There are many different types of bottles and nipples available—you may need to try a few different brands before you find the combination that works best for you and your baby. Check nipples regularly for signs of wear, and replace them often.

Feed your baby when he seems hungry, and listen to his cues. Mix your baby's formula in 2- or 3-ounce (56–85 gram) servings for the first few weeks, and gradually increase the amount as you become familiar with your baby's eating patterns and appetite.

Always hold your baby during feeding times. Don't leave a baby unattended feeding from a propped bottle. Mealtimes provide a great opportunity for snuggling and bonding with your baby.

Never put your baby to bed with a bottle—it's a choking hazard, and formula pooling in your baby's mouth can lead to tooth decay in older babies and toddlers. Also, don't give your baby juice in a bottle unless your child's doctor says it's okay.

Common Feeding Questions

Whether you've decided to breast-feed or bottle-feed, it's likely that you'll have a few questions or concerns about feeding your baby.

Is my baby eating enough?

Babies grow at different rates, and at times you may wonder whether your baby is getting enough nutrients to develop properly. To help determine whether your baby is eating enough, follow the schedule of regular postnatal checkups so that your baby can be weighed and measured. Also, you probably will be changing at least 4 to 6 wet diapers each day (or 6 to 8, if you use cloth diapers)—this can be a good indicator that your baby is getting enough to eat. If you see yellowish crystals in a wet diaper, contact your baby's doctor— these can signal inadequate fluid intake or dehydration.

Each baby is different, but on average, a newborn consumes about 1.5 to 2 ounces every 2 to 3 hours.

Does my baby have an allergy?

Some bottle-fed babies may be sensitive to the cow's-milk protein in their formula. If your baby suddenly becomes fussy or colicky, your baby's doctor may suggest switching to a soy-based formula or a special hypoallergenic preparation.

A breast-fed baby may have an allergic or sensitivity reaction after the mother consumes certain foods or drinks. If you think your baby has had such a reaction, call your baby's doctor and avoid eating or drinking anything your baby cannot tolerate.

When should I introduce solid foods?

Wait until your baby is 4 to 6 months old before introducing solids. Feeding solids earlier than this can increase the chances of your baby developing food allergies. Watch for signs of readiness, such as your baby's tongue-thrust reflex subsiding and your baby beginning to reach for other people's food. Always start with baby cereal on a spoon for 1 to 2 months before advancing to fruits and vegetables. And don't add cereal to your baby's bottle unless your child's doctor instructs you to do so.

Don't expect your baby to eat a lot at this stage. Solid foods are more for recreation and practice than for nutrition during the first year of your baby's life—almost all the nutrition your baby receives should be from breast milk, commercially prepared formula, or a combination of the two.

Is it safe to microwave my baby's bottles?

The microwave can create dangerous hot spots in bottles of formula or breast milk. If you use a microwave for this purpose, make sure the formula or breast milk in the bottle is well-mixed after microwaving, and that the bottle and contents are not overheated. In the case of breast milk, microwaving will also change the composition of the milk, destroying some of its protective properties. Instead, warm your baby's bottles in a pan of hot water and test the temperature by squirting a drop or two on your hand before feeding your baby.

Section 22.2

How to Feed Babies and Toddlers

This section includes "Helping Your Baby Grow (6–11 Months)" and "Helping Your Toddler Learn about Food (1–2 Years)," from Bright Futures Nutrition Family Fact Sheets, © 2002 National Center for Education in Maternal and Child Health (NCEMCH) and Georgetown University. Used with permission.

Helping Your Baby Grow (6–11 Months)

As babies grow, they eat more food and a greater variety of foods. Here are answers to important questions you may have about your baby's nutrition.

What can I expect my baby to do as she grows?

At about 4 to 6 months of age, your baby will:

- begin to eat solid foods, such as iron-fortified infant cereal and pureed or strained fruits and vegetables.
- bring objects to her mouth.
- explore foods with her mouth.

At 7 to 9 months of age, your baby will:

- try to grasp foods, such as toast, crackers, and teething biscuits, with all fingers and pull them toward her palm.
- move food from one hand to the other.

At 9 to 11 months of age, your baby will:

- reach for pieces of food and pick them up between her thumb and forefinger.
- try to hold a cup.
- pick up and chew soft pieces of food.

When and how should I introduce solid foods?

- Introduce solid foods when your baby can sit with support and has good head and neck control.
- Offer iron-fortified rice cereal as the first solid food, because it is least likely to cause an allergic reaction, such as a rash. Offer a small amount (for example, 1 or 2 teaspoons) of one new food at a time. Wait 7 days or more to see how your baby tolerates the new food before introducing the next new food.
- Introduce solid foods in this order: iron-fortified infant cereal, fruits and vegetables, and meats.
- Do not add honey to food, water, or infant formula because it can be a source of spores that cause botulism, which can poison your baby.
- Do not add cereal to bottles, and do not use "baby food nursing kits" (which let solid food filter through the bottle nipple along with the liquid).

When should I give my baby cow's milk?

- Continue to feed your baby breast milk or iron-fortified infant formula for the first year.

- Cow's milk, goat's milk, and soy milk are not recommended until after your baby's first birthday.

How can I protect my baby's teeth from tooth decay?

- Serve 100% fruit juice in a cup in small amounts, about 4 ounces per day.

- Do not serve juice in a bottle. Juice served in a bottle can cover your baby's teeth with sugar for long periods of time and contribute to tooth decay (early childhood caries).

- Do not put your baby to bed with a bottle or allow him to have a bottle whenever he wants.

- Clean your baby's gums and teeth twice a day. Use a clean, moist washcloth to wipe his gums. Use a small, soft toothbrush (without toothpaste) and water to clean his teeth.

When should I wean my baby from the bottle?

- As your baby begins to eat more solid foods and drink from a cup, she can be weaned from the bottle.

- Begin to wean your baby gradually, at about 9 to 10 months. By 12 to 14 months, most babies can drink from a cup.

How can I prevent my baby from choking?

- Avoid foods that may cause choking, such as hard candy, mini marshmallows, popcorn, pretzels, chips, spoonfuls of peanut butter, nuts, seeds, large chunks of meat, hot dogs, raw carrots, raisins and other dried fruits, and whole grapes.

- Do not add cereal to your baby's bottle.

Should I give my baby sweets?

- Do not give your baby sweets, such as candy, cake, or cookies, during the first 12 months. He needs to eat healthy foods for growth and development.

Helping Your Toddler Learn about Food (1–2 Years)

Toddlers are unpredictable. The foods they like one day may be different the next. Here are answers to important questions you may have about your toddler's nutrition.

What can I expect my child to do as he grows?

At 1 to 1½ years of age, your child will:

- grasp and release foods with his fingers.
- be able to hold a spoon, but will not be able to use it very well.
- be able to use a cup, but will have difficulty letting go of it.
- want foods that others are eating.

At 1½ to 2 years old your child will:

- eat less than babies and children 2 years and older.
- like to eat with his hands.
- have favorite foods.
- get distracted easily.

At 2 years of age, your child will:

- be able to hold a cup.
- be able to chew more foods.
- have definite likes and dislikes.

How can I make mealtimes enjoyable?

- Be patient and understanding when your child makes a mess while she learns to feed herself—this is normal.
- Serve healthy foods for meals and snacks at scheduled times, but allow for flexibility.
- Use your child's favorite plate, bowl, cup, and eating utensils.
- Create a relaxed setting for meals (for example, turn off the television).

I am struggling with my child over food. Is this normal?

- Your child may struggle with you over food in an attempt to make his own decisions and become independent. Struggling over food may make him even more determined.
- Keep in mind that you are responsible for what, when, and where your child eats. Let your child decide whether to eat and how much.

- Continue to serve a new food even if your child has rejected it. It may take several times before your child accepts the food.

What should my child eat?

- At mealtime, offer small portions of what the rest of your family is eating (for example, bread, pasta, or rice; fruits and vegetables; cheese or yogurt; and cooked lean meat, poultry, fish, or eggs).

- Children under 2 usually eat small portions. Offer small portions (for example, 1 or 2 tablespoons) and let your child ask for more if she is still hungry.

- Offer your child food every 2 to 3 hours for a meal or snack.

What should my child drink?

- Your child should drink about 2 cups (16 ounces) of whole milk per day. Drinking more than this can reduce your child's appetite for other healthy foods.

- Until age 2, do not give your child low-fat or fat-free milk. He needs the extra fat in whole milk for growth and development.

- Offer 100% fruit juice in small amounts, about 4 to 6 ounces per day. Drinking more than this can reduce your child's appetite for other healthy foods.

- Serve juice in a cup, not a bottle. Juice served in a bottle can cover your child's teeth with sugar for long periods of time and contribute to tooth decay (early childhood caries).

- Your child may not tell you when he is thirsty. Make sure he drinks plenty of water throughout the day, especially between meals and snacks.

How can I prevent my child from choking?

- For children younger than 3, avoid foods that may cause choking, such as hard candy, mini marshmallows, popcorn, pretzels, chips, spoonfuls of peanut butter, nuts, seeds, large chunks of meat, hot dogs, raw carrots, raisins and other dried fruits, and whole grapes.

- Children ages 3 to 5 years may eat these foods if you are prepared to make them safer. For example, cut hot dogs in quarters lengthwise and then into small pieces, cut whole grapes in half lengthwise, chop nuts finely, chop raw carrots finely or into thin strips, and spread peanut butter thinly on crackers or bread.

- Have your child sit while eating. Eating while walking or running may cause her to choke.

- Keep things calm at meal and snack times. If your child becomes overexcited, she may choke.

- Do not let your child eat in a moving car. If she chokes while you are driving, you will not be able to help her.

How can I encourage my child to be physically active?

- Encourage active, spur-of-the-moment play, such as jumping and skipping.

- Play together (for example, play hide and seek or kick a ball). It is a great way to spend time with your child.

- Limit the time your child spends watching television and videotapes to 1 to 2 hours per day.

Additional Information

American Dietetic Association
120 S. Riverside Plaza, Suite 2000
Chicago, IL 60606-6995
Toll-Free: 800-877-1600
Fax: 312-899-4899
Website: http://www.eatright
.org/Public
E-mail: hotline@eatright.org

La Leche League International
P.O. Box 4079
Schaumburg, IL 60168-4079
Toll-Free: 800-525-3243
Phone: 847-519-7730
Fax: 847-519-0035
TTY: 847-592-7570
Website: http://
www.lalecheleague.org

USDA Food and Nutrition Information Center
10301 Baltimore Ave.
Beltsville, MD 20705-2351
Phone: 301-504-5719
Fax: 301-504-6409
TTY: 301-504-6856
Website: http://www.nal.usda.gov/
fnic
E-mail: fnic@nal.usda.gov

Note: This is general information and is not a substitute for talking with your baby's health professional about your particular concerns about your baby.

Section 22.3

Failure to Thrive

This information was provided by KidsHealth, one of the largest resources online for medically reviewed health information written for parents, kids, and teens. For more articles like this one, visit www.KidsHealth.org, or www.TeensHealth.org. © 2005 The Nemours Center for Children's Health Media, a division of The Nemours Foundation.

The first few years of life are a time when most children gain weight and grow much more rapidly than they will later on. Sometimes, however, babies and children do not meet expected standards of growth. Although many of these children are normal, with the child simply falling at the lower end of the growth chart, others are considered to have "failure to thrive."

This is a general diagnosis, with many possible causes. Common to all the cases, though, is the failure to gain weight and grow as expected. So, diagnosing and treating a child who fails to thrive focuses on identifying any underlying problem and promoting weight gain. From there, doctors and the family work together to get the child back into a healthy growth pattern.

What Is Failure to Thrive?

Although it has been recognized for more than a century, failure to thrive lacks a precise definition, in part because it describes a condition rather than a specific disease. Children who fail to thrive don't receive or are unable to take in or retain adequate nutrition to gain weight and grow as expected. The condition is common in babies born prematurely, usually in conjunction with other medical problems linked to prematurity.

But full-term infants can also fail to thrive. Whereas the average-term baby doubles its birth weight by 6 months and triples it at 1 year, these children often do not meet those marks. "The typical picture has been one of a child who starts out plump and growing well but over time begins to fall off, particularly in weight gain," says Jay A. Perman, M.D., professor and chairman of the department of pediatrics at the

University of Maryland. After a while, linear growth (height) slows as well.

If the condition progresses, the undernourished child may become apathetic and irritable, and may not reach milestones like sitting up, walking, and talking at the usual age. Most diagnoses of failure to thrive are made in infants and toddlers in the first few years of life, a crucial period of physical and mental development. After birth, a child's brain grows as much in the first year as it will grow during the rest of the child's life. Poor nutrition during this period can have permanent negative effects on a child's mental development in some cases.

What Causes Failure to Thrive?

Failure to thrive can have a number of different underlying causes. Some children fail to thrive because of an illness or medical disorder. If a child has trouble eating—owing to prematurity or a cleft lip or palate, for example—he may not take in enough calories to get adequate nutrition.

Conditions involving the gastrointestinal system like gastroesophageal reflux, chronic diarrhea, cystic fibrosis, chronic liver disease, and celiac disease can also result in failure to thrive. With reflux, the esophagus may become so irritated that the child refuses to eat because it hurts. Persistent diarrhea can interfere with the body's ability to hold on to the calories from food that is eaten. Cystic fibrosis, chronic liver disease, and celiac disease are conditions that limit the body's ability to absorb nutrients. These are known as malabsorptive disorders: the infant may eat a lot, but his body does not absorb and retain enough of that food. Celiac disease results from a sensitivity to a dietary protein found in wheat and certain other grains. The immune system's abnormal response to this protein causes damage to the lining of the intestine, interfering with its ability to absorb nutrients.

An intolerance of milk protein can put an entire class of food out of reach, restricting the child's diet and occasionally leading to failure to thrive. Infections (parasites, urinary tract infections, tuberculosis, etc.) place great demands on the body and force it to use nutrients rapidly, sometimes bringing about short- or long-term failure to thrive. Inborn errors of metabolism can also limit a child's capacity to make the most of calories consumed. Metabolic disorders might make it difficult for the body to break down, process, or derive energy from food, or they can cause a buildup of toxins during the breakdown process, which can make the child feed poorly or vomit.

A host of additional medical causes—including neurologic, cardiac, endocrine, and respiratory ones—can be suspects as well. In some cases, doctors are unable to pinpoint a specific cause. In others, they may not identify a medical problem but find that parents' attitudes or behaviors are causing the failure to thrive. Some parents restrict the amount of calories they give their infants. They may fear their child will get fat or put him on a limited diet similar to one they follow. Other children fail to thrive as a result of neglect: the parents simply do not feed them enough.

Although in the past doctors tended to categorize cases of failure to thrive as either organic (caused by an underlying medical disorder) or inorganic (caused by caregiver actions), they are less likely to make such sharp distinctions today. That's because medical and behavioral causes often appear together. For instance, if a baby has severe reflux and is reluctant to eat, feeding times can be stressful for a caregiver. She may become tense and frustrated, and this may make it difficult for her to sustain attempts to feed the child adequate amounts of food.

Diagnosis

Many babies go through brief periods when their weight gain plateaus or they even lose a little weight. These are normal intervals of development. However, if a baby does not gain weight for three consecutive months during the first year of life, the doctors usually become concerned.

Doctors diagnose failure to thrive by plotting the child's weight, length, and head circumference—which are measured at each well-baby exam—on standard growth charts. Children who fall below a certain weight range for their age or who drop down two or more percentile curves on the weight chart over a short period of time will likely be evaluated further to determine if there is a problem. A complete blood count, urinalysis, and various blood chemical and electrolyte tests can be helpful in the search for underlying medical problems. If the doctor suspects a particular disease or disorder as a possible cause, he or she may perform specific tests to identify that condition.

To determine whether the child is receiving enough food, the child's doctor (sometimes with the help of a dietitian) will do a calorie count after asking the parents what the child eats every day. And talking to the parents can help a doctor identify any problems at home, such as neglect, poverty, household stress, or difficulty during feedings.

Treatment

Children with failure to thrive need the help of their parents and a doctor. Sometimes an entire medical team will work on the child's case. In addition to the child's primary doctor, the team might include a nutritionist to evaluate the child's dietary needs and an occupational or speech therapist to help the caregiver and child develop successful feeding behaviors and address any sucking or swallowing problems the child might have. Because treatment of failure to thrive involves treating any disease or disorder causing the problem, specialists such as a cardiologist, neurologist, or gastroenterologist may also be part of the care team. Particularly in cases of nonorganic failure to thrive, a social worker and a psychologist or other mental health professional may help address problems in the child's home environment and provide any needed support for the child's caregiver.

Luckily, simple cases of poor nutrition can be tackled noninvasively, according to Dr. Perman. The doctor will recommend high-calorie foods and place the child on a high-density formula like PediaSure. Usually the treatment can be carried out at home, with frequent follow-up visits to the doctor's office or clinic.

More severe cases may call for tube feedings, which can also take place at home. Once a tube that runs from the nose into the stomach is put in place, the child is usually fed at night, so as not to interfere with his activities or limit his desire to eat during the day. (About half of a child's caloric needs can be delivered at night through a continuous drip, Dr. Perman says.) Once he is more adequately nourished, he will feel better and will probably start to eat more on his own. At that point, the tube can be removed.

A child with extreme failure to thrive may need to be hospitalized, where he can be fed and monitored continuously. During this time, any possible underlying causes of the condition are evaluated and treated appropriately. This also gives the treatment team the opportunity to observe first-hand the caregiver's feeding technique and the interaction between caregiver and child during feedings and at other times.

The duration of treatment varies significantly from case to case. Weight gain takes time, so several months may pass before a child is back in the normal range for his age. Children who require hospitalization usually stay for 10 to 14 days or more to bring them out of danger, but it can be many months until the symptoms of severe malnutrition are no longer present. Failure to thrive caused by a chronic illness or disorder may have to be monitored periodically and treated for even longer, perhaps for a lifetime.

Does My Child Have Failure to Thrive?

If you are worried that your child is failing to thrive, remember that there are many reasons why he might be slower to gain weight other than failure to thrive. For instance, breast-fed babies often gain weight more slowly than bottle-fed infants in the early going. Genetics also play a big role in weight gain, so if you and your spouse are slim, your baby may not put on pounds quickly.

As a guideline, babies usually eat eight to twelve times in a 24-hour period (a couple of ounces every few hours) in the first weeks after birth. By the time they are 2 to 3 months old, the number of feedings has dropped to six to eight, but the amount they eat each time has increased. At 4 months, about 30 ounces a day provides sufficient nutrition for most infants.

If your baby has regular well-child checkups, your child's doctor will have plenty of opportunities to identify a problem. As mentioned, the doctor can recognize failure to thrive by plotting a child's measurements on standard growth charts, so be sure your child is measured at each regular checkup. You can also periodically check your baby's weight at home. Weight gain that levels off for more than a few weeks, trouble feeding, and apathy about eating are all possible warning signs.

When to Call Your Child's Doctor

If you notice a drop in weight gain or your baby does not want to eat, get in touch with your child's doctor. A major change in eating pattern also warrants a call to the doctor. Toddlers and other kids may have days and sometimes weeks when they show little interest in eating, but that should not happen in infants.

If you have trouble feeding your baby, your child's doctor can offer some advice. When a child does not eat readily, parents tend to become frustrated and feel they are not taking care of their child well. "Do not let mealtimes become a war zone," advises Dr. Perman. That will magnify the problem and increase the stress for both you and your baby. Instead, make things easy on yourself and consult your child's doctor. With the doctor's help, mealtime can be much more enjoyable.

Chapter 23

Healthy Eating for Children

Chapter Contents

Section 23.1

Helping Children Eat Well

"Nutrition: Healthy Eating Tips: Healthy Children, Healthy Choices,"
Centers for Disease Control and Prevention (CDC), updated April 2005.

Parents Are in Charge

As a parent, your responsibility is to buy healthy groceries and serve nutritious food to your growing children. Start by establishing a routine, even if it is difficult at first. This means a set time for breakfast, lunch, dinner, and snacks. Once you have a routine for meals and snacks, meal times are more relaxed. Most children are happier on a schedule and become hungry at regular times. You'll feel happier about your parenting job when the family has a routine.

- Be consistent. Children need a meal routine just as they need a bedtime routine. Plan for three meals and two snacks each day. Serve a vegetable or fruit at every meal. Fruits and vegetables are great for snacking too.

- Instead of rewarding your child with food, reward them with attention (hugs, kisses, and smiles) and playful activities.

Money-Saving Ideas for Better Health

- Avoid arguments about high-fat, high-sugar foods by not bringing them into the house. Leave the candy, soft drinks, chips, and cookies at the store.

- Serve water when your child is thirsty. Water is cheap and healthy.

Portion Size for Young Children 2–6 Years Old

Serve child-sized portions, and let your child ask for more. Here are some examples of child-sized portions:

- 1/3 to 1/2 cup of frozen veggies

- 1 or 2 little cooked broccoli spears
- 1/2 cup of tomato sauce
- 5 to 7 cooked baby carrots
- 1/3 to 1/2 cup of melon
- 5 to 7 strawberries
- 1/2 cup of apple sauce
- 1 small tangerine
- 1/3 to 1/2 cup of frozen or fresh berries
- 1 cup (8 fl. oz.) low-fat yogurt or nonfat milk
- 1/3 to 1/2 cup of macaroni-and-cheese, rice, pasta, or mashed potatoes
- 2 oz. hamburger
- 1/4 cup ground meat such as turkey or pork, browned and drained
- 1 or 2 drumsticks

Television Time

Tired of hearing your children beg for sugary, high-fat foods? They may be influenced by too many commercials.

- Limit the amount of time your children watch TV to less than 2 hours a day.
- Remove the TV from your child's room.
- Find fun activities to do inside and outside your home: play hopscotch, jump rope, walk the dog, play hide-and-seek, or build an obstacle course in the hall.

Eat at Home

Part of having a healthy family includes spending time together. The family meal is a great way for everyone to get together, have a conversation, and eat together.

- Serving meals at home requires planning. Before you do your shopping, sit down and plan your meals for the week. Make a list of all the ingredients you'll need to prepare healthy, balanced meals. When fatigue kicks in and you want dinner on the table fast, your menu is already planned and the ingredients are right on hand.

- Make sure to always include low-fat or nonfat dairy products, fruit, and vegetables.

- Limit the amount of processed ready-to-eat snacks you buy (such as potato chips or cookies). Prepackaged and processed foods are usually higher in calories and fats and often more expensive. For the price of a large bag of chips or a box of cookies you can buy the following items:

  - 2 pounds of apples

  - 1 pound of bananas

  - 1 pound of carrots

  - 3 pounds of potatoes

  - 1 pound of peppers

- Simplify your schedule for better quality of life. Say no to lessons, teams, and commitments that don't interest you or your child. If you or your child are feeling overwhelmed, consider limiting the number of organized activities to one per child per season.

- Children thrive on routine. Routine meals, naps, outdoor play, and bedtime can make for a happy child who comes to the table rested and hungry for the food you have prepared.

To serve a healthy and balanced meal at home, choose a variety of foods from several food groups. Children need to eat a variety of different foods every day.

Getting Children Involved

An easy way to get children to try new foods is to get them involved in meals. Here are some age-appropriate suggestions.

3-Year-Olds Can

- Wipe table tops.
- Scrub and rinse fruit and vegetables.
- Wash and tear lettuce.
- Snap green beans.

- Bring ingredients from one place to another.
- Mix ingredients and pour liquids.
- Knead and shape yeast dough.
- Put things in the trash.
- Shake liquids in a covered container.

4-Year-Olds Can Also

- Peel oranges or hard cooked eggs.
- Mash bananas with a fork.
- Set a table.
- Cut parsley or green onions with kid-safe scissors.

5-year-Olds Can Also

- Measure ingredients.
- Use an egg beater or whisk.

Tips for Helping Picky Eaters

- Parents are role models. Set a good example by eating healthy foods yourself. Buy and try new fruits and vegetables. Drink water between meals. Set an eating routine at home for your meals and snacks. Your children will learn by your good example.

- Don't expect your child to like something new the first time. Offer it again in a week. It usually takes several tries before children are willing to try new foods.

- Place a small amount of each food on your children's plates. Let them ask for more.

- It is normal for children to explore foods. Young children often touch or smell the food on their plate.

- Children thrive on routine. Stick to a feeding routine, as you do a bedtime routine. Your child is less likely to be tired or fussy at mealtimes.

- Offer healthy foods. Your child soon learns these are the foods in your home and will eventually eat.

Section 23.2

Fiber and Your Child

Few children—even the most nutrition conscious—would say they crave a good fiber-rich meal. Although the thought of fiber might elicit gags and groans in kids of all ages, a plethora of appetizing foods are actually good sources of fiber—from many fruits to whole grain cereals. And your child is probably eating them without even knowing it.

Not just for the senior-citizen crowd, foods that are good sources of fiber are beneficial because they're filling and, therefore, discourage overeating—even though fiber itself adds no calories. Plus, when combined with drinking adequate fluids, eating high-fiber fare helps move food through the digestive system and protect against gut cancers and constipation. It may also lower LDL cholesterol (bad cholesterol) as well as help prevent diabetes and heart disease.

Figuring Out Fiber

Listed on food labels under total carbohydrates, dietary fiber is found in plant foods like fruits, vegetables, and grains. Some of the best sources are:

- whole grain breads and cereals (which have more fiber than white bread and white rice);
- apples;
- oranges;
- bananas;
- berries;
- prunes;
- pears;

- green peas;
- legumes (split peas, soy, lentils, etc.);
- artichokes;
- almonds.

A high-fiber food has 5 grams or more of fiber per serving and a good source of fiber is one that provides 2.5 to 4.9 grams per serving. Here's how some fiber-friendly foods stack up:

- ½ cup (118 milliliters) of cooked navy beans (9.5 grams of fiber)
- ½ cup (118 milliliters) of cooked lima beans (6.6 grams)
- 1 medium baked sweet potato with peel (4.8 grams)
- 1 whole wheat English muffin (4.4 grams)
- ½ cup (118 milliliters) of cooked green peas (4.4 grams)
- 1 medium raw pear with skin (4 grams)
- ½ cup (118 milliliters) of raw raspberries (4 grams)
- 1 medium baked potato with skin (3.8 grams)
- ¼ cup (59 milliliters) of oat bran cereal (3.6 grams)
- 1 ounce (28 grams) of almonds (3.3 grams)
- 1 medium raw apple with skin (3.3 grams)
- ½ cup (118 milliliters) of raisins (3 grams)
- ¼ cup (59 milliliters) of baked beans (3 grams)
- 1 medium orange (3 grams)
- 1 medium banana (3 grams)
- ½ cup (118 milliliters) canned sauerkraut (3 grams)

A simple way to determine how many grams of fiber your child should be consuming each day is to add 5 to your child's age in years (i.e., a 5-year-old should get about 10 grams of fiber). After the age of 15, kids (and adults) need about 20 to 25 grams of fiber per day.

Making Fiber Part of Your Family's Diet

Although many kids often cringe at the mere mention of fiber, they're probably eating fiber every day without even realizing that it's so good for them. And there are plenty of creative, fun, and even tasty ways to incorporate—even sneak—these fiber-rich foods into your child's diet.

Breakfast

- Make oatmeal (a whole grain) part of your kids' morning meals.
- Opt for whole wheat or other whole grain cereals that list ingredients such as whole wheat or oats as one of the first few items on the ingredient list.
- Make pancakes with whole grain (or buckwheat) pancake mix and top with apples, berries, or raisins.
- Serve bran or whole grain waffles topped with fruit.
- Offer whole wheat bagels or English muffins, instead of white toast.
- Serve whole grain cereals. Many popular cereals are made with whole grains, but try to choose ones that have less sugar than some of the excessively sweet whole grain cereal offerings.
- Top fiber-rich cereal with apples, oranges, berries, or bananas. Add almonds to pack even more fiber punch.
- Mix your child's favorite cereal with a fiber-rich one or top it with a tablespoon of bran.

Lunch and Dinner

- Make sandwiches with whole grain breads (rye, oat, or wheat), instead of white.
- Make a fiber-rich sandwich with whole grain bread, peanut butter, and bananas.
- Serve whole grain rolls with dinner, instead of white rolls.
- Use whole grain spaghetti and other pastas, instead of white.
- Serve wild or brown rice with meals, instead of white rice. Add beans (kidney, black, navy, and pinto) to rice dishes for even more fiber.
- Spice up salads with berries, almonds, chickpeas, cooked artichokes, and beans (kidney, black, navy, or pinto).
- Use whole grain (corn or whole wheat) soft taco shells or tortillas to make burritos or wraps. Fill them with eggs and cheese

for breakfast; turkey, cheese, lettuce, tomato, and light dressing for lunch; and beans, salsa, taco sauce, and cheese for dinner.

- Add lentils or whole grain barley to your child's favorite soups.

- Create mini-pizzas by topping whole wheat English muffins or bagels with pizza sauce, low-fat cheese, mushrooms, and chunks of grilled chicken.

- Add bran to meatloaf or burgers. (The trick is not to add too much bran, or the food will taste like sawdust and your family might catch on.)

- Serve sweet potatoes, with the skins, as tasty side dishes. Regular baked potatoes, with the skins, are good sources of fiber, too.

- Top low-fat hot dogs or veggie dogs with sauerkraut and serve them on whole wheat hot dog buns.

- Include fresh fruit as part of your child's packed school lunch. Pears, apples, bananas, oranges, and berries are all high in fiber.

Snacks and Treats

- Bake cookies or muffins using whole wheat flour, instead of regular. Or use some whole wheat and some regular flour, so that the texture of your baked treats won't be drastically different from what your child is used to.

- Add raisins, berries, bananas, or chopped or pureed apples to the mix for even more fiber. Add bran to baking items such as cookies and muffins.

- Top whole wheat crackers with peanut butter or low-fat cheese.

- Offer popcorn—a whole grain food—as a mid-day treat or while your child watches TV or movies. Aim for popcorn without lots of added fat or sugar. (However, only give popcorn to kids over 4 years old because the popular snack can be a choking hazard.)

- Top ice cream, frozen yogurt, or regular yogurt with whole grain cereal, berries, or almonds for some added nutrition and crunch.

- Serve apples topped with peanut butter.

- Make fruit salad with pears, apples, bananas, oranges, and berries. Top with almonds for added crunch. Serve as a side dish with meals or alone as a snack.

- Make low-fat breads, muffins, or cookies with canned pumpkin.

- Leave the skins on when giving your child fruits and veggies as snacks or as part of a meal.

However you choose to incorporate fiber into your child's regular diet, don't push fiber on your family. Instead of introducing high-fiber foods and ingredients into your child's meals and snacks immediately, make gradual changes that will add up to a diet that's higher in fiber over time.

And it's not all about making your child try to like foods—from prunes to bran, from split peas to lima beans—that many kids often find unappealing. Just offer your family plenty of things they likely never imagined are good sources of fiber—fruits like pears and berries, vegetables like beans and peas, and whole grain breakfast cereals that they're probably already getting as their regular diet. Not only will your child be getting the fiber he or she needs, you'll be setting the tone for a lifetime of healthy eating.

Section 23.3

School Lunches

This information was provided by KidsHealth, one of the largest resources online for medically reviewed health information written for parents, kids, and teens. For more articles like this one, visit www.KidsHealth.org, or www.TeensHealth.org. © 2004 The Nemours Center for Children's Health Media, a division of The Nemours Foundation.

Buying lunch at school may be the first time your child gets to call the shots about which foods he or she will eat. The good news is that school lunches have improved over the years, both in taste and nutrition. A recent study shows these meals meet the standards for protein, vitamins, calcium, and iron, but still exceed recommendations for fat. Some schools also have made an effort to serve better dishes, such as grilled chicken sandwiches and salads.

The downside is obvious: In the typical school cafeteria, your child can still choose an unhealthy mix of foods, taking advantage of the less nutritious fare often available a la carte or in the vending machine. For instance, a child might decide to buy the same kid-pleasing entrée, such as a hot dog, day after day.

A Lunchtime Opportunity

Use school lunches as a chance to steer your child toward good choices. You can't force a child, but you can make it easier to eat healthy. Especially with younger kids, start by explaining how a nutritious lunch will give them the energy to finish the rest of the school day and enjoy after-school activities. Here are some other steps to take:

- Look over the cafeteria menu with your child. Ask what a typical lunch includes and which meals he or she particularly likes. Recommend items that are healthier, but be willing to allow your child to buy favorite lunch items occasionally, even if that includes a hot dog.

- Ask about foods like chips, soda, and ice cream. Find out if and when these foods are available at school.

- Encourage your child to pack a lunch, at least occasionally. If you do it right, this can put you back in the driver's seat and help you to ensure that your child is getting a nutritious midday meal.

Healthier Alternatives

Encourage your child to choose cafeteria meals that include fruits, vegetables, lean meats, and whole grains, such as wheat bread instead of white. Also, avoid fried foods when possible and choose milk or water as a drink.

If you're helping your child pack a lunch, start by brainstorming foods and snacks that he or she would like to eat. In addition to old standbys, such as peanut butter and jelly, try pitas or wrap sandwiches stuffed with grilled chicken or veggies. Try soups and salads, if your child is willing, and don't forget last night's leftovers as an easy lunch box filler.

You also can take your child's current lunch and perform a lunch makeover. Here are some suggestions for small changes that do make a nutritional difference.

Table 23.1. Lunch Makeover

Instead of:	Consider:
Higher-fat lunch meats	Lower-fat deli meats, such as turkey
White bread	Whole grain breads (wheat, oat, multigrain)
Mayonnaise	Light mayonnaise or mustard
Fried chips and snacks	Baked chips, air-popped popcorn, trail mix, veggies and dip
Fruit in syrup	Fruit in natural juices or fresh fruit
Cookies and snack cakes	Trail mix, yogurt, or homemade baked goods such as oatmeal cookies or fruit muffins
Fruit drinks and soda	Milk, water, or 100% fruit juice

And here's how two lunches stack up, after a typical lunch received a nutritional upgrade.

Table 23.2. Comparison of Typical Lunch and Nutritional Lunch

Typical lunch	Nutritional upgrade	Why it's better
Beef bologna on white, 980 calories	Lean turkey on whole wheat, 725 calories	Less fat and more fiber, 255 fewer calories
Mayonnaise, 48 g fat	Lettuce and mustard, 13.5 g fat	Less fat and fewer calories, 34.5 fewer grams of fat
Potato chips, 13.5 g saturated fat	Carrots and celery with light dressing, 2.5 g saturated fat	Less fat and two additional vegetable servings, 11 fewer grams of saturated fat
Fruit cup in light syrup, 125 g carbohydrates	Fresh grapes, 120 g carbohydrates	Fewer calories and more fiber, 5 fewer grams of carbohy-drates
Chocolate sandwich cookies, 59 g sugar	Homemade trail mix, 52 g sugar	Less fat and more fiber, 7 fewer grams of sugar
Fruit punch drink, 3 g fiber	Skim milk, 13 g fiber	Fewer calories, less sugar, plus calcium, 10 more grams of fiber

Prepackaged lunches for kids are popular and convenient, but they're also expensive and can be less than nutritious. Instead, create your own packable lunch using healthier ingredients. Consider these components and pack them in plastic containers, resealable plastic bags, or colorful plastic wrap:

- cold-cut roll ups (lean, low-fat turkey, ham, or roast beef; lower-fat cheese; and flour tortillas)

- cold pizza (shredded mozzarella cheese; pizza sauce; flour tortilla, English muffin, or mini pizza shell)

- cracker sandwiches (whole grain crackers filled with cream cheese or peanut butter and jelly)

- peanut butter and celery sticks

231

- veggie sticks with low-fat dip or dressing

- 100% fruit juice box

- optional dessert (choose one): flavored gelatin, low-fat pudding, oatmeal raisin cookie, graham crackers, fresh fruit

Don't forget to involve the kids in the process so that healthier lunches can become a goal they can strive for, too.

Safe Packing

A packed lunch carries the added responsibility of keeping the food safe to eat. That means keeping hot foods hot and cold foods cold. One study found that fewer than a third of parents included a cold pack when packing yogurt, deli-meat sandwiches, and other foods that need refrigeration.

Here are some suggestions to keep foods safe when packing your child's lunches:

- Wash your hands first.

- Use a thermos for hot foods.

- Use cold packs or freeze some foods and drinks overnight. They'll thaw in the lunch box.

- Wash out lunch boxes every day or use brown paper lunch bags that can be discarded.

- Toss in some moist towelettes to remind kids to wash their hands before eating—and to clean themselves up afterward.

Chapter 24

Why Milk Matters for Children and Teens

Good nutrition is important for good health and can help protect against many diseases later in life. However, one important nutrient many kids and teens do not get enough of is calcium, found mainly in milk and dairy products; dark green, leafy vegetables; and foods with added calcium. Calcium is a nutrient that helps to make bones and teeth strong and healthy. It is used in building bone mass and also helps to reduce the risk of bone fracture due to osteoporosis, a condition where bones become fragile and can break easily.

How Do We Build Strong Bones?

Our bodies continually remove and replace small amounts of calcium from our bones. If your body removes more calcium than it replaces, your bones will become weaker and have a greater chance of breaking. By getting the recommended amount of calcium, you can help your bones stay strong.

Calcium needs are highest during the childhood and teen years, because bones are growing fast then and calcium must be added into bones to make them strong. Most of the calcium that makes bones strong is added by the age of 17. By eating and drinking foods that are good sources of calcium, children and teens can help store this important nutrient in their bones for later in life. As adults, calcium

"Why Milk Matters Now for Children and Teens," National Institute of Child Health and Human Development (NICHD), NIH Publication No. 00-4864, January 2001.

is lost. The more calcium that is in the bones when loss begins, the less likely it is that bones will become fragile and fracture easily.

How Much Calcium Do Kids Need?

Nutrition guidelines recommend that children ages 4–8 get 800 milligrams (mg) of calcium per day, or about 2 servings of Milk Group foods daily. Teens and young adults, ages 9–18, need more calcium because their bones are growing more than at other times of life. They should have 1,300 mg of calcium per day, or about 3 servings of Milk Group foods daily. One 8-ounce glass of milk has about 300 mg of calcium, so just a few glasses can go a long way towards getting the calcium needed each day.

How Do I Know How Much Calcium a Food Has?

Food labels can tell you how much calcium is in one serving of a food. Look at the % Daily Value (DV) next to the calcium number on the food label.

- Try to eat and drink foods with 20% or more DV for calcium (like milk). These foods are good sources of calcium.

- Foods with less than 5% DV for calcium only give you a small amount of what you need each day.

- For most adults, 100% DV = 1,000 mg of calcium. But children ages 9–18 need extra calcium. This age group needs 1,300 mg (130 DV), an additional 300 mg of calcium each day. That means an extra 8-ounce glass of milk or extra servings of another calcium-rich food.

How Much Calcium Do Kids Get?

Unfortunately, most children and teens do not meet calcium recommendations. National nutrition surveys show that only 19% of teen girls and 52% of teen boys get the recommended amounts of calcium. In fact, teenage girls only average about 740 mg of calcium per day, well below the amount needed for their normal growth and development.

Where Is the Calcium?

Low-fat and fat-free milk and dairy products, such as cheese and yogurt, are excellent sources of calcium. In addition to having lots of calcium, milk and dairy products provide other essential nutrients, all necessary for good bone health and development. These include phosphorus, magnesium, and added vitamin D in milk. Other sources of calcium include dark green, leafy vegetables, such as kale, and foods like broccoli, soybeans, tofu processed with calcium, orange juice with calcium added, and other calcium-fortified foods.

What Kind of Milk Is Best?

Fat-free (skim) and low-fat (1%) milk and dairy products are excellent choices because they make it easy to get enough calcium without adding a lot of extra fat and saturated fat to the diet. For example, a glass of whole milk contributes 25% of your total saturated fat for the day, while a glass of low-fat milk contributes only 7.5% of the total saturated fat. There are now a variety of milk products available including different levels of fat and even different flavors but an 8-oz glass (1 cup) of any variety still contains about 300 mg of calcium.

However, babies under one year old should drink only breast milk or iron-fortified formula. Children ages one to two should drink whole milk rather than reduced fat varieties because some fats are necessary for their early growth and development. Between ages two and five, parents should gradually transition children to low-fat or fat-free milk. Beginning at age 2, children should get most of their calories from grain products; fruits; vegetables; low-fat dairy products; and beans, lean meat, poultry, fish, or nuts.

Can Everyone Drink Milk?

Lactose, the sugar found in milk and dairy foods, can cause abdominal discomfort in some people. A person with lactose intolerance has trouble digesting lactose. Lactose intolerance is not common among infants and young children, but can occur in older children, adolescents, and adults. It is more common among people of African-American, Hispanic, Asian, American Indian, and Alaskan Native descent.

For people with lactose intolerance, milk is often better digested when drunk in small amounts and when combined with other foods, such as cereal with milk. In addition, many people can eat dairy foods such as cheeses or yogurt, which cause fewer symptoms. Recent studies also show that many people who are lactose intolerant can drink two to three 8 oz glasses of milk each day without getting any symptoms. Also, lactose-free milk products are now available in most stores and there are pills and drops that make it easier to digest milk and dairy products that have lactose in them.

Some people, however, are allergic to milk and dairy products and should not eat them. For those people who cannot have any milk, calcium can come from non-dairy sources like dark green, leafy vegetables such as kale, or foods like broccoli, lime-treated tortillas, and tofu processed with calcium. There are also foods with added calcium, such as calcium-fortified orange juice, soy beverages, and some cereals. Getting calcium from food is recommended, but calcium supplements can also be a way to add necessary calcium.

Solving the Calcium Crunch

Getting enough calcium is important for building strong bones and ensuring future health. Here are three things you can do to help get enough calcium and keep bones and teeth strong.

1. Think of ways to incorporate milk and other calcium rich foods into meals and snacks. For example, top a baked potato with broccoli and low-fat cheese, or dunk baby carrots into low-fat yogurt dip.

2. Keep foods with calcium in the house and put them on the table during meals and snacks.

3. Keep drinking milk throughout your life, and be sure to eat and drink other foods with calcium. These foods should be an important part of the diet your whole life long.

Additional Information

National Institute of Child Health and Human Development (NICHD)
Milk Matters Clearinghouse
P.O. Box 3006
Rockville, MD 20847
Toll-Free: 800-370-2943
Fax: 301-496-7101
Website: http://www.nichd.nih.gov/milk

Chapter 25

Nutrition for Teens

Chapter Contents

Section 25.1

Making Healthy Food Choices

Excerpted from "Take Charge of Your Health," Weight-Control Information Network (WIN), National Institute of Diabetes and Digestive and Kidney Diseases (NIDDK), NIH Publication No. 01-4328, December 2001.

As a teenager, you are going through a lot of changes. Your body is changing and growing. Have you noticed that every year, you can't seem to fit into your old shoes anymore? Or that your favorite jeans are now tighter or 3 inches too short? Your body is on its way to becoming its adult size.

Along with your physical changes, you are also becoming more independent. You are starting to make more choices about your life. You are relying less on your parents and more on yourself and your friends when making decisions. Some of the biggest choices that you face are those about your health. Why should you care about your health? Well, there are lots of reasons—like feeling good, looking good, and getting stronger. Doing well in school, work, or other activities (like sports) is another reason. Believe it or not, these can all be affected by your health. Healthy eating and being active now may also help prevent diabetes, high blood pressure, heart disease, osteoporosis, stroke, and some forms of cancer when you are older.

Some teenagers are not very physically active and some do not get the foods that their growing bodies need. Now is the time to take charge of your health by eating better and being more physically active. Even small changes will help you look and feel your best.

Family Matters

Even if health problems run in your family, it doesn't mean that you will have the same problems. To learn more about your health, start by looking at your family. Are your parents, brothers, or sisters overweight? Do any of them have health problems related to their weight, such as type 2 diabetes? Your family's gene pool, eating habits, and activities can all play a role in your health and the way you look.

Type 2 diabetes is increasing in adolescents and teenagers who are overweight. Diabetes means that blood glucose (blood sugar) is too high. Diabetes is serious. It can hurt your eyes, kidneys, heart and blood vessels, gums, and teeth. Even if members of your family have type 2 diabetes or other health problems, it doesn't mean that you will have the same problems. To lower your chances of developing them, eat healthy foods, get moving, and talk to your family or health care provider if you are concerned about your weight or health.

You Are What You Eat!

Take a look at your eating habits. What you eat, where you eat, and why you eat are important to your health. As a teen, you need to eat a variety of foods that give you the nutrients your growing body needs. Eating better and being more active can make you feel better and think more clearly.

What do you eat?

If you eat a lot of burgers and fries or pizza loaded with toppings—plus an extra helping of dessert—your diet is probably not balanced. There's nothing wrong with eating these foods—you just need to eat smaller amounts and balance them with other foods.

Where do you usually eat?

If you eat in places such as your room or in front of the TV, you may want to change that habit. Eating while doing other things makes it easy to lose track of how much you've already eaten. By eating meals and snacks at a table, you can pay more attention to what you're eating so that you don't overeat. (If you want to snack while watching TV, take a small amount of food with you—such as a handful of pretzels or a couple of cookies—not the whole bag.)

Why do you eat?

To see if you need to change your eating habits, let's look at why you eat. For most people, the following are reasons to eat:

- Time of day
- Hunger
- Food looks tempting

- Everyone else is eating
- Boredom, frustration, nervousness, or sadness

The best reason to eat is because your body tells you that you are hungry. If you are eating when you are not hungry, try doing something else to get food off of your mind. Call a friend, exercise, read, or work on a craft. These activities can help you to cut back on eating when you are feeling bored, upset, or stressed.

What Counts as a Serving?

To improve your eating habits, each day try to eat the suggested number of servings from each food group in the Food Guide Pyramid. A range of servings is given for each group. The smaller number is for people who consume about 1,600 calories a day, such as inactive women. The larger number is for those who eat about 2,800 calories a day, such as teenage boys, active men, and very active women.

Bread, Cereal, Rice, and Pasta Group (6–11 Servings)

- 1 slice of bread
- 1 ounce of ready-to-eat cereal
- ½ cup of cooked cereal, rice, or pasta

Vegetable Group (3–5 Servings)

- 1 cup of raw leafy vegetables
- ½ cup of other vegetables—cooked or chopped raw
- ¾ cup of vegetable juice

Fruit Group (2–4 Servings)

- 1 medium apple, banana, or orange
- ½ cup of chopped, cooked, or canned fruit
- ¾ cup of fruit juice

Milk, Yogurt, and Cheese Group (2–3 Servings)

- 1 cup of milk or yogurt
- 1½ ounces of natural cheese

- 2 ounces of processed cheese (1 ounce is about the size of your thumb)

Meat, Poultry, Fish, Dry Beans, Eggs, and Nuts Group (2–3 Servings)

- 2–3 ounces of cooked lean meat, poultry, or fish (3 ounces is about the size of a deck of cards)
- ½ cup of cooked dry beans or 1 egg counts as 1 ounce of lean meat
- 2 tablespoons of peanut butter or 1/3 cup of nuts counts as 1 ounce of meat

Let's Talk about Health

- Get moving. Activity can make you stronger and more flexible.
- Eat healthy every day. Choose fruits, vegetables, breads, cereals, lean meat, poultry, fish, dry beans, and low-fat or nonfat milk and cheeses.
- Eat slowly. You will be able to tell when you are full before you eat too much.
- Eat less fats, oils, and sweets. Butter, margarine, oils, candy, high-fat salad dressings, and soft drinks offer little or no protein, vitamins, or minerals.
- Eat when you are hungry. Your body will tell you when it's hungry. Snacking is okay, but try to go for a variety of nutritious snacks.

Healthy Snack Attack Choices

- Baked potato chips or tortilla chips with salsa
- Pretzels (lightly salted or unsalted)
- Bagels with tomato sauce and low-fat cheese
- Flavored rice cakes (like caramel or apple cinnamon)
- Popcorn—air popped or low-fat microwave
- Veggies with low-fat or fat-free dip
- Low-fat cottage cheese topped with fruit or spread on whole-wheat crackers

- Ice milk, low-fat frozen or regular yogurt (add skim milk, orange or pineapple juice, and sliced bananas or strawberries to make a low-fat milk shake)

- Frozen fruit bars

- Vanilla wafers, gingersnaps, graham crackers, animal crackers, fig bars, raisins

- Angel food cake topped with strawberries or raspberries and low-fat whipped cream

- String cheese

Staying Healthy and Happy

Being a teenager can be tough, and sometimes teens who are healthy try to lose weight even though they don't need to. You may feel a lot of pressure to look a certain way. Acting on this pressure may lead to eating disorders like anorexia nervosa or bulimia nervosa. Anorexia nervosa is a form of self-starvation where a person does not eat enough food to keep healthy and does not maintain a healthy weight. Bulimia nervosa is when a person eats a lot of food and then vomits or uses other methods, such as fasting or over-exercising, to avoid gaining weight after overeating.

If you are concerned about your eating habits or the way you look, it's important to talk to someone you trust. Try talking to a parent, friend, doctor, teacher, or counselor at your school. Being happy with who you are and what you look like is important for a healthy body and mind. You don't have to be an athlete, supermodel, or movie star to like who you are and to stay fit and healthy. You can take charge of your health by making small changes in your eating and physical activity habits. These changes will help you feel and look better now and be healthier for the rest of your life.

Section 25.2

Healthy Dining Hall Eating

This information was provided by TeensHealth, one of the largest resources online for medically reviewed health information written for parents, kids, and teens. For more articles like this one, visit www.Teens
Health.org, or www.KidsHealth.org. © 2004 The Nemours Center for
Children's Health Media, a division of The Nemours Foundation.

Maybe you started out with healthy goals at dinnertime: some
steamed vegetables with your lasagna, a heaping bowl of greens from
the salad bar. But as you headed to a table, the fries caught your eye.
Then you decided you'd better hit the desserts now, because who knows
what will be left when you're done with dinner?

Sound familiar? You're away at college, and your parents are no
longer looking over your shoulder to make sure you eat your vegetables. This and many other new freedoms might feel great, but they
may not be good news for your body.

While some students stock up on fruits and vegetables in the dining hall, most fill their trays with things they like without paying
much attention to what their bodies need. Even someone with the best
intentions probably finds it difficult to resist the less-healthy options.

Your waistline's not the only thing at stake, either. The foods you
choose affect your energy, concentration, and memory, because your
body and brain need the right nutrition to function properly. So before you reach for a cup of coffee or another slice of pizza, remember
that the right choices from the different food groups will help you feel
your best.

What Does Your Body Need?

Nutritional requirements vary from person to person, depending
on age, sex, size, level of activity, and other factors. For specific recommendations suited to your needs, talk to a doctor, registered dietitian,
or your student health office or nutritional counselor at your university. In general, however, your diet should provide you with a balance
of protein, dairy products, carbohydrates, vegetables, and fruits.

Many nutritional experts recommend that the majority of a person's diet come from grains, vegetables, and whole fruit. Whole grain carbohydrates—such as brown rice and whole grain breads, cereals, and pasta—are better choices than their more processed counterparts (like white bread and regular pasta) because they retain more vitamins, minerals, and fiber. When choosing vegetables and fruits, select fresh or frozen ones over canned if possible, as canned vegetables and fruits sometimes contain lots of added salt or sugar. And even though fruit and vegetables are often referred to as one food group, don't skip your vegetables in favor of fruit. (You should actually eat more vegetables than fruit for an ideal balance.)

Protein is another essential part of any diet that should not be overlooked. You can get protein from meat, fish, poultry, eggs, or non-animal sources such as beans and nuts. Dairy products like cheese, yogurt, and milk also provide protein, as well as much-needed calcium. Eating a few servings of low-fat dairy such as yogurt or skim milk and 2 to 3 servings of additional lean protein-rich foods every day will give you nutritional benefits without too much fat and cholesterol. Snack foods high in sugar, oils, and other fats don't need to be completely eliminated, but they should only play a small role in your overall diet.

Snack Attacks

Sometimes, though, those fatty or sugary foods are just what you crave. When you've been up for hours studying, you might look to sugar, a fried treat, or caffeine because you think they'll give you a boost. Plus, they're readily available and easy to grab. But you may want to consider healthier alternatives that can give you more energy with fewer negative consequences. Step one is to drink plenty of water rather than caffeinated beverages. Caffeine may provide a short-term fix, but the more you consume, the more you'll grow to depend on it. Staying hydrated can generally give you more energy than quick caffeine fixes.

If you need a solid snack, consider a lean munchie like popcorn. Or if you're really hungry, a combination of protein and carbohydrates will satisfy you longer than high-fat or sugary snacks. Try an apple and peanut butter, yogurt mixed with low-fat granola, or a tortilla with cheese, heated in the microwave and topped with salsa.

Meeting Special Dietary Needs

Eating well is difficult for everyone, but some people face an even greater challenge than others. Like lots of students, Brian, a sophomore at the University of Virginia and a vegetarian, sometimes finds it tough to focus on nutrition. "The dining halls try to serve veggie stuff, but a lot of the time it looks pretty unappealing," he says. "Sometimes it's downright nasty, and you can't find many other options." That means on some days he ends up eating peanut butter and jelly for three meals in a row—and lots of cookies.

Yet Brian is no stranger to nutrition and taking care of his body. He's an avid runner and became a certified personal trainer in high school. To make up for his occasional ruts, he works hard to give his body the variety of food it needs. In particular, he pays attention to his vitamin B_{12} intake—a vitamin that vegetarians get from eggs and cheese and non-vegetarians can find in meat. Because Brian has little money to supplement his dining hall meal plan, he always grabs a healthy snack for later, usually a ripe piece of fruit.

Vegetarians and students with food allergies, medical conditions like diabetes, or special religious requirements may find it harder to get by in a dining hall, but most schools make an effort to meet their needs. Dining hall meals typically feature several choices for a main course, one of which is usually vegetarian. Vegetarian meals can often help meet the needs of both vegetarians and students with religious requirements. Another option is to make a meal out of side dishes. Combine a baked potato topped with low-fat cheese, some steamed vegetables, and peanut butter or low-fat cream cheese on wheat toast for a filling meal. Sample salad, soup, fruit, yogurt, pasta, and other foods for more selections.

If you have special dietary requirements—especially medical ones—you may need to talk to the manager of the dining hall or to someone in student services to request certain foods. Students with food allergies need to know the ingredients that go into the dishes they enjoy—not to mention they have to be careful about ensuring that foods haven't been cross-contaminated with possible allergens like nuts or shellfish. Most schools offer nutrition counseling through dining services or the student health center. Check your school's telephone directory for information.

Overcoming Common Dining Hall Mistakes

Even when they know what their bodies need, the most attentive diners can still make mistakes while filling their plates. For the best results at mealtime, follow a few simple guidelines.

Take the right approach to food. Don't feel guilty if you have a burger or a piece of cake. Instead of thinking of foods as bad or good, most experts say moderation is the key. No food is off-limits—just pay attention to the size of the portions you take and how often you eat that food. Try not to get caught up in counting every calorie. It's more important to concentrate on getting the nutrients you need by eating a wide variety of food and including plenty of fruits, vegetables, grains, and lean proteins.

Check your fluids. Sometimes it's easy to confuse hunger and thirst. You may think you're hungry when your body actually needs more liquid. Be sure you stay hydrated throughout the day—and several cups of coffee or servings of soda don't count. The caffeine in sodas and coffee is a diuretic (which means it makes you urinate more) and can actually sap your body of fluid. Instead, drink plenty of water.

Go for variety. Frozen yogurt tastes great, but it shouldn't be the staple of your diet. Try not to eat the same one or two foods all the time or always take three of your food groups from the dessert counter. It's healthier to focus on getting a variety of fruits, vegetables, proteins, carbohydrates, and fats. A salad of raw vegetables, dark leafy greens, and beans, topped with some nuts and fruit, delivers the different nutrients your body needs. Or add some chicken and a little cheese to a green salad and you have a whole meal. (Plus, this is a great way to help you get the USDA-recommended five servings of fruits and vegetables a day.)

Watch your portions. What is a serving size, and does it really matter? Absolutely. Our bodies can't always tell us when enough is enough: One study found that people given larger portions tend to eat more food, no matter how hungry they are. So pay attention to what you're eating and stop when you start to feel full.

An appropriate portion varies depending on a person's age, gender, and activity level. But if you're concerned about your weight and you're not able to fit in a lot of extra exercise you may want to stick to the following guidelines:

- Keep protein portions about the size of your palm.

- A portion of milk is around 8 fluid ounces (about 237 milliliters).

- A grain portion is the equivalent of two pieces of bread or half a bagel.

- Limit nuts and other snack foods to a few tablespoons.

- Fill up on vegetables—the least caloric food group.

Don't linger. Dining halls are like endless buffets—you can sit for hours, and the longer you sit the more you can eat. Try to avoid hanging out in the dining hall for too long so you don't eat more than your body needs.

Stock up on healthy snacks. Most dining halls will let you take fruit or other healthy snacks with you when you leave. Slip an apple or an orange into your bag to help you resist the late-night lure of the vending machine later on.

Beyond the dining hall, learning more about nutrition can help you make better choices about what you put in your body. Talk to a nutrition counselor or someone on the school's health services staff for suggestions. When you turn to the Web for facts, choose carefully. Some sites concentrate on nutritional fads or promote information that is incorrect. Your school's website may be a good place to start. Many universities offer online health and nutrition information tailored to students.

As you educate yourself about nutrition, making smart choices in the dining hall will become second nature. While you're paying attention to food, think about fitness, too. Make an effort to work in at least 30 minutes of moderate exercise each day (like walking, jogging, swimming, or working out at the gym). Pairing exercise with healthy foods will help fuel both your body and your mind.

Section 25.3

Weight Control for College Students

This information was provided by TeensHealth, one of the largest resources online for medically reviewed health information written for parents, kids, and teens. For more articles like this one, visit www.Teens
Health.org, or www.KidsHealth.org. © 2004 The Nemours Center for
Children's Health Media, a division of The Nemours Foundation.

Beating the Freshman 15

Everyone's heard warnings about the "freshman 15," but is it true
that many college students pack on 15 pounds during their first year
at school? Recent studies find that some first-year students are indeed
likely to gain weight. Researchers at Cornell University found that students gained an average of 4 pounds during the first 12 weeks of their
freshman year—a rate of gain that is 11 times higher than the typical weight gain for 17- and 18-year-olds.

Not everyone is destined to gain the full frosh 15, though: A multi-
year study by researchers at Tufts University found that, on average, men
gain 6 pounds and women gain 4.5 during their first year of college.

What's Behind First-Year Weight Gain?

College offers many temptations. You're on your own and free to
eat what you want, when you want it. You can pile on the portions in
the dining hall, eat meals of french fries and ice cream, and indulge
in sugary and salty snacks to fuel late-night study sessions. In addition, you may not get as much exercise as you did in high school.

College is also a time of change, and the stress of acclimating to
school can trigger overeating. People sometimes eat in response to
anxiety, homesickness, sadness, or stress, and all of these can be part
of adapting to being away at school.

Should I Worry about the Weight?

Some weight gain is normal as an adolescent body grows and metabolism shifts, but pronounced or rapid weight gain may become a
problem. Weight gain that pushes you above your body's normal range

carries health risks. People who are overweight are more likely to have high blood pressure, high cholesterol, breathlessness, and joint problems. People who are overweight when they're younger have a greater likelihood of being overweight as adults. Poor diet and exercise habits in college can start you on a path that could later lead to heart disease, type 2 diabetes, or obesity, and may increase your risk for developing certain cancers.

Unhealthy food choices also won't give you the balance of nutrients you need to keep up with the demands of college. You may notice that your energy lags and your concentration and memory suffer. The Tufts study found that most students earn failing marks when it comes to good nutrition: Almost 70% of students get fewer than the recommended five servings of fruits and vegetables each day.

College-age adults are still building bone mass, and bone health is influenced by diet, fitness, and other factors. Smoking and alcohol interfere with calcium absorption (along with their other harmful effects), whereas eating calcium-rich foods (like dairy products) and doing weight-bearing exercises (like running) help build bone mass. Cola, often a staple of late-night studying, also interferes with the absorption of calcium. The Tufts study found that women who drink more than three 12-ounce servings of a cola soda each day have lower bone density in their hips than their peers who drink less than one serving.

If you do gain weight, don't freak out. Take a look at your eating and exercise habits and make adjustments. The Cornell study found that only 174 extra calories a day accounted for the extra 4 pounds mentioned, so cutting out one can of soda or a midnight snack and being more active will help you get back on track. It may be tempting to go for the easy fix, like skipping meals or trying the latest fad diet, but these approaches don't generally work to keep weight off in the long run.

How Can I Avoid Gaining Weight?

The best way to beat first-year weight gain is to prevent it altogether. Good habits like a balanced diet, regular exercise, and getting enough sleep can do more than keep the pounds off—they can also help you stay healthy and avoid problems down the line. Adopting some simple practices can have a big impact today and years from now.

Take a Sound Approach to Eating

In addition to avoiding eating when you're stressed, studying, or watching TV, there are several steps you can take to adopt a healthy food attitude:

- eat slowly

- eat at regular times

- keep between-meal snacking to a minimum

- choose a mix of nutritious foods

- pick lower-fat options when you can, such as low-fat milk instead of whole milk or light salad dressing instead of full-fat dressing

- watch the size of your portions (not too much or too little)

- resist going back for additional servings

- steer clear of vending machines and fast food

- keep healthy snacks like fruit on hand in your room

- replace empty-calorie soft drinks with water or other healthier beverages

Be aware of your attitude toward food, too—does it preoccupy you? If you find yourself fixating on food or feeling guilty about what you eat, talk to your doctor or ask someone at the student health center for advice.

Learn about Nutrition

Many schools have nutrition counselors. If yours does not, you can talk to someone on the student health services staff about nutrition and how to make good choices in the dining hall.

Take Control of Your Lifestyle

Keep an eye on your alcohol consumption. Not only can excess drinking lead to health problems, but beer and alcohol are high in calories and can cause weight gain. (Why do you think it's called a beer belly?) If you're going to drink, do it in moderation.

Smoking is another culprit. Although cigarettes may suppress your appetite, smoking can make exercise and even normal activity such as walking across campus or climbing stairs more difficult—not to mention causing heart and lung problems and increasing your risk of cancer.

Many smokers who quit find they have more energy, so battle the extra pounds by exercising. You can avoid gaining weight and increase your chances of quitting if you do. If you want to stop smoking, you don't have to go it alone. Someone at your student health center can direct you to smoking-cessation programs and give you the tips and support you need to quit.

Get Enough Exercise and Sleep

Students in the Tufts study who said they exercised at least 3 days a week were more likely to report better physical health, as well as greater happiness, than those who did not exercise. They were also more likely to report using their time productively.

Reaping the benefits of exercise does not have to be as difficult as it might seem. Try to work 30 minutes of moderate exercise into your schedule each day (like walking, jogging, swimming, or working out at the gym) and you'll feel and see the results. For other options, check out biking or hiking trails or sign up for a martial arts class. Attending a class on a regular schedule may motivate you to stick with your fitness goals.

If you don't like organized forms of exercise, you can also work 30 minutes of exercise into your daily schedule by walking briskly across campus instead of taking the bus, taking the stairs instead of the elevator, or cycling to class. And take time—even just a few minutes, here and there—to move around and stretch when you've been sitting for a long time, such as during study sessions.

Getting enough sleep can help keep stress under control. Although sleep can't banish stress entirely, it can help you feel up to meeting the challenges of college without giving in to unhealthy habits.

Although it may seem difficult to work 7 or 8 hours of sleep into your schedule every day, make sleep a priority. Here are some ways to make the most of your sleep:

- keep a regular sleeping schedule by getting up and going to bed at about the same time every day

- don't nap too much

- avoid caffeine in the evening

- avoid exercising, watching TV, or listening to loud music before bed

Gaining weight during the first year of college is not inevitable. You may have your ups and downs, but a few simple changes to your daily routine can help you fend off excess weight while keeping you physically and mentally healthy.

Chapter 26

Women's Nutrition Issues

Chapter Contents

Section 26.1

Eating during Pregnancy

This information was provided by KidsHealth, one of the largest resources online for medically reviewed health information written for parents, kids, and teens. For more articles like this one, visit www.KidsHealth.org, or www.TeensHealth.org. © 2004 The Nemours Center for Children's Health Media, a division of The Nemours Foundation.

To eat well during pregnancy you must do more than simply increase how much you eat. You must also consider what you eat. Although you need about 300 extra calories a day—especially later in your pregnancy, when your baby grows quickly—those calories should come from nutritious foods so they can contribute to your baby's growth and development.

Why It's Important to Eat Well when You're Pregnant

Do you wonder how it's reasonable to gain 25 to 35 pounds (on average) during your pregnancy when a newborn baby weighs only a fraction of that? Although it varies from woman to woman, this is how those pounds may add up:

- 7.5 pounds—average baby's weight
- 7 pounds—your body's extra stored protein, fat, and other nutrients
- 4 pounds—your extra blood
- 4 pounds—your other extra body fluids
- 2 pounds—breast enlargement
- 2 pounds—enlargement of your uterus
- 2 pounds—amniotic fluid surrounding your baby
- 1.5 pounds—the placenta

Of course, patterns of weight gain during pregnancy vary. It's normal to gain less if you start out heavier and more if you're having twins or triplets—or if you were underweight before becoming pregnant. More important than how much weight you gain is what makes up those extra pounds.

When you're pregnant, what you eat and drink is the main source of nourishment for your baby. In fact, the link between what you consume and the health of your baby is much stronger than once thought. That's why doctors now say, for example, that no amount of alcohol consumption should be considered safe during pregnancy.

The extra food you eat shouldn't just be empty calories—it should provide the nutrients your growing baby needs. For example, calcium helps make and keep bones and teeth strong. While you're pregnant, you still need calcium for your body, plus extra calcium for your developing baby. Similarly, you require more of all the essential nutrients than you did before you became pregnant.

A Nutrition Primer for Expectant Mothers

Whether or not you're pregnant, a healthy diet includes proteins, carbohydrates, fats, vitamins, minerals, and plenty of water. The Food Guide Pyramid helps you determine how many servings of each kind of food to eat every day. Eating a variety of foods in the proportions indicated is a good step toward staying healthy.

Food labels can tell you what kinds of nutrients are in the foods you eat. The letters RDA, which you find on food labeling, stand for recommended daily allowance, or the amount of a nutrient recommended for your daily diet. When you're pregnant, the RDAs for most nutrients are higher.

Some of the most common nutrients you need and the foods that contain them are shown in Table 26.1.

Scientists know that your diet can affect your baby's health—even before you become pregnant. For example, recent research shows that folic acid helps prevent neural tube defects (including spina bifida) from occurring during the earliest stages of fetal development—so it's important for you to consume plenty of it before you become pregnant and during the early weeks of your pregnancy.

Even though lots of foods, particularly breakfast cereals, are fortified with folic acid, doctors now encourage women to take folic acid supplements before and throughout pregnancy (especially for the first 28 days). Be sure to ask your doctor about folic acid if you're considering becoming pregnant.

Calcium is another important nutrient for pregnant women. Because your growing baby's calcium demands are high, you should increase

Table 26.1. Nutrients Needed during Pregnancy and Foods that Contain Them

Protein
Needed for: cell growth and blood production
Best sources: lean meat, fish, poultry, egg whites, beans, peanut butter, tofu

Carbohydrates
Needed for: daily energy production
Best sources: breads, cereals, rice, potatoes, pasta, fruits, vegetables

Calcium
Needed for: strong bones and teeth, muscle contraction, nerve function
Best sources: milk, cheese, yogurt, sardines or salmon with bones, spinach

Iron
Needed for: red blood cell production (needed to prevent anemia)
Best sources: lean red meat, spinach, iron-fortified whole grain breads and cereals

Vitamin A
Needed for: healthy skin, good eyesight, growing bones
Best sources: carrots, dark leafy greens, sweet potatoes

Vitamin C
Needed for: healthy gums, teeth, and bones; assistance with iron absorption
Best sources: citrus fruit, broccoli, tomatoes, fortified fruit juices

Vitamin B$_6$
Needed for: red blood cell formation; effective use of protein, fat, and carbohydrates
Best sources: pork, ham, whole grain cereals, bananas

Vitamin B$_{12}$
Needed for: formation of red blood cells, maintaining nervous system health
Best sources: meat, fish, poultry, milk (Note: vegetarians who don't eat dairy products need supplemental B$_{12}$)

Vitamin D
Needed for: healthy bones and teeth; aids absorption of calcium
Best sources: fortified milk, dairy products, cereals, breads

Folic acid
Needed for: blood and protein production, effective enzyme function
Best sources: green leafy vegetables, dark yellow fruits and vegetables, beans, peas, nuts

Fat
Needed for: body energy store
Best sources: meat, whole-milk dairy products, nuts, peanut butter, margarine, vegetable oils (Note: limit fat intake to 30% or less of your total daily calorie intake)

your calcium consumption to prevent a loss of calcium from your own bones. Your doctor will also likely prescribe prenatal vitamins for you, which contain some extra calcium.

Your best food sources of calcium are milk and other dairy products. However, if you have lactose intolerance or dislike milk and milk products, ask your doctor about a calcium supplement. (Signs of lactose intolerance include diarrhea, bloating, or gas after eating milk or milk products. Taking a lactase capsule or pill, or using lactose-free milk products may help.) Other calcium-rich foods include sardines or salmon with bones, tofu, broccoli, spinach, and calcium-fortified juices and foods.

Doctors don't usually recommend starting a strict vegan diet when you become pregnant. However, if you already follow a vegetarian diet, you can continue to do so during your pregnancy—but do it carefully. Be sure your doctor knows about your diet. It's challenging to get the nutrition you need if you don't eat fish and chicken, or milk, cheese, or eggs. You'll likely need supplemental protein and may also need to take vitamin B_{12} and D supplements. To ensure that you and your baby receive adequate nutrition, consult a registered dietitian for help with planning meals.

What Do Food Cravings during Pregnancy Mean?

You've probably known women who craved specific foods during pregnancy, or perhaps you've had such cravings yourself. Researchers have tried to determine whether a hunger for a particular type of food indicates that a woman's body lacks the nutrients that food contains. Although this isn't the case, it's still unclear why these urges occur.

Some pregnant women crave chocolate, spicy foods, fruits, and comfort foods, such as mashed potatoes, cereals, and toasted white bread. Other women crave non-food items, such as clay and cornstarch. The craving and eating of non-food items is known as pica. Consuming things that aren't food can be dangerous to both you and your baby. If you have urges to eat non-food items, notify your doctor.

But following your cravings is fine, as long as you crave foods and these foods contribute to a healthy diet. Frequently, these cravings diminish about 3 months into the pregnancy.

What Should You Avoid Eating and Drinking during Pregnancy?

As mentioned earlier, avoid alcohol. No level of alcohol consumption is considered safe during pregnancy. Also, check with your doctor before you take any vitamins or herbal products. Some of these can be harmful to the developing fetus.

And although many doctors feel that one or two 6- to 8-ounce cups per day of coffee, tea, or soda with caffeine won't harm your baby, it's probably wise to avoid caffeine altogether if you can. High caffeine consumption has been linked to an increased risk of miscarriage, so limit your intake or switch to decaffeinated products.

When you're pregnant, it's also important to avoid food-borne illnesses, such as listeriosis and toxoplasmosis, which can be life-threatening to an unborn baby and may cause birth defects or miscarriage. Foods you'll want to steer clear of include:

- soft, unpasteurized cheeses (often advertised as fresh) such as feta, goat, Brie, Camembert, and blue cheese;
- unpasteurized milk, juices, and apple cider;
- raw eggs or foods containing raw eggs, including mousse and tiramisu;
- raw or undercooked meats, fish, or shellfish;
- processed meats such as hot dogs and deli meats (these should be well-cooked).

If you've eaten these foods at some point during your pregnancy, try not to worry too much about it now; just avoid them for the remainder of the pregnancy. If you're really concerned, talk to your doctor.

You'll also want to avoid eating shark, swordfish, king mackerel, or tilefish, as well as limit the amount of other kinds of fish that you eat. Although fish and shellfish can be an extremely healthy part of your pregnancy diet (they contain beneficial omega-3 fatty acids, and are high in protein and low in saturated fat), these types of fish may contain high levels of mercury. Because mercury can cause damage to the developing brain of a fetus or growing child, the U.S. Food and Drug Administration (FDA) and the U.S. Environmental Protection Agency (EPA) say that these fish should not be eaten at all by pregnant women, women who may become pregnant, nursing mothers, and young children.

Mercury, which occurs naturally in the environment, can also be released into the air through industrial pollution and can accumulate in streams and oceans where it turns into methylmercury in the water. The methylmercury builds up in fish, especially larger fish that eat other smaller fish.

If you're pregnant and eat shark, swordfish, king mackerel, or tilefish, even occasionally, it's a good idea to stop. Although almost all fish and shellfish contain small amounts of mercury, you can enjoy some with lower mercury levels (shrimp, canned light tuna, salmon, pollock, and catfish) in moderation (no more than 12 ounces a week, say the FDA and EPA). Because albacore (or white) tuna or tuna steaks are higher in mercury than canned light tuna, it's recommended that you eat no more than 6 ounces a week.

Avoiding Some Common Problems

Because the iron in prenatal vitamins and other factors may cause constipation during pregnancy, it's a good idea to consume more fiber than you did before you became pregnant. Try to eat about 20 to 30 grams of fiber a day. Your best sources are fresh fruits and vegetables and whole grain breads, cereals, or muffins.

Some people also use fiber tablets or drinks or other high-fiber products available at your pharmacy, but check with your doctor before trying them. (Don't use laxatives while you're pregnant unless your doctor advises you to do so. And avoid the old wives' remedy—castor oil—because it can actually interfere with your body's ability to absorb nutrients.)

If constipation is a problem for you, your doctor may prescribe a stool softener. Be sure to drink plenty of fluids, especially water, when increasing fiber intake, or you can make your constipation worse. One of the best ways to avoid constipation is to get more exercise. You should also drink plenty of water between meals each day to help soften your stools and move food through your digestive system. Sometimes hot tea, soups, or broth can help. Also, keep dried fruits handy for snacking.

Some pregnant women find that broccoli, spinach, cauliflower, and fried foods give them heartburn or gas. You can plan a balanced diet to avoid these foods. Carbonated drinks also cause gas or heartburn for some women, although others find they calm the digestive system.

If you're frequently nauseated, eat small amounts of bland foods, like toast or crackers, throughout the day. If nothing else sounds good, try cereal with milk or a sweet piece of fruit. To help combat nausea, you can also:

- Take your prenatal vitamin before going to bed after you've eaten a snack—not on an empty stomach.

- Eat a small snack when you get up to go to the bathroom early in the morning.

- Suck on hard candy.

How Can You Know If You're Eating Well during Pregnancy?

The key is to eat foods from the different food groups in approximately the recommended proportions. If nausea or lack of appetite cause you to eat less at times, don't worry—it's unlikely to cause fetal harm because your baby gets first crack at the nutrients you consume. And although it's generally recommended that a woman of normal weight gain approximately 25 to 35 pounds during pregnancy (most gain 4 to 6 pounds during the first trimester and 1 pound a week during the 2nd and 3rd trimesters), don't fixate on the scale. Instead, focus on eating a good variety and balance of nutritious foods to keep both you and your baby healthy.

Section 26.2

What You Need to Know about Mercury in Fish

"What You Need to Know about Mercury in Fish and Shellfish," U.S. Food and Drug Administration (FDA) and Environmental Protection Agency (EPA), March 2004.

Fish and shellfish are an important part of a healthy diet. Fish and shellfish contain high-quality protein and other essential nutrients, are low in saturated fat, and contain omega-3 fatty acids. A well-balanced diet that includes a variety of fish and shellfish can contribute to heart health and children's proper growth and development. So, women and young children in particular should include fish or shellfish in their diets due to the many nutritional benefits.

However, nearly all fish and shellfish contain traces of mercury. For most people, the risk from mercury by eating fish and shellfish is not a health concern. Yet, some fish and shellfish contain higher levels of mercury that may harm an unborn baby or young child's developing nervous system. The risks from mercury in fish and shellfish depend on the amount of fish and shellfish eaten and the levels of mercury in the fish and shellfish. Therefore, the U.S. Food and Drug Administration (FDA) and the U.S. Environmental Protection Agency

(EPA) are advising women who may become pregnant, pregnant women, nursing mothers, and young children to avoid some types of fish and eat fish and shellfish that are lower in mercury.

By following these three recommendations for selecting and eating fish or shellfish, women and young children will receive the benefits of eating fish and shellfish and be confident that they have reduced their exposure to the harmful effects of mercury.

1. Do not eat shark, swordfish, king mackerel, or tilefish because they contain high levels of mercury.

2. Eat up to 12 ounces (2 average meals) a week of a variety of fish and shellfish that are lower in mercury.

    -   Five of the most commonly eaten fish that are low in mercury are shrimp, canned light tuna, salmon, pollock, and catfish.

    -   Another commonly eaten fish, albacore (white) tuna has more mercury than canned light tuna. So, when choosing your two meals of fish and shellfish, you may eat up to 6 ounces (one average meal) of albacore tuna per week.

3. Check local advisories about the safety of fish caught by family and friends in your local lakes, rivers, and coastal areas. If no advice is available, eat up to 6 ounces (one average meal) per week of fish you catch from local waters, but don't consume any other fish during that week.

Follow these same recommendations when feeding fish and shellfish to your young child, but serve smaller portions.

Frequently Asked Questions about Mercury in Fish and Shellfish

What is mercury and methylmercury?

Mercury occurs naturally in the environment and can also be released into the air through industrial pollution. Mercury falls from the air and can accumulate in streams and oceans and is turned into methylmercury in the water. It is this type of mercury that can be harmful to your unborn baby and young child. Fish absorb the methylmercury as they feed in these waters, and so it builds up in them. It builds up more in some types of fish and shellfish than others, depending on what the fish eat, which is why the levels vary.

I'm a woman who could have children, but I'm not pregnant—so why should I be concerned about methylmercury?

If you regularly eat types of fish that are high in methylmercury, it can accumulate in your blood stream over time. Methylmercury is removed from the body naturally, but it may take over a year for the levels to drop significantly. Thus, it may be present in a woman even before she becomes pregnant. This is the reason why women who are trying to become pregnant should also avoid eating certain types of fish.

Is there methylmercury in all fish and shellfish?

Nearly all fish and shellfish contain traces of methylmercury. However, larger fish that have lived longer have the highest levels of methylmercury because they've had more time to accumulate it. These large fish (swordfish, shark, king mackerel, and tilefish) pose the greatest risk. Other types of fish and shellfish may be eaten in the amounts recommended by FDA and EPA.

What about fish sticks and fast food sandwiches?

Fish sticks and fast food sandwiches are commonly made from fish that are low in mercury.

The advice about canned tuna is in the advisory, but what's the advice about tuna steaks?

Because tuna steak generally contains higher levels of mercury than canned light tuna, when choosing your two meals of fish and shellfish, you may eat up to 6 ounces (one average meal) of tuna steak per week.

What if I eat more than the recommended amount of fish and shellfish in a week?"

One week's consumption of fish does not change the level of methylmercury in the body much at all. If you eat a lot of fish one week, you can cut back for the next week or two. Just make sure you average the recommended amount per week.

Where do I get information about the safety of fish caught recreationally by family or friends?

Before you go fishing, check your Fishing Regulations Booklet for information about recreationally caught fish. You can also contact your local health department for information about local advisories. You need to check local advisories because some kinds of fish and shell-fish caught in your local waters may have higher or much lower than average levels of mercury. This depends on the levels of mercury in the water in which the fish are caught. Those fish with much lower levels may be eaten more frequently and in larger amounts.

Additional Information

U.S. Food and Drug Administration (FDA)
Seafood Information and Resources
5600 Fishers Lane
Rockville, MD 20857
Toll-Free: 888-723-3366
Website: http://www.cfsan.fda.gov/seafood1.html

U.S. Environmental Protection Agency(EPA)
Fish Advisory Program
1200 Pennsylvania Ave., N.W.
Washington, DC 20460
Website: http://www.epa.gov/ost/fish

Section 26.3

Women Should Adjust Nutrition after Menopause

As children, we all heard our parents say, "Eat your fruits and vegetables—they'll make you healthy and strong." It was good advice then and could be life-saving today, especially for women. Poor nutrition is implicated as a contributing factor in 5 of the 10 leading causes of death in women—coronary heart disease, cancer, stroke, diabetes, and diseases of the liver and kidneys. It is also a key factor in osteoporosis (thinning of the bones), putting women especially at risk for fractures of the hip, wrist, back, and other bones.

As female baby boomers enter midlife in record numbers, more and more of them are becoming aware of the link between what they eat and their health and longevity, says Joan Pleuss, RD, MS, CDE, CD. She is Bionutrition Research Manager at the Medical College of Wisconsin's General Clinical Research Center.

"Women, especially as they reach menopause, need to reassess their nutrition," Pleuss says. "As we age, a number of issues emerge that require changes in the nutrients we need." For example, metabolism starts to slow down in midlife, she says. Bone mass begins to decrease, and bones become more brittle. Exposure to sunlight triggers vitamin D synthesis in the skin, but older women don't convert sunlight into essential vitamin D as efficiently as they did when they were younger, nor do they process another essential vitamin—B_{12}—as well as they once did.

Good Diet Best, but Some Supplements Can Help

Nevertheless, Pleuss says, women of all ages should strive to get the nutrients they need the old-fashioned way—"by eating a healthy diet with servings from all food groups."

The federal government's *Dietary Guidelines for Americans* describe a healthful diet this way: "Start with plenty of breads, cereals, rice, pasta, vegetables, and fruits. Add 2 to 3 servings from the milk group and 2 to 3 servings from the meat group. Remember to go easy on fats, oils, and sweets, the foods in the small tip of the Pyramid," it says, referring to the government's Food Guide Pyramid.

Pleuss realizes that few Americans actually fulfill those recommended guidelines, since the typical American diet is too high in fat and sugar, and too low in fiber, fruit, and vegetables. In addition to altering their diets, women often need to increase their physical activity level and add supplementary vitamins and minerals. "I think a multivitamin is a good idea for all women," she says. "Older women have increased need for additional calcium, vitamin D, and vitamin B_{12}. Taking a multivitamin together with good food choices ensures women that they are meeting the current dietary recommendations."

Calcium

After 50, women need more calcium than women 25 to 50 require, Pleuss says. "The recommended amount of calcium for post-menopausal women to maintain bone strength is between 1,200 and 1,500 milligrams a day—the same amount girls and young women need to build bones."

In dietary form, older women can fulfill their increased demands for calcium by drinking enough milk (an 8-ounce glass contains 300 milligrams of calcium). They can also get 300 milligrams of calcium by eating an 8-ounce cup of yogurt or 1 to 2 ounces of cheese. Some brands of orange juice are fortified with calcium, in the same amount per serving as milk, yogurt, or cheese.

Vitamin D

Women 50 to 70 years old should consume 400 international units (IU) of vitamin D daily, Pleuss says. Women over 70 need even more; the recommended amount is 600 IU daily.

Most multivitamins provide 100% of the recommended amount of vitamin D. A glass of milk provides 100 IU of vitamin D, but vitamin D is not available in yogurt or cheese. Pleuss also recommends that women choose low-fat or non-fat milk, yogurt, and cheese. Cardiovascular disease and some cancers are thought to be related to diets that are too high in fat. Obesity and overweight may account for 20% of all cancer deaths in U.S. women and 14% in U.S. men, American Cancer Society researchers said in a study published in April 2003 in the *New England Journal of Medicine*.

Vitamin B$_{12}$

It is recommended that older women get 2.4 micrograms of vitamin B$_{12}$ daily, Pleuss says. "This vitamin is present in all animal products, but in a form the body needs to break down—and that process is less efficient in older women." Most multivitamins provide at least 2 micrograms of vitamin B$_{12}$.

"Women's" Foods and Vitamins Not Needed

What about those vitamins and other foods—cereals, muffins, even sports drinks—that are targeted toward women? "They can provide some benefit, especially those that add calcium to the diet," Pleuss says. "But they're not necessary, and they tend to be fairly expensive." Many also contain iron and folate, nutrients that are needed in greater quantities for women in their child-bearing years. Also, some "foods for women" may be surprisingly high in fat, salt (sodium), and sugar. Excess fat and sugar can lead to weight gain and might cause women to eat fewer healthful foods. Overweight increases the risk of diabetes, heart disease, and some cancers. Eating less salt decreases the chance of developing high blood pressure.

"Compare food labels," Pleuss recommends. "Remember it's whole grains, fruits, vegetables, legumes, and dairy products that are found to provide the health benefits."

Make sure to carefully evaluate vitamin labels, too, she cautions. Many supplements are tailored to meet the needs of adults in the middle age range, and might not be appropriate for older adults. For instance, older women should avoid vitamins with iron unless a physician recommends the extra iron intake. (From about age 50 and on, women need less iron than those under 50, but even some vitamins marketed to older people have more iron than needed for that age group.)

In addition, keep in mind that various units are used to measure different supplements—for instance, vitamin B$_{12}$ is measured in micrograms, vitamin C is measured in milligrams, and vitamin E is measured in International Units. This can be confusing, so compare labels thoroughly.

Soy Products

Many of today's "foods for women" contain soy, which is being studied for its ability to help prevent cardiovascular disease by lowering the so-called bad cholesterol, or LDL—low density lipoprotein. Some older adults add niacin to raise their good cholesterol (HDL, or high density lipoprotein); however adding supplemental niacin should be avoided unless prescribed by a physician, since extremely high doses are needed to be effective and can have side effects.

Soy also "has a weak estrogenic effect," Pleuss says. Phytoestrogens—chemicals found in plants such as soy—can mimic the human hormone estrogen. It's unknown at this point whether the similarities between the estrogen-like substances present in soy has the potential to stimulate estrogen-dependent human breast cancer cells.

Until more is known, women who have had estrogen-influenced breast cancer should use soy in moderation. As for soy's ability to reduce hot flashes after menopause, Pleuss says: "A lot of studies are being done. So far, results are showing that soy may have modest effects on reducing hot flashes, but the results are inconclusive."

Use Herbals Cautiously

As for herbal remedies for women's health, Pleuss says there are no general recommendations. Some women try black cohosh for relief of hot flashes, but Pleuss says this herb should not be taken for longer than six months. Some women take valerian to thwart insomnia; Pleuss said she tried it and it actually kept her awake.

Some herbs can interfere with or intensify the action of blood thinners and others drugs, she warns, so patients should always ask a health practitioner before taking any herbal products. Patients facing surgery must quit taking certain herbal medications two weeks before the operation.

The bottom line for women's nutritional requirements? "Eating a variety of foods, supplemented by a multivitamin, is the best way to get the nutrients we need," Pleuss says.

Chapter 27

Dietary Health for Adults over Fifty

Chapter Contents

Section 27.1

Nutrition after Fifty

Excerpted from "Nutrition After Fifty: Tips and Recipes,"
© 2002 American Institute for Cancer Research. Reprinted with permission.

Turning 50, 60, 70, or even 80 is not what it used to be. Americans are living longer and enjoying life more than ever. One desire we all share is to feel good and stay healthy. This section can show you how good nutrition and a healthy lifestyle can add vitality to your years and help you reduce the risk of cancer and other diseases. It is written for people age 50 and over. It also contains plenty of general information and practical strategies for those of any age who would like to lower their risk for chronic illness and feel better than ever.

How to Stay Healthy

When it comes to your cancer risk and overall health, the foods you choose have a major impact. There is still much to learn about nutrition and aging, but scientists are continually finding answers.

We know that plant substances found in vegetables and fruits can help prevent the cell damage that, over time, can lead to the weakening of body tissues such as skin, organs, and vessels, and diseases such as cancer. Getting enough calcium and vitamin D can help prevent osteoporosis, the leading cause of bone fractures in older adults. The B vitamins folate, B_6 and B_{12} may help reduce the risk of heart disease and stroke. Early studies show these vitamins could possibly delay a decline in brain activities like concentration, reason, and memory that may come with age. In addition, researchers are also discovering that it is never too late to reap the benefits of exercise. That is true even for people in their 80s and 90s, who have been shown to increase their muscle mass, strength, and independence by strength training.

By adopting sensible diet and exercise habits, you can enjoy the rewards of a longer, healthier life. Make change easier by taking it one step at a time. Seek out support, build on your successes, and enjoy the benefits you will receive from doing positive things for your health.

Focus on Plant-Based Foods

Many of us grew up as meat and potatoes people. As a result, eating more plant-based foods is probably a new idea. In our lifetimes, a wealth of information has come to light about the ways in which foods can affect our health. We know that by choosing to eat more foods that come from plants and fewer that come from animals, we can benefit our health in many ways, including helping to prevent cancer and heart disease, maintain a healthy weight, and promote digestion.

Work toward filling at least two-thirds of your plate with vegetables, fruits, whole grains, and beans, and one-third or less with fish, poultry, or lean meat. Try adapting favorite recipes to include larger amounts of plant-based foods and smaller amounts of meat or poultry. Try new recipes from the newspaper, cooking magazines, television cooking programs, or Internet websites. You might even want to enroll in a healthy cooking class to taste and learn to prepare a variety of plant-based dishes.

Fill Up on Vegetables and Fruits

When it comes to vegetables and fruits, think variety and think abundance. These two food groups are two of your best dietary defenses against cancer and other diseases. In fact, experts estimate that simply eating at least five servings of vegetables and fruits each day could decrease overall cancer rates by 20 percent. Fruits and vegetables contain antioxidants and other phytochemicals that are potent cancer fighters. Phytochemicals, literally "plant chemicals," are found in all plants; most have been discovered in only the last 10 years. Some phytochemicals are antioxidants that can deactivate cell-damaging molecules in the body, and thereby slow tissue weakening, aging, and cancer development.

Did you know that fitting more servings of vegetables and fruits into your day could be easy? Try these ideas:

- **Make breakfast count.** In addition to your cereal or toast, start the day with a glass of 100% fruit juice and mixed berries stirred into low-fat or nonfat yogurt. Or combine juice, fruit, and yogurt in a blender for a quick, healthy breakfast shake.

- **Pack a fruit or veggie snack** for a day's outing. Bring along dried fruits, like apples, apricots, prunes, or raisins. Stash a snack-size can of peaches or pears packed in fruit juice (and a plastic spoon) in your bag.

- **Add vegetables to your everyday meals.** Add carrots, peppers, broccoli, sliced mushrooms, or zucchini to pasta sauce. Top a baked potato with salsa. Lessen the layer of cheese on your pizza and load it with vegetables like tomatoes, onions, green peppers, broccoli, and spinach.

- **Choose fruit for dessert.** Top low-fat frozen yogurt with sliced strawberries. Slice ripe peaches onto graham crackers. Have a baked apple sprinkled with cinnamon.

- **Look beyond the usual.** Try different varieties of melons, potatoes, or greens. Make a fruit salad with mango, papaya, kiwi, pineapple, or other fruits that are new to you. Create a new vegetable salad with Belgian endive, radicchio, cherry tomatoes, and yellow bell peppers.

- **Make it easy on yourself.** The convenience of frozen and canned vegetables and fruits makes them an easy addition to many meals. Veggies and fruits are frozen right after harvesting and contain similar nutrient levels to fresh produce. Canned products are preserved after being lightly cooked. They are also a very nutritious choice. Be sure to rinse canned veggies before using to wash off excess sodium. Also, choose fruit canned in its own juice.

Go Easy on Red Meat and Fats

If you eat red meat, try to limit portions to three ounces or less a day—about the size of a deck of cards. Too much red meat probably increases the risk of cancers of the colon and rectum, and possibly does the same for cancers of the breast, prostate, pancreas, and kidney.

The type of fat found mainly in animal products like meat, milk, cheese, eggs, butter, and lard is called saturated fat. There are many reasons to avoid eating a diet high in saturated fat, and high in fat in general. This type of diet possibly increases the risk of cancers of the lung, colon, rectum, breast, prostate, and endometrium. It also increases heart disease risk. Fat in general is high in calories. Excess fat and calories can lead to weight gain, which itself increases the risk of some forms of cancer, particularly endometrial cancer. Obesity also heightens risk for heart disease, type 2 diabetes, and high blood pressure.

Eating some fat is important for health, but certain fats are healthier than others. Vegetable oils like olive or canola are your best choices because they are high in monounsaturated fat and low in saturated fat. When choosing a spread, look for a soft tub margarine or squeeze spread that includes little saturated and no *trans* fat. *Trans* fat acts like saturated fat in the body. It may increase the risk of heart disease and other illnesses. The softer the spread, the less *trans* fat it will contain. There are several spreads that are saturated and *trans* fat-free available—try to find one you like.

When baking, sometimes there is no substitute for butter, stick margarine, or shortening. If you like the taste of your favorite cake and cookie recipes, and there are no simple ways to make them more healthful, don't change them. Just save these snack foods for special occasions and savor them in small portions. Focus instead on making healthier choices of the oils and spreads you eat every day.

Keep Weight in Check

Carrying around extra pounds can slow you down. It also affects your health—increasing your chances of developing heart disease, diabetes, high blood pressure, joint problems, and some cancers.

Did you know as you get older, your body may need fewer calories to maintain its weight? Use these tips to help you reach a healthy weight:

- **Set yourself up for success.** Fill your fridge and cupboards with mostly plant-based foods. Keep nutritious foods such as vegetables, fruits, whole grains, and beans where they are easy to find. Keep higher-calorie treats out of sight or, better yet, out of the house.

- **Pay attention to portions.** Eating too much of anything— even low-fat or fat-free foods—can affect your weight. Find serving size information on the Nutrition Facts panel of a food label. Get out your measuring cups and see what one portion looks like on your plate. This will give you an accurate idea of how much you are eating.

- **Cut down on fat.** Fat is high in calories. Try lower-fat versions of higher-fat foods, such as dressings, spreads, milk, and cheese. Be aware, however, that low-fat or fat-free products may contain added sugar for flavor, so calorie levels may still be high. Read the nutrition labels of the foods you choose. If you eat meat, make sure it is lean. Discard the skin from poultry. Sauté vegetables in minimal oil or use broth, water, or cooking spray to cut down on fat.

- **Drink up.** A glass of sparkling mineral water, low sodium tomato juice, tea, or cup of broth-based soup before your meal may help you feel less hungry when your entrée is served. Also, all adults should aim for eight glasses of water or other nonalcoholic fluid daily.

• **Enjoy what you eat.** Eat slowly and savor every bite. Healthy eating can be delicious. And when you know you are eating for good health, you can feel true satisfaction after a meal.

• **Keep active to help burn calories** and stay healthy.

Flavor Your Foods

Americans consume more salt and high-sodium foods than is good for our health. You may be surprised to hear that most of the sodium in the American diet comes from processed foods such as soups, sauces, meats, frozen dinners, chips, and crackers. Foods with no salty taste may still be high in sodium. And for some people, too much sodium may worsen high blood pressure and increase the risk of stroke. Diets high in salted foods, and foods preserved in salt can increase the risk for stomach cancer—although this cancer is rare in the United States.

To cut down on salt, read food labels and look for low-sodium versions of your favorite processed foods. Also, think fresh. Fresh foods have less sodium than commercially canned or frozen foods. You can prepare your foods with less salt—avoid adding salt to cooking water and taste your food before salting. Flavor your foods with an abundance of fresh and fragrant herbs, spices, salsas, chutneys, and healthful sauces. Experiment in the kitchen. Invite friends over for a delicious, flavorful dinner.

Did you know the senses of taste and smell decline with age? Medications can also affect how food tastes. As the senses get duller, food can start to lose its flavor and appeal. Try these tips to give foods a boost:

• **Vary the texture and temperature of foods** at one meal. For instance, top smooth low-fat yogurt with crunchy cereal. Enjoy a cool fruit salad and sorbet following a hot and spicy Mexican burrito.

• **Use color to maximize eye appeal.** Add red and yellow pepper strips to a mixed green salad; sprinkle red paprika on white potatoes; create a rainbow fruit salad with red and green grapes, honeydew and cantaloupe chunks, strawberries, and blueberries.

274

- **Intensify the flavor.** Use seasonings, spices, and herbs instead of salt and fat for flavor. As an added bonus, herbs and spices contain health-protective phytochemicals. To start, use 3/4 teaspoon of fresh herbs (or 1/4 teaspoon dried) per serving, until you get a feel for the amount that suits your taste.

Choose Moderation when Drinking Alcohol

You may have read that moderate amounts of alcohol may help protect against heart disease. Drinking alcohol, however, can increase the risk of liver, mouth, and throat cancers as well as possibly breast and colon cancers. While reasonable amounts of alcohol may enhance the enjoyment of meals, drinking to excess can impair judgment, which can lead to accidents and injury. Alcohol can also interfere with the effectiveness of some medications.

It is important to weigh for yourself the risks and benefits of drinking alcohol. The American Institute for Cancer Research (AICR) recommends avoiding alcohol. If you decide to drink, limit alcoholic beverages to no more than two drinks a day for men, and one for women.

Supplement Your Diet Wisely

As your body ages, your nutritional needs change. For example, your body absorbs less vitamin B_{12} from the food you eat. Your skin's ability to produce vitamin D from sunlight also decreases. In addition, some studies show that more vitamin E may help reduce your risk of heart disease.

For these reasons, many health experts advise older people to take a 100% Recommended Daily Allowance (RDA) multivitamin and mineral supplement once a day. Basic supplementation can help prevent deficiencies caused by aging and may add extra protection against disease. Be sure to discuss any dietary supplement with your doctor first.

Taking more than a multivitamin, however, is not recommended. High doses of single vitamins and minerals can have adverse effects. Science indicates that these substances work in the body as a team. Too much of one can create an imbalance.

Whether you decide to take a supplement or not, it is still important to eat a wide variety of vegetables and fruits every day as part of a mostly plant-based diet. Vegetables and fruits contain vitamins, minerals, fiber, and phytochemicals that help protect your health and fight disease. While scientists are still discovering and learning about all the protective substances in vegetables and fruits, eating whole foods is a sure way to get them.

Did you know food, alcohol, and dietary supplements may interact with drugs, changing the effectiveness of the drug or the way nutrients are absorbed in your body?

Keep your doctor and pharmacist informed of all the over-the-counter and prescription drugs you take and any vitamin, mineral, or herbal supplements you are using. Ask about interactions between these substances and food or alcohol. Take medications only as directed and adhere to any warnings found on the label. If you're unable to read the drug name or understand the instructions on the label, ask for assistance or ask the pharmacist for a copy with larger size type.

Beware of interactions between common drugs and foods, including the following:

- Aspirin and ibuprofen should be taken with meals, since these drugs can irritate the stomach.

- Do not take the antibiotic tetracycline, or its derivatives (except doxycycline), at the same time as dairy foods or calcium supplements. The calcium in these products can block the absorption of the drug.

- Vitamin K can make the blood clot faster, so if you are on a blood-thinning medication, like Coumadin, avoid large amounts of foods that are high in vitamin K, such as kale, spinach, and other greens, parsley, broccoli, and brussel sprouts; eating small amounts of these foods is fine. Avoid alcohol if you use a blood thinning medication.

- If you are taking an antidepressant that functions as a monoamine oxidase (MAO) inhibitor such as isocarboxazid, phenelzine sulfate, or tranylcypromine, it is important that you avoid foods high in tyramine. Eating aged cheeses, sausages like salami, herring, liver, red wine, and beer could lead to a deadly change in blood pressure—ask your doctor for a complete list of foods to avoid and about the use of other alcoholic drinks.

- If you use gout medication such as allopurinol, it is important to drink at least 10 to 12 glasses of water a day and to avoid alcohol.

- Grapefruit juice (but not other citrus juices) changes the way the body processes some medications, including certain cholesterol-lowering drugs and blood pressure medications. If you like to drink grapefruit juice, check with your doctor about any possible reactions with prescription medications.

Store and Prepare Food Safely

With increased age comes an increased risk for food borne illness. This may be due to an aging immune system or an existing health problem. For some, poor eyesight and difficulty cleaning the kitchen may add to this risk.

Common Age-Related Health Questions

As we get older, many of us lead active, independent lives, while others are confronted with medical or lifestyle situations that make it harder to adopt healthy habits. Not all of us will face the same challenges. The questions and answers that follow may help you find solutions to some of yours—and help you take control of your health.

My mouth is sore and I'm having problems chewing. What should I do?

You may experience a sore mouth for many reasons, including gum disease, poor-fitting dentures, or soreness caused by a medication or medical treatment. Choose foods that have a soft or creamy texture. Here are some examples of nutritious foods that are easier to chew:

- baked or mashed sweet potatoes
- cooked vegetables or vegetable juice
- very ripe, canned, mashed or puréed fruit
- cooked pasta, couscous, barley, or hot cereal
- tofu, cooked or canned beans, low-fat refried beans or hummus
- yogurt, pudding, milk shakes, or soft low-fat cheese
- cooked and chopped lean meat, chicken, fish, scrambled eggs, peanut butter, or almond butter

These things are also good ideas:

- Visit your dentist and have your teeth checked. If you wear dentures, make sure they fit properly. Keep in mind that changes in your weight can affect the fit of your dentures.
- Drink fluids with meals to make chewing and swallowing easier.

I don't feel like eating. I've lost my appetite and I'm losing weight, which I don't need to do. Any suggestions?

There are many reasons for a loss of appetite, including illness, depression, pain, and some medications. Discuss your loss of appetite with your physician. Poor nutrition prevents proper healing and can bring on fatigue. If it causes you to become underweight, you also have a greater chance of suffering from falls or bone fractures.

To perk up your appetite, try these tips:

- Make mealtimes appealing. Choose foods with vibrant colors and pleasant aromas that permeate the room. Set an attractive table, even if you're the only one eating. Use a tablecloth or place mats and colorful dishes or napkins. Put flowers on the table, play soft music, and relax while you're eating.

- Stimulate your appetite with a pre-meal walk.

To help prevent weight loss, try these tips:

- Eat more frequent, smaller meals, about four to six a day.

- Eat regularly, at specific times of the day.

- Keep high-calorie foods on hand. Snack on crackers with peanut or almond butter, eat dried fruit, or enjoy a bagel or English muffin with fruit preserves or a tasty bean spread. Add grated cheese to pasta dishes or to a baked potato stuffed with veggies.

- Drink higher-calorie beverages like milk, juice, or fruit and yogurt shakes more often than coffee, tea, or diet sodas.

- Prepare hot cereal and soup with milk instead of water.

- Consider a commercial liquid supplement. Speak with your doctor or a registered dietitian for assistance in choosing a liquid supplement or other foods that can help you gain weight or prevent further weight loss. Also, check with your doctor about taking vitamin and mineral supplements. Keep in mind, however, that supplements are not a substitute for eating healthfully.

I've been constipated lately. What can I do?

There are several simple ways to relieve constipation:

- Eat plenty of fiber-rich foods, such as vegetables, fruits, whole grains, legumes, and bran cereal. If you're not used to eating high-fiber foods, add them slowly to your diet and drink extra water to avoid abdominal discomfort.

- Drink plenty of water. Fluids keep the fiber moving in your body and add bulk to stools, making elimination easier. Aim for at least 8 cups of water or other fluids a day.

- Keep active. It helps to keep your body regular.

- Do not make laxatives a habit. Heavy use of laxatives can make your body depend on them, which could eventually prevent your system from working on its own.

- If constipation is more than an occasional problem, speak with your doctor.

I have diverticulosis. What should I eat?

A low-fiber diet can lead to constipation and pressure in the colon, which causes pouches (diverticula) to form at weak spots. This condition is known as diverticulosis.

Eat a high-fiber diet full of vegetables, fruits, whole grains, and beans to control your condition or prevent diverticulosis altogether.

Until recently, many doctors suggested that people with diverticulosis avoid foods with small seeds, like tomatoes and berries. It was thought that particles could lodge in the pouches and cause inflammation. Research now questions the need for this restriction.

If the pouches become inflamed, diverticulitis occurs. Medical treatment is necessary to prevent complications from the abdominal pain and fever. During this time, often a liquid diet is needed. However, once the inflammation has cleared, you should eat a high-fiber diet again.

My arthritis is bothering me and I don't have the energy to cook as much as I used to. Do you have any ideas on preparing quick and easy meals for one?

Here are a few ideas for making easy meals in minutes:

- Do not do all of the work yourself. Pre-cut, frozen stir-fry vegetables; pre-cooked and pre-sliced chicken strips; and pre-washed, pre-cut salad greens can save you effort and energy in the kitchen. (Read labels to avoid products high in sodium.) Heat the vegetables with the meat or chicken strips and add low sodium soy sauce for an easy stir-fry. Or create a tasty chef's salad by topping the salad greens with chicken or meat and low-fat cheese and dressing. Enjoy with a whole grain roll.

279

- Make more than one serving of pasta or rice and save the extra for another day. Add cooked vegetables, canned beans, and a prepared low fat, low sodium pasta sauce for a nutritious one-dish meal.

- Add leftover vegetables and chicken or lean meat to reduced sodium canned soups. Have a whole wheat roll and low-fat milk or pudding to round out the meal.

- Make it easier on yourself to prepare a meal. Sit while you work. Make sure cooking utensils and equipment are easily accessible. Keep appliances on the counter and pots and pans on lower shelves.

- Cook a few dishes when you have the time and energy, and freeze in meal-size portions to reheat in a hurry.

- If cooking gets too difficult or you become too ill to leave your home, you may qualify for home-delivered meals. Call your local Office on Aging and ask about the Meals on Wheels program.

I don't like to eat by myself. How can I make up for missing meals?

Instead of missing meals, explore opportunities for making meal-times more social.

- Call a friend or relative and designate a specific day each week to go out to eat. If the restaurant portion is too large, split it with your companion, or take part of it home and refrigerate it promptly for tomorrow's lunch or dinner.

- Organize a monthly potluck dinner with some friends or neighbors. Ask everyone to bring a dish to share. To make it more interesting, have the dinner in a different person's home each month.

- Call your local senior center or Office on Aging to find out about community lunch programs for older adults. It is a great way to socialize and enjoy a nutritious meal.

I take my meals at the dining center of my adult residence community. How can I make healthy choices when I'm not the cook?

It is possible to eat very healthfully, even if you're not in charge of the cooking. Follow these tips for smart meal selection:

- Choose dishes that are plant-based. That means two-thirds or more of the plate is covered with vegetables, fruits, whole grains, and beans, and one-third or less is covered with meat, chicken, or fish. In general, mixed dishes such as pastas and stir-fries are mostly plant-based. If necessary, request that a special plate be made for you that has less meat and more plant-based foods.

- If offered soup, opt for selections with vegetables such as minestrone, vegetable noodle, or tomato.

- Always request a vegetable salad with your meal, if available.

- Ask for whole grain bread or rolls to accompany your meal.

- Select 100% fruit juice such as orange, grapefruit, cranberry, or prune juice for your beverage rather than a fruit drink or punch.

- Often, dessert selections include a fruit cup. On most days, pass up the cheesecake in favor of fruit. Or have a few bites of the cheesecake and save the fruit for a healthy snack later.

Additional Information

American Institute for Cancer Research
1759 R Street N.W.
Washington, DC 20009
Toll-Free: 800-843-8114
Phone: 202-328-7744
Fax: 202-328-7226
Website: http://www.aicr.org
E-mail: aicrweb@aicr.org

Administration on Aging
330 Independence Ave. S.W.
Washington, DC 20201
Toll-Free Eldercare Locator: 800-677-1116
Phone: 202-619-7501
Website: http://www.eldercare.gov
E-mail:
eldercarelocator@spherix.com

USDA Food and Nutrition Information Center
10301 Baltimore Ave.
Beltsville, MD 20750-2351
Phone: 301-504-5719
Fax: 301-504-6409
TTY: 301-504-6856
Website: http://www.nal.usda.gov/fnic
E-mail: fnic@nal.usda.gov

Section 27.2

Nutrition Tips for a Healthy Heart

This section includes: Excerpts from "How to Keep Your Heart Healthy," *FDA Consumer*, November-December 2003, U.S. Food and Drug Administration (FDA), Pub No. FDA 04–1333C rev., revised May 2004. And, "High Doses of Vitamin E Supplements Do More Harm Than Good," reproduced with permission from http://www.americanheart.org. © 2004 American Heart Association.

How to Keep Your Heart Healthy

One of the reasons that some people may shrug off the possibility of developing heart disease is that it is a gradual, lifelong process that people cannot see or feel. About the size of a fist, the heart muscle relies on oxygen and nutrients to continually pump blood through the circulatory system. In coronary artery disease, the most common type of heart disease, plaque builds up in the coronary arteries, the vessels that bring oxygen and nutrients to the heart muscle. As the walls of the arteries get clogged, the space through which blood flows narrows. This decreases or cuts off the supply of oxygen and nutrients, which can result in chest pain or a heart attack. Damage can result when the supply is cut off for more than a few minutes. It is called a heart attack when prolonged chest pain or symptoms (20 minutes or more) are associated with permanent damage to the heart muscle.

Every year, more than 1 million people have heart attacks, according to the National Heart, Lung, and Blood Institute (NHLBI). About 13 million Americans have coronary heart disease, and about half a million people die from it each year.

Take Charge of Your Health

Because of advances in medicine and technology, people with heart disease are living longer, more productive lives than ever before. But prevention is still the best weapon in the fight against heart disease. As with anything in life, there are no guarantees. You could do all the right things and still develop heart disease because there are so many factors involved. But by living a healthier life, you could delay heart disease for years or minimize its damage. Whether you are already healthy, are at high risk for heart disease, or have survived a heart attack, the advice to protect your heart is the same.

Get moving and maintain a healthy weight. Exercise improves heart function, lowers blood pressure and blood cholesterol, and boosts energy. Being overweight forces the heart to work harder.

The general recommendation from the NHLBI is to get at least 30 minutes of moderate physical activity on most, and preferably all, days of the week. You do not need to run a marathon or buy an expensive gym club membership to get the necessary exercise. The 30 minutes also do not have to be done all at once, but can be broken up into 10-minute intervals throughout your day.

Talk with your doctor about what form of exercise is best for you. Those with severe heart disease, for example, are advised against strenuous exercise.

Stick to a nutritious, well-balanced diet. This advice might make you groan if your usual lunch consists of cheeseburgers with french fries or pizza slices topped with sausage. But the good news is that diet is not an all-or-nothing affair.

A heart-healthy diet means a diet that is low in fat, cholesterol, and salt, and high in fruits, vegetables, grains, and fiber. "But it doesn't mean that you can never have pizza or ice cream again," Bolger says. You could start by telling yourself that you will eat a big leafy green salad first, and then you will have one slice of cheese pizza, not three slices with sausage. "Or if you must have a burger, don't get your usual order of french fries," Bolger suggests. "That alone cuts hundreds of calories."

Experts point out that a heart-healthy diet should be the routine. That way, when you have high-fat food every now and then, you're still on track. Making a high-fat diet the routine is asking for trouble.

Look at the Nutrition Facts label on the foods you buy for guidance. The general rule of thumb is that foods that provide 5 percent of the daily value (DV) of fat or less are low in fat, and foods that are labeled as providing 20 percent or more of the daily value are high in fat.

Control your blood pressure. About 50 million American adults have high blood pressure, also called hypertension. The top number of a blood pressure reading, called the systolic pressure, represents the force of blood in the arteries as the heart beats. The bottom number, called diastolic pressure, is the force of blood in the arteries as the heart relaxes between beats. High blood pressure makes the heart work extra hard and hardens artery walls, increasing the risk of heart disease and stroke. A blood pressure level of 140 over 90 mm Hg (millimeters of mercury) or higher is considered high. The NHLBI recently set a new pre-hypertension level of any reading above 120 over 80 mm Hg.

Poor eating habits and physical inactivity both contribute to high blood pressure. According to the NHLBI, table salt increases average levels of blood pressure, and this effect is greater in some people than in others. The National Institutes of Health's DASH diet (Dietary Approaches to Stop Hypertension) is rich in fruits, vegetables, and low-fat dairy foods, and low in total and saturated fat. The DASH diet also reduces red meat, sweets, and sugary drinks, and it is rich in potassium, calcium, magnesium, fiber, and protein.

It is important to keep on top of your blood pressure levels through regular doctor visits. High blood pressure disproportionately affects racial and ethnic minority groups, including blacks, Hispanics, and American Indians/Alaska Natives. The condition is known as a silent killer because there are no symptoms. If lifestyle changes alone do not bring your blood pressure within the normal range, medications may also be needed.

Control blood cholesterol. Cholesterol is a fat-like substance in the blood. High levels of triglycerides, another form of fat in the blood, can also indicate heart disease risk.

As with blood pressure, eating a low-fat, low-cholesterol diet and engaging in physical activity can lower cholesterol levels. Your body turns saturated fats into cholesterol. The higher your cholesterol level, the more likely it is that the substance will build up and stick to artery walls.

The only way to find out your cholesterol levels is to go to a doctor and have a blood test after fasting for nine to 12 hours. A lipoprotein profile will reveal your total cholesterol, which is measured in milligrams (mg) of cholesterol per deciliter (dL) of blood. Total cholesterol less than 200 mg/dL is desirable, 200–239 mg/dL is borderline high, and 240 mg/dL or more is high.

People ages 20 and older should have cholesterol measured at least once every five years. If lifestyle changes alone do not adequately budge cholesterol levels, medications may be needed.

Prevent and manage diabetes. About 17 million people in the United States have diabetes, and heart disease is the leading cause of death of those with the disease. According to the American Diabetes Association (ADA), 2 out of 3 people with diabetes die from heart disease or stroke.

Diabetes is a disease in which the body does not properly produce or use insulin. Insulin is a hormone needed to convert sugar, starches, and other nutrients into energy. Another 16 million Americans have pre-diabetes, a condition in which blood glucose levels are higher than normal, but not high enough to be diagnosed as diabetes. Genetics and lifestyle factors such as obesity and physical inactivity can lead to diabetes.

One in three people who have diabetes do not know they have it. See a doctor if you have any diabetes symptoms which include frequent urination, excessive thirst, extreme hunger, unusual weight loss, increased fatigue, irritability, and blurry vision.

The American Heart Association Reports That High Doses of Vitamin E Supplements Do More Harm Than Good

Reproduced with permission from http://www.americanheart.org. © 2004 American Heart Association.

Daily vitamin E doses of 400 international units (IU) or more can increase the risk of death and should be avoided, researchers reported at the American Heart Association's Scientific Sessions November 10, 2004.

In animal and observational studies, vitamin E supplementation was shown to prevent cardiovascular disease and cancer. However, other studies suggested that high doses could be harmful.

To determine if there is a dose response, researchers examined different doses of vitamin E supplements and risk of death from any cause. They studied death rates in published clinical trials comparing vitamin E supplementation to placebo and included findings from 14 studies, from 1993 to 2004. Doses ranged from 15 to 2000 IU/day, and average intake was about 400 IU a day.

"Increasing doses of vitamin E were linked to an increase in death," said lead author Edgar R. Miller, M.D., Ph.D., associate professor of medicine at Johns Hopkins University in Baltimore, Maryland.

According to the analysis, there is no increased risk of death with a dose of 200 IU per day or less, and there may even be some benefit. However, an increased risk was found at amounts above 200 IU per day and significant risk of death was found starting at 400 IU a day.

285

Those who take greater than 400 IU of vitamin E a day are about 10 percent more likely to die than those who do not, researchers said. "Many people who take vitamin E supplements take between 400 and 800 IU in a single capsule," said Miller.

The confusion for many, said Miller, is that some doctors have recommended vitamin E supplementation based on studies suggesting that it is beneficial for specific illnesses. One study in people with a history of prior heart attack showed that vitamin E use correlated with a lower risk of having a second event. In another trial, patients with end-stage kidney disease seemed to benefit. However, in both of these studies (in fact, in seven of the eight high-dose vitamin E trials in this analysis) the patients on vitamin E supplementation were more likely to die than those in the placebo group.

"Typically, we get about 6–10 IU per day of vitamin E in our diets. Vegetable oils, nuts, and green leafy vegetables are the main dietary sources of vitamin E. Supplementation can increase intake by 100-fold," said Miller. Researchers said the current U.S. dietary guidelines

Table 27.1. Heart Smart Substitutions

Instead of:	Do this:
whole or 2 percent milk and cream	use 1 percent or skim milk
fried foods	eat baked, steamed, boiled, broiled, or microwaved foods
lard, butter, palm and coconut oils	cook with unsaturated vegetable oils such as corn, olive, canola, safflower, sesame, soybean, sunflower, or peanut
fatty cuts of meat	eat lean cuts of meat or cut off the fatty parts
one whole egg in recipes	use two egg whites
sauces, butter, and salt	season vegetables with herbs and spices
regular hard and processed cheeses	eat low-fat, low-sodium cheeses
salted potato chips	choose low-fat, unsalted tortilla and potato chips, unsalted pretzels and popcorn
sour cream and mayonnaise	use plain low-fat yogurt, low-fat cottage cheese, or low-fat or light sour cream

do not recommend vitamin E supplementation, but indicate that the upper tolerable limit of intake is 1000 IU per day.

These findings parallel the findings of beta-carotene supplementation trials. Two major studies showed that beta-carotene supplementation results in an increased risk for lung cancer and death. And, as a result, "you will never see beta-carotene supplements recommended again," he said.

There is room for more research, however, on the effects of 200 IU or less per day of vitamin E and how low doses taken in combination with other vitamins might positively affect death rates, he said. "The big questions that need to be answered are: What is the dose? And how low a dose—in what combination—would be most useful?" Miller said.

Additional Information

American Heart Association
7272 Greenville Ave.
Dallas, TX 75231
Toll-Free: 800-AHA-USA-1 (242-8721)
Website: http://www.americanheart.org

National Heart, Lung, and Blood Institute
P.O. Box 30105
Bethesda, MD 20824-0105
Toll-Free: 800-575-WELL (575-9355)
Phone: 301-592-8573
Fax: 301-592-8563
TTY: 240-629-3255
Website: http://www.nhlbi.nih.gov/health/hearttruth
E-mail: nhlbiinfo@nhlbi.nih.gov

Section 27.3

Importance of Water Consumption

Excerpts from "More Than One in Three Older Americans May
Not Drink Enough Water," *Nutrition Insight 27*, September 2002,
U.S. Department of Agriculture (USDA).

Whether drunk from the tap or a bottle or eaten in foods, water
has important health benefits. Insufficient consumption can lead to
muscle spasm, renal dysfunction, increased risk of bladder cancer, and
even death.

Importance of Water Consumption

Water is the most abundant and essential component or macronutrient in the human body. It comprises, on average, about 60% of total body weight for young adults and about 50% for the elderly. Various
body components account for different percentages of the body's water content; generally, water constitutes 65% to 75% of muscle weight
and 50% of body fat weight. The proportion of body water is generally smaller in females, the elderly, and the obese because of the
smaller portion of muscle mass in these populations.

The human body cannot store water; therefore, fluid must be replaced and kept in balance daily. Body water turnover rate is estimated
to be 4% of total body weight to maintain normal body functions, which
include excretion of body waste and evaporation from the lungs and
skin. Recommendations for adequate water intake by adults are generally based upon several factors: humidity, temperature, altitude,
exercise status, and use of diuretic medications.

Dehydration in the Elderly

Dehydration occurs when water balance is negative; that is, intake
of water is less than its loss. This issue is especially pertinent to older
adults when total available body water has decreased because of losses
in muscle mass, changes in the cells as people age, less efficient kidney function, and reduced thirst sensation. Thirst is usually the most

important mechanism used to increase water consumption. When the volume of body water decreases, thirst signals the brain and triggers the person to consume fluids. Older adults, compared with other segments of the population, have impaired responses to reduced body water; thus, they are most vulnerable to dehydration.

Recommendations for Water Intake

For adults whose energy expenditure and environmental exposure are average, the Food and Nutrition Board recommends 1 ml of water per kilocalorie expenditure (or, at 237 ml per eight fluid ounces, 4.2 glasses per 1,000 kilocalories) as a general guideline for total water consumption. Chernoff recommends a total fluid intake of 30 ml/kg body weight (or 0.06 glasses per pound of body weight) and with a minimum of 1,500 ml (6.3 glasses) per day. This criterion was used to assess the adequacy of water intake by the elderly U.S. population.

Conclusion

Based on the analysis data and the particular criterion used, more than one in three Americans over the age of 60 may not be consuming enough total water from all sources.

In addition to drinking plenty of plain water every day, eating foods with a high moisture content—such as fruits and vegetables—could be a good way to increase total water consumption. Water constitutes 90% of most fruits and vegetables and about 50% of meats and cheese.

Valtin suggests that caffeinated drinks (e.g., coffee and soft drinks) and alcoholic beverages may also count towards daily consumption of fluid. However, because of the diuretic effects of these types of beverages, additional plain water should be consumed to replace the water that is lost.

Further investigation of the recommendation for optimal water consumption by older adults should focus on different physiological needs. For example: Living arrangements, physical activity, and medications can affect water consumption and physiological needs. In addition, intakes of electrolytes can also affect the hydration status of a person.

Section 27.4

Checklist to Determine Nutritional Health

"Determine Your Nutritional Health," developed in 2003 and distributed by the Nutrition Screening Initiative, a project of: American Academy of Family Physicians, The American Dietetic Association, and The National Council on the Aging, Inc. The Nutrition Screening Initiative is funded in part by a grant from Ross Products Division of Abbott Laboratories, Inc. Reprinted with permission.

The Nutrition Checklist is based on the following warning signs. Use the word "determine" to remind you of the warning signs.

Disease

Any disease, illness, or chronic condition which causes you to change the way you eat, or makes it hard for you to eat, puts your nutritional health at risk. Four out of five adults have chronic diseases that are affected by diet. Confusion or memory loss that keeps getting worse is estimated to affect one out of five or more of older adults. This can make it hard to remember what, when, or if you've eaten. Feeling sad or depressed, which happens to about one in eight older adults, can cause big changes in appetite, digestion, energy level, weight, and well-being.

Eating Poorly

Eating too little and eating too much both lead to poor health. Eating the same foods day after day or not eating fruit, vegetables, and milk products daily will also cause poor nutritional health. One in five adults skip meals daily. Only 13% of adults eat the minimum amount of fruit and vegetables needed. One in four older adults drink too much alcohol. Many health problems become worse if you drink more than one or two alcoholic beverages per day.

Tooth Loss and/or Mouth Pain

A healthy mouth, teeth, and gums are needed to eat. Missing, loose, or rotten teeth or dentures which don't fit well or cause mouth sores make it hard to eat.

Economic Hardship

As many as 40% of older Americans have incomes of less than $6,000 per year. Having less, or choosing to spend less, than $25–30 per week for food makes it very hard to get the foods you need to stay healthy.

Reduced Social Contact

One-third of all older people live alone. Being with people daily has a positive effect on morale, well-being, and eating.

Multiple Medicines

Many older Americans must take medicines for health problems. Almost half of older Americans take multiple medicines daily. Growing old may change the way we respond to drugs. The more medicines you take, the greater the chance for side effects such as in increased or decreased appetite, change in taste, constipation, weakness, drowsiness, diarrhea, nausea, and others. Vitamins or minerals when taken in large doses act like drugs and can cause harm. Alert your doctor to everything you take.

Involuntary Weight Loss or Gain

Losing or gaining a lot of weight when you are not trying to do so is an important warning sign that must not be ignored. Being overweight or underweight also increases your chance of poor health.

Needs Assistance in Self Care

Although most older people are able to eat, one of every five have trouble walking, shopping, buying, and cooking food, especially as they get older.

Elder Years above Age 80

Most older people lead full and productive lives. But as age increases, risk of frailty and health problems increase. Checking your nutritional health regularly makes good sense.

Part Four

Lifestyle and Nutrition

Chapter 28

The Healthy Eating Index: Dietary Patterns of Americans

Healthful eating is essential for development and well-being. In the United States today, some dietary patterns are associated with 4 of the 10 leading causes of death (coronary heart disease, certain types of cancer, stroke, and type 2 diabetes) (U.S. Department of Health and Human Services [DHHS], 2000). A healthful diet, however, can reduce major risk factors for chronic diseases such as obesity, high blood pressure, and high blood cholesterol (USDA and DHHS, 2000). Studies have shown an increase in mortality associated with overweight and obesity resulting from poor eating habits (DHHS, 2001). Major improvements in the health of the American public can, therefore, be made by improving people's dietary patterns.

To assess the dietary status of Americans and monitor changes in these patterns, the U.S. Department of Agriculture's (USDA) Center for Nutrition Policy and Promotion (CNPP) developed the Healthy Eating Index (HEI). CNPP's HEI has been computed with 1989–90 and with 1994–96 data. The HEI is a summary measure of the overall quality of people's diets (broadly defined in terms of adequacy, moderation, and variety).

This chapter presents information from the HEI for 1999–2000. The HEI is calculated for the general population and selected subgroups. A comparison of the 1999–2000 HEI with the HEI of earlier years examines possible trends in the diets of Americans. The Healthy

Excerpted from "The Healthy Eating Index: 1999–2000," U.S. Department of Agriculture, December 2002.

295

Eating Index measures overall diet quality, but does not necessarily reflect over-consumption.

Data used are from the Federal Government's 1999–2000 National Health and Nutrition Examination Survey, which is nationally representative and contains information on people's consumption of foods and nutrients.

Overall HEI Score

The mean HEI score for the U.S. population was 63.8 for 1999–2000. During 1999–2000, most people's (74 percent) diets needed improvement. Ten percent of the population had a good diet, and 16 percent had a poor diet.

Components of the Healthy Eating Index

The Healthy Eating Index score is the sum of 10 components, each representing different aspects of a healthful diet:

- **Components 1–5** measure the degree to which a person's diet conforms to serving recommendations for the five major food groups of the Food Guide Pyramid: grains (bread, cereal, rice, and pasta), vegetables, fruits, milk (milk, yogurt, and cheese), and meat (meat, poultry, fish, dry beans, eggs, and nuts).

- **Component 6** measures total fat consumption as a percentage of total food energy (calorie) intake.

- **Component 7** measures saturated fat consumption as a percentage of total food energy intake.

- **Component 8** measures total cholesterol intake.

- **Component 9** measures total sodium intake.

- **Component 10** examines variety in a person's diet.

Table 28.1. Healthy Eating Index Rating, U.S. Population, 1999–2000

Diet Classification	HEI Score	Percent of U.S. Population
Good	Greater than 80	10%
Needs improvement	51–79	74%
Poor	Less than 51	16%

Each component of the Index has a maximum score of 10 and a minimum score of zero. Intermediate scores were computed proportionately. The maximum overall score for the 10 components combined is 100. High component scores indicate intakes close to recommended ranges or amounts; low component scores indicate less compliance with recommended ranges or amounts. An HEI score over 80 implies a good diet, an HEI score between 51 and 80 implies a diet that needs improvement, and an HEI score less than 51 implies a poor diet.

The fruits component of the HEI had the lowest mean score for the U.S. population (3.8); the milk component, the second lowest score (5.9). For the other HEI components, average scores were generally between 6 and 6.7. Overall, 69 percent of people had a maximum score of 10 for cholesterol—that is, they met the dietary recommendation, and 55 percent had a maximum score for variety. For the other HEI components, only 17 to 41 percent of the population met the dietary recommendations on a given day.

HEI Scores of Selected Segments of the Population

HEI scores varied by demographic and socioeconomic characteristics of the U.S. population. (The results discussed here are statistically significant.) During 1999–2000:

- Females had a slightly higher HEI score than did males (64.5 vs. 63.2).

Table 28.2. HEI Component Scores 1999–2000 on a Scale of Zero to Ten

Component	Mean Score
Cholesterol	7.7
Variety	7.7
Total fat	6.9
Grains	6.7
Meat	6.6
Saturated Fat	6.5
Vegetables	6.0
Sodium	6.0
Milk	5.9
Fruits	3.8

- Children age 2 to 3 had the highest average HEI score (75.7) among all age/gender groups.

- As children aged, their HEI scores declined.

- Non-Hispanic Whites had a higher average HEI score than did non-Hispanic Blacks (64.2 vs. 61.1).

- Native-born Americans had a lower HEI score than did members of the U.S. population born in Mexico or other countries (63.5 vs. 66 and 65.7).

HEI scores generally increased as the level of education and income increased. For example, people with household income below the poverty threshold had an average HEI score of 61.7. By comparison, people with household income over 184 percent of the poverty threshold had an average HEI score of 65. However, regardless of selected characteristics, the average HEI score indicated that people's diets needed improvement.

Trends in the HEI

The diets of Americans have slightly improved from 1989 to 1999–2000 but have not changed since 1996. In 1989, the HEI score for all people 2 years old and over was 61.5, compared with 63.8 in 1996 and 1999–2000. Saturated fat and variety scores increased steadily while sodium scores decreased steadily over the three periods. These findings provide a better understanding of the types of dietary changes needed to improve people's eating patterns.

Additional Information

USDA Food and Nutrition Information Center
10301 Baltimore Ave.
Beltsville, MD 20750-2351
Phone: 301-504-5719
Fax: 301-504-6409
TTY: 301-504-6856
Website: http://www.nal.usda.gov/fnic
E-mail: fnic@nal.usda.gov

The full report, *Healthy Eating Index: 1999–2000* can be viewed at http://www.usda.gov/cnpp/Pubs/HEI/HEI99-00report.pdf

Chapter 29

The New American Plate: Transition Your Meals for Better Health

Proportion: What's on the New American Plate?

When thinking about the New American Plate, use this general rule of thumb: Plant foods like vegetables, fruits, whole grains, and beans should cover two-thirds (or more) of the plate. Fish, poultry, meat, or low-fat dairy should cover one-third (or less) of the plate. The plant foods on the plate should include one or more vegetables or fruits in addition to whole grain products like brown rice, kasha, whole wheat bread, or pasta.

Plenty of Vegetables and Fruits

We should all make sure to eat at least five servings of vegetables and fruits each day. Research suggests that this one change in eating habits could prevent at least 20 percent of all cancers. Vegetables and fruits provide vitamins, minerals, and phytochemicals (natural substances found only in plants) that protect the body's cells from damage by cancer-causing agents. They can stop cancer before it even starts. A number of phytochemicals may also interfere with cancer cell growth.

By including fruits or vegetables at every meal, it is easy to reach five—or even more—servings a day. (Remember, a standard serving of vegetables or fruit is usually only 1/2 cup.) It is also important to eat a variety of these healthful foods. That way, you get the widest possible array of protective nutrients and phytochemicals. Be sure to include vegetables that are dark green and leafy, as well as those deep orange in color. Also include citrus fruits and other foods high in vitamin C. Juice does count toward your "five or more" goal, but most of your servings should come from solid fruits and vegetables.

Other Plant-Based Foods

In addition to fruits and vegetables, the American Institute on Cancer Research (AICR) recommends eating at least seven servings of other plant-based foods each day. This includes whole grains such as brown rice, barley, quinoa, whole grain breakfast cereal, oatmeal, whole wheat bread, and legumes (peas and dried beans, including lentils, kidney, garbanzo, and black beans).

Make sure to include whole grains in your meal choices each day. They are higher in fiber and phytochemicals than refined grains like white bread and white rice.

The Second Reason for Eating Plant-Based Foods

One reason, then, for increasing the proportion of vegetables, fruits, whole grains, and beans on your plate is to help reduce risk of cancer and other chronic diseases. A second reason is that substituting plant-based foods for foods rich in fat will help you manage your weight. Most plant foods contain a lot of fiber and water. They fill you up and make you feel satisfied. They are also low in calories. So when you've stopped eating, you've consumed fewer calories than if you had eaten fatty foods.

So eating fruits, vegetables, whole grains, and beans means a full stomach on fewer calories. That makes it an important tool for managing your weight as well as reducing cancer risk. That is a happy coincidence, because any plan you adopt to manage your weight should also help reduce risk of chronic disease. Getting thin and dying young needn't go hand in hand.

Meat on the Side

If you eat red meat like beef, pork, or lamb, choose lean cuts and limit yourself to no more than 3 ounces cooked (4 ounces raw) per day. That is about the size of a deck of cards. Findings from AICR's expert report show that diets high in red meat probably increase the risk of colon cancer.

Research on the impact of poultry, fish, and game is not as extensive, so no specific limits have been set. Just keep portions small enough that you have room to eat an abundance of vegetables, fruits, whole grains, and beans.

Reverse the traditional American plate, and think of meat as a side dish or condiment rather than the main ingredient. It can be as simple as preparing your favorite, store-bought brown rice or grain mix and topping it with steamed green beans, carrots, yellow squash, and an ounce or two of cooked chicken.

Making the Transition

When adjusting your meals to include more plant-based foods, even the smallest change can provide real health benefits. Every new vegetable, fruit, whole grain, or bean that finds its way onto your plate contributes disease-fighting power. And all the fat and calories you save may make a real difference on your waistline.

Many other benefits come from increasing the amount of plant-based foods on your plate. Learning about new foods, tasting new flavors, trying new recipes—the New American Plate allows you to enjoy an endless combination of nutritious foods that leave you well satisfied.

As you make the transition toward the New American Plate, it helps to evaluate your current eating habits. Just how close is the plate in front of you to a New American Plate? Take a look at the following examples.

Three Strategies for Weight Loss

1. Eat a greater proportion of plant foods.

2. Watch the size of your portions.

3. Keep physically active.

Stage 1: The Old American Plate

The typical American meal is heavy on meat, fish, or poultry. Fully half of the plate is loaded down with a huge (8–12 oz.) steak. The remainder is filled with a hearty helping of buttery mashed potatoes and peas. Although this meal is a home style favorite, it is high in fat and calories and low in phytochemicals and fiber. A few changes, however, will bring it closer to the New American Plate.

Stage 2: A Transitional Plate

This meal features a more moderate (4–6 oz.) serving of meat. A large helping of green beans prepared with your favorite herbs and the addition of a filling whole grain (seasoned brown rice) increases the proportion of nutritious, plant-based foods. This plate is on the right track, but does not yet take advantage of all the good-tasting foods the New American Plate has to offer.

Stage 3: A Better Plate

A modest 3-ounce serving of meat (fish, poultry, or red meat) fits AICR's guideline for cancer prevention. This better plate also features a wider variety of foods, resulting in a diverse assortment of cancer-fighting nutrients. Two kinds of vegetables help increase the proportion of plant-based foods. A healthy serving of a tasty whole grain (brown rice, barley, kasha, bulgur, millet, or quinoa) completes the meal.

Stage 4: The New American Plate

In a one-pot meal such as stir fry, you can reduce the animal food and increase the plant-based ingredients without even noticing the difference. This New American Plate is bursting with colorful vegetables, hearty whole grains, and cancer-fighting vitamins, minerals, and phytochemicals. Fish, poultry, or red meat is used as a condiment, adding a bit of flavor and substance to the meal. Plates like this include the delicious possibilities—the new tastes, colors, and textures—that can be found on the New American Plate.

Additional Information

American Institute for Cancer Research
1759 R Street N.W.
Washington, DC 20009
Toll-Free: 800-843-8114
Phone: 202-328-7744
Fax: 202-328-7226
Website: http://www.aicr.org
E-mail: aicrweb@aicr.org

Chapter 30

Healthy Eating Alone

Food tastes better when there is someone sitting across the table. A good part of the pleasure of eating comes from enjoying others' company during a meal.

People living alone often neglect to eat nutritious meals because there is less incentive to cook. Those who eat alone often select diets that are below par in recommended nutrients. They may graze through the day, or indulge at one meal and skip others because they have no one to eat with.

To make the most of eating alone, try the following ideas.

- **The eyes have it:** Add pizazz to dining by dressing up the table with a placemat, flowers, candles, and other special touches to remind you that eating can be a pleasant, leisurely experience. Eat colorful meals. A plate containing several colors looks more appetizing. Sliced red tomatoes, green peas, and orange carrot sticks with browned meat makes a more appealing meal than white or brown foods.

- **Texture tips:** Eat crispy or shredded low-sugar cereals in yogurt for breakfast. Include different textures within the same meal— soft, chewy, crisp, and firm. Adapt the textures to chewing ability. Even those who need a softer diet can try soft vegetables or fruits.

"Healthy Eating Alone" by Laurel L. Kubin, August 2004, is reprinted with permission from Colorado State University Cooperative Extension, http://www .ext.colostate.edu. © 2004 Colorado State University Cooperative Extension.

- **Enjoy companionship:** Those who live alone can invite a friend over for dinner, eat out once a week with friends, plan lunches with others, or visit a senior center at lunchtime. Prepare a new recipe each week and invite friends over for a tasting party or potluck meal. When dining out alone, choose restaurants that serve family style with large groups of customers seated at the same table. You may end up with good company.

- **Convenience counts:** Buy prepackaged mixed salad greens and salad bar vegetables, especially green peppers, spinach, broccoli, carrots, and tomatoes. Salads made with these are great sources of vitamins A and C. Add salad bar vegetables to stir-fry meals. Combine a prepackaged frozen entree with fresh or frozen vegetables and fresh fruits. Watch the entree label for sodium and fat content. When you cook, make a large batch of food and freeze leftovers in small portions for later.

- **Breakfast bonus:** Even if you are in a hurry or do not feel hungry, take time for breakfast. Spread a thin layer of peanut butter on whole wheat toast and add sliced fruit. Eat near a window and watch the sunrise or birds in the trees. Use your best dishes and feel special.

Chapter 31

Family Meals

Good nutrition and a balanced diet will help your child grow up healthy. Whether your kid is a toddler or a teen, you can take steps to improve nutrition and encourage smart eating habits. Five of the best strategies are:

1. Have regular family meals.
2. Serve a variety of healthy foods and snacks.
3. Be a role model by eating healthy yourself.
4. Avoid battles over food.
5. Involve kids in the process.

But it's not easy to take these steps when everyone is juggling busy schedules and convenience food, such as fast food, is so readily available. Here are some suggestions to help you incorporate all five strategies into your routine.

Family Meals

Family meals are a comforting ritual for both parents and kids. Children like the predictability of family meals and parents get a

This information was provided by KidsHealth, one of the largest resources online for medically reviewed health information written for parents, kids, and teens. For more articles like this one, visit www.KidsHealth.org, or www.Teens Health.org. © 2004 The Nemours Center for Children's Health Media, a division of The Nemours Foundation.

chance to catch up with their kids. Kids who take part in regular family meals are also:

- more likely to eat fruits, vegetables, and grains;
- less likely to snack on unhealthy foods;
- less likely to smoke, use marijuana, or drink alcohol.

In addition, family meals offer the chance to introduce your child to new foods and find out which foods your child likes and which ones he or she doesn't like.

Teens may turn up their noses at the prospect of a family meal—not surprising because they're trying to establish independence. Yet studies find that teens still want their parents' advice and counsel, so use mealtime as a chance to reconnect. Also, consider trying these strategies:

- Allow your teen to invite a friend to dinner.
- Involve your teen in meal planning and preparation.
- Keep mealtime calm and congenial—no lectures or arguing.

What counts as a family meal? Any time you and your family eat together—whether it's takeout food or a home-cooked meal with all the trimmings. Strive for nutritious food and a time when everyone can be there. This may mean eating dinner a little later to accommodate a child who is at sports practice. It can also mean setting aside time on the weekends, such as Sunday brunch, when it may be more convenient to gather as a group.

Stocking Up on Healthy Foods

Kids, especially younger ones, will eat mostly what's available at home. That's why it's important to control the supply lines—the foods that you serve for meals and have on hand for snacks. Follow these basic guidelines:

- **Work fruits and vegetables into the daily routine**, aiming for the goal of 5 servings a day.

- **Make it easy for your child to choose healthy snacks** by keeping fruits and vegetables on hand and ready to eat. Other good snacks include yogurt, peanut butter and celery, or whole grain crackers and cheese.

- **Serve lean meats and other good sources of protein**, such as eggs and nuts.

- **Choose whole grain breads and cereals** so your child gets more fiber.

- **Limit fat intake** by avoiding deep-fried foods and choosing healthier cooking methods, such as broiling, grilling, roasting, and steaming.

- **Limit fast food and other low-nutrient snacks**, such as chips and candy. But don't completely ban favorite snacks from your home. Instead, make them "once-in-a-while" foods, so your child doesn't feel deprived.

- **Limit sugary drinks**, such as soda and fruit-flavored drinks. Serve water and milk instead.

By drinking milk, kids also boost their intake of calcium, which is important for healthy bones. That means 800 milligrams (mg) a day for kids ages 6 to 8, and 1,300 mg a day after age 9. To reach the 1,300 mg goal, your child could have:

- 1 cup (237 milliliters) of milk (300 mg of calcium);

- 1 cup (237 milliliters) of calcium-fortified orange juice (300 mg of calcium);

- 2 ounces (57 grams) of cheese (300 mg of calcium);

- 1 cup (237 milliliters) of yogurt (315 mg of calcium);

- ½ cup (118 milliliters) of cooked white beans (120 mg of calcium).

How to Be a Role Model

The best way for you to encourage healthy eating is to eat well yourself. Kids will follow the lead of the adults they see every day. By eating fruits and vegetables and not overindulging in the less nutritious stuff, you'll be sending the right message.

Another way you can be a good role model is by limiting portions and not overeating. Talk about your feelings of fullness, especially with younger children. You might say, "This is delicious, but I'm full, so I'm going to stop eating." At the same time, parents who are always dieting or complaining about their bodies may foster these same negative feelings in children. Try to keep a positive approach when it comes to food.

307

Don't Battle over Food

It's easy for food to become a source of conflict. Well-intentioned parents might find themselves bargaining or bribing kids so they eat the healthy food in front of them. A better strategy is to give kids some control, but to also limit the kind of foods available at home.

Kids should decide if they're hungry, what they will eat from the foods served, and when they're full. Parents control which foods are available to the child, both at mealtime and between meals. Here are some guidelines to follow:

- **Establish a predictable schedule of meals and snacks**. Kids like knowing what to expect.

- **Don't force kids to clean their plates**. Doing so teaches kids to override feelings of fullness.

- **Don't bribe or reward kids with food**. Avoid using dessert as the prize for eating the meal.

- **Don't use food as a way of showing love**. When you want to show love, give them a hug, some of your time, or praise.

Get Kids Involved

Most kids will enjoy making the decision about what to make for dinner. Talk to them about making choices and planning a balanced meal. Some children may even want to help shop for ingredients and prepare the meal. At the store, help your child look at food labels to begin understanding nutritional values.

In the kitchen, select age-appropriate tasks so your child can play a part without getting injured or feeling overwhelmed. And at the end of the meal, don't forget to praise the chef.

School lunches can be another learning lesson for kids. More importantly, if you can get them thinking about what they eat for lunch, you may be able to help them make positive changes. A good place to start may be at the grocery store, where you can shop together for healthy, packable foods.

There's another important reason why kids should be involved: It can help prepare them to make good decisions on their own about the foods they want to eat. That's not to say that your child will suddenly want a salad instead of french fries, but the mealtime habits you help create now can lead to a lifetime of healthier choices.

Chapter 32

Vegetarianism

Definition

A vegetarian diet is one that excludes all or most animal products, particularly a diet that excludes any food that requires the death of an animal. There are many variations, including the following:

- **Vegan:** Diet consists of only foods of plant origin.

- **Lacto-vegetarian:** Diet consists of plant foods plus some or all dairy products.

- **Lacto-ovovegetarian:** Diet consists of plant foods, dairy products, and eggs.

- **Semi- or partial vegetarian:** Diet consists of plant foods and may include chicken or fish, dairy products, and eggs. Excludes red meat.

Function

A vegetarian diet may be adopted for a variety of reasons, including religious, moral or political beliefs, economics, or the desire to consume a more healthful diet.

The American Dietetic Association states that a well-planned vegetarian diet can be consistent with good nutritional intake. Dietary recommendations vary with the type of vegetarian diet.

For children and adolescents these diets require special planning, because it may be difficult to obtain all the nutrients required for growth and development. Nutrients that may be lacking in a vegetarian's diet are protein, vitamin B_{12}, vitamin D, riboflavin, calcium, zinc, and iron.

Eating protein, which is made up of smaller chemicals called amino acids, is necessary for good health. There are two types of proteins: complete and incomplete. Complete proteins contain adequate amounts of the essential amino acids needed for health and are found in animal products such as meats, milk, fish, and eggs.

Incomplete proteins contain all of the essential amino acids, but not in adequate amounts. These proteins generally have one amino acid in insufficient quantity, referred to as the limiting amino acid. Grains and beans are sources of incomplete proteins.

You do not have to eat animal products to get complete proteins in your diet. You can mix two incomplete proteins or an incomplete protein with a complete protein to get all the essential amino acids in adequate amounts. Some combinations are milk and cereal, peanut butter and bread, beans and rice, beans and corn tortillas, and macaroni and cheese.

Integrating the vegetarian style of eating into a non-vegetarian diet is recommended for individuals wishing to choose a healthier diet. For example, a person may choose to simply eat meat less frequently.

Recommendations

Vegetarian diets that include some animal products (lacto-vegetarian and lacto-ovovegetarian) are nutritionally sound. Vegan diets require careful planning in order to obtain adequate amounts of required nutrients. The following are recommendations for feeding vegetarian children.

- Breast milk or formula should be the basis of the diet until one year of age.

- Milk or a fortified soy formula should be used.

- Fat should not be limited for a child less than two years of age.

- For children not drinking milk or a fortified substitute, the following nutrients may be limited: calcium, protein, vitamin D, riboflavin. These children may need a vitamin and mineral supplement.

- Vitamin B_{12} must be supplemented if no animal products are consumed.

- Adequate iron intake is difficult to achieve if meat is not consumed. Good sources of iron include prunes and prune juice, fortified cereals and grain products, raisins, and spinach.

Note: Any specialized diet, particularly for children but also for adults, should be reviewed by a registered dietitian prior to the start of the diet to ensure that it meets all nutritional needs.

Chapter 33

Eating Well while Eating Out

You know the importance of eating well, but how are you supposed to do so when your schedule is so demanding that you're hardly ever at home? Read this chapter to find out how people make healthy food choices while eating out.

If I Eat Well at Home, What's Wrong with Splurging when I Eat Out?

A slice of pizza once in a while won't do you any harm, but if pizza (or any fast food) is all you eat, that can lead to problems. The most obvious health threat of eating too much fast food is weight gain—or even obesity. Teens are more at risk than ever of developing type 2 diabetes, a disease that's linked to being overweight and used to affect only adults. But weight gain isn't the only problem. Too much fast food can drag a person's body down in other ways. Because the food we eat affects all aspects of how the body functions, eating the right (or wrong) foods can influence any number of things, including:

- mental functioning;
- emotional well-being;

This information was provided by TeensHealth, one of the largest resources online for medically reviewed health information written for parents, kids, and teens. For more articles like this one, visit www.TeensHealth.org, or www.Kids Health.org. © 2004 The Nemours Center for Children's Health Media, a division of The Nemours Foundation

- energy;
- strength;
- weight;
- future health.

According to the U.S. Food and Drug Administration (FDA), what's important is a person's average food intake over a few days—not just in a single meal. So if you eat a meal consisting of only junk food, try to balance it with healthier foods the rest of that day and the next.

One thing you may want to watch out for when eating out (or even in) is your soda consumption. Colas and other sodas not only contain a lot of sugar, which can cause you to gain weight, they can also interfere with a person's calcium absorption. Because even the sugar-free versions can cause this problem, it's best to limit soda intake.

Eating on the Go

Eating at a fast food restaurant, the mall, or even the cafeteria may not sound healthy. But it's actually easier than you think to make good choices in these kinds of situations. Cafeterias and fast food places now offer healthy choices that are also tasty, like grilled chicken salads. There are two pointers to remember that can help you make wise choices when eating out:

- Our bodies (and our taste buds) need variety. Look for meals that contain a balance of lean proteins (like fish, chicken, or beans if you're a vegetarian), fruits and vegetables (fries and potato chips don't qualify as veggies), and complex carbohydrates like whole grain breads. That's why a turkey sandwich on whole wheat (with fixings) is a better choice than a burger on a white bun.

- Watch your portion sizes. The portion sizes of American foods have increased over the past few decades so that we are now eating way more than we need. The average size of a hamburger in the 1950s was just 1.5 ounces, compared to our supersize version weighing in at 8 ounces today.

The Food Guide Pyramid can help guide you in building a variety of foods into your daily diet. It also helps you learn what constitutes a healthy portion size of different foods.

Here are some more suggestions to keep in mind when you're eating away from home.

At a Restaurant

Most restaurant portions are way larger than the average serving of food. Ask for half portions, share an entrée with a friend, or take half of your dish home. Here are some other restaurant survival tips:

- Ask for sauces and salad dressings on the side and use them sparingly.

- Use salsa and mustard instead of mayonnaise or oil.

- Ask for olive or canola oil instead of butter, margarine, or shortening.

- Use nonfat or low-fat milk instead of whole milk or cream.

- Order baked, broiled, or grilled (not fried) lean meats including turkey, chicken, seafood, or sirloin steak.

- Salads and vegetables make healthier side dishes than french fries. Use a small amount of sour cream instead of butter if you order a baked potato.

- Choose fresh fruit instead of sugary, high-fat desserts.

At the Mall or Fast Food Place

It's tempting to pig out while shopping, but with a little planning, it's easy to eat healthy foods at the mall. Here are some choices:

- single slice of veggie pizza

- grilled, not fried, sandwiches (for example, a grilled chicken breast sandwich)

- small hamburger

- bean burrito

- baked potato

- side salad

- frozen yogurt

Resist the temptation to supersize your meals. This can add up to 25% more fat and calories. The American Dietetic Association also recommends that when you have a craving for something unhealthy, try sharing the food you crave with a friend.

In the School Cafeteria

The suggestions for eating in a restaurant and at the mall apply to cafeteria food as well. Add vegetables and fruit whenever possible, and opt for leaner, lighter items. Go easy on the high-fat, low-nutrition items, such as mayonnaise, fried foods, and heavy salad dressings.

You might want to consider packing your own lunch occasionally. Here are some lunch items that pack a healthy punch:

- sandwiches with lean meats or fish, like turkey, chicken, tuna (made with low-fat mayo), lean ham, or lean roast beef. For variety, try other sources of protein, like peanut butter, hummus, or meatless chili.

- low-fat or nonfat milk, yogurt, or cheese

- any fruit that's in season

- raw baby carrots, green and red pepper strips, tomatoes, or vegetable juice

- whole grain breads, pita, bagels, or crackers

It can be easy to achieve a healthy diet, even on the run. If you develop the skills to make healthy choices now, your body will thank you later. And the good news is you don't have to eat perfectly all the time. It's okay to splurge every once in a while, as long as your diet is generally good.

Chapter 34

Alcohol Use and Nutrition

Alcohol Use Information from Dietary Guidelines for Americans

The hazards of heavy ethanol (alcohol) intake have been known for centuries. Heavy drinking increases the risk of liver cirrhosis, hypertension, cancers of the upper gastrointestinal tract, injury, and violence (USDA, HHS, 2000). A recent analysis found that alcohol use is the third leading actual cause of mortality in the United States, after tobacco use and poor diet and/or inactivity (Mokdad et al., 2004).

Relationship between Moderate Alcohol Intake and Health

In middle-aged and older adults, a daily intake of one to two alcoholic beverages is associated with the lowest all-cause mortality. Compared with nondrinkers, adults who consume one to two alcoholic beverages per day appear to have lower risk of coronary heart disease (CHD), but women who consume one alcoholic beverage per day appear to have a slightly higher risk of breast cancer.

Relationships of alcohol consumption with major causes of death do not differ for middle-aged and elderly Americans. However, among

This chapter includes excerpts from "Ethanol," from *Report of the Dietary Guidelines Advisory Committee on the Dietary Guidelines for Americans, 2005,* U.S. Department of Health and Human Services (HHS) and U.S. Department of Agriculture (USDA); and excerpts from "Relationships between Nutrition, Alcohol Use, and Liver Disease," by Charles S. Lieber, M.D., M.A.C.P., *Alcohol Research and Health,* Volume 27, Number 3, 2003.

younger people alcohol consumption appears to provide little, if any, health benefit, and is associated with a higher risk of traumatic injury and death.

A daily intake of one to two alcoholic beverages is not associated with inadequate intake of macronutrient or micronutrients, or with overall dietary quality. Nonetheless, alcoholic beverages supply calories but few nutrients. The energy contribution from alcoholic beverages varies widely. Specifically, some alcoholic beverages, such as dessert wines and mixed drinks, provide almost three times as many calories as do the standard drink portions: 12 oz. of beer, 5 oz. of wine, or 1.5 oz. of distilled spirits. For those who choose to drink an alcoholic beverage, it is advisable to consume it with meals to slow alcohol absorption.

Adverse Effects of Moderate Alcohol Consumption

The Committee reviewed evidence regarding adverse effects of moderate alcohol consumption (National Institute on Alcohol Abuse and Alcoholism [NIAAA], 2003).

Trauma. According to the NIAAA report (2003), studies on relationships of alcohol with injuries from falls and with violence and/or abuse frequently do not distinguish between moderate and excessive drinking. Studies of acute effects of alcohol show that even moderate-dose consumption compromises brain performance in terms of error detection, processing speed, and response time. Low levels of drinking and blood alcohol content below 0.08 percent increase the risk of driving-related accidents. Thus, there are compelling temporary reasons not to drink alcohol, such as when planning to drive, operate machinery, or take part in activities that require attention, skill, or coordination.

Hepatic effects. Alcohol abuse is the leading cause of liver-related mortality in the United States, accounting for at least 40 percent, and perhaps as many as 90 percent, of cirrhosis deaths (CDC, 1993; Vong and Bell, 2004). Lower levels of alcohol intake can result in liver function abnormalities short of cirrhosis. For example, moderate alcohol consumption may potentiate the carcinogenic potency of other hepatotoxins (NIAAA, 2003).

Young age. Children or adolescents should not consume alcohol. Alcohol consumption increases the risk of traumatic injury, which is the number one cause of death in this age group. Animal data on alcohol-related structural changes in the brain, while less compelling, illustrates why drinking is inappropriate for adolescents (Land and Spear, 2004; Markwiese et al., 1998). "Designer drinks" (i.e., newer alcohol products that tend to target young adults) are of recent concern because of their possible effect on underage drinking.

Pregnancy (including the first few months of pregnancy—often before the pregnancy is recognized). Moderate drinking during pregnancy may have behavioral or neurocognitive consequences in the offspring. Heavy drinking during pregnancy can produce a range of behavioral and psychosocial problems, malformations, and mental retardation in the offspring (NIAAA, 2003).

Breastfeeding. The level of alcohol in breast milk mirrors the mother's blood alcohol content. Low or moderate alcohol consumption does not enhance lactational performance and actually may decrease infant milk consumption. Recent data indicate that alcohol consumption while breast-feeding has adverse effects on the infant's feeding and behavior (NIAAA, 2003).

Other conditions. The NIAAA review also provides documentation that alcohol consumption should be avoided by individuals who cannot restrict their drinking to moderate levels, individuals taking medications that can interact with alcohol, and persons with specific medical conditions, such as liver disease (NIAAA, 2003).

Reasons to Not Drink Alcoholic Beverages

Abstention is an important option; approximately one in three American adults does not drink alcohol. Moreover, studies suggest adverse effects at even moderate alcohol consumption levels in specific individuals and situations, as previously described.

People who should not drink include the following groups:

- Individuals who cannot restrict their drinking to moderate levels

- Children and adolescents

- Individuals taking prescription or over-the-counter medications that can interact with alcohol

- Individuals with specific medical conditions (e.g., liver disease)

Situations where alcohol should be avoided:

- Women who may become pregnant or who are pregnant
- Women who are breast-feeding
- Individuals who plan to drive, operate machinery, or take part in other activities that require attention, skill, or coordination

What is the relationship between consuming four or fewer alcoholic beverages daily and obesity?

Available data on the relationship between alcohol consumption and weight gain/obesity are sparse and inconclusive. There are contradictory findings at the higher end of the spectrum (i.e., 3 to 4 drinks per day) that may relate to fundamental limitations of the cross-sectional study design. At moderate drinking levels (i.e., up to one drink per day for women, up to one drink per day for men), there is no apparent association between alcohol intake and obesity.

Summary

A daily intake of one to two alcoholic beverages is associated with the lowest all-cause mortality and a low risk of CHD among middle-aged and older adults. Among younger people, however, alcohol consumption appears to provide little, if any, health benefit; alcohol use among young adults is associated with a higher risk of traumatic injury and death. Thus, the Committee recommends that if alcohol is consumed, it should be consumed in moderation, and only by adults. Moderation is defined as the consumption of up to 1 drink per day for women and up to 2 drinks per day for men; and 1 drink is defined as 12 oz of regular beer, 5 oz of wine (12 percent alcohol), or 1.5 oz of 80-proof distilled spirits. A number of situations and conditions call for the complete avoidance of alcoholic beverages.

Relationships between Nutrition, Alcohol Use, and Liver Disease

Many alcoholics are malnourished, either because they ingest too little of essential nutrients (e.g., carbohydrates, proteins, and vitamins) or because alcohol and its metabolism prevent the body from properly absorbing, digesting, and using those nutrients. As a result, alcoholics frequently experience deficiencies in proteins and vitamins, particularly vitamin A, which may contribute to liver disease and other serious alcohol-related disorders. Nutritional approaches can help prevent or ameliorate alcoholic liver disease. For example, a complete balanced diet can compensate for general malnutrition. Administration of antioxidants (e.g., precursors of the endogenous antioxidant glutathione) can help the body eliminate reactive oxygen molecules and other reactive molecules generated from abnormal lipid breakdown. New agents currently are being studied as promising nutritional supplements for alcoholics with liver disease.

A complex interplay exists between a person's alcohol consumption and nutritional status. Many people, including light-to-moderate drinkers who consume one to two glasses or less of an alcoholic beverage per day, consider those beverages a part of their normal diet and acquire a certain number of calories from them. When consumed in excess, however, alcohol can cause diseases by interfering with the nutritional status of the drinker. For example, alcohol can alter the intake, absorption into the body, and utilization of various nutrients. In addition, alcohol exerts some harmful effects through its breakdown (i.e., metabolism) and the resulting toxic compounds, particularly in the liver, where most of the alcohol metabolism occurs (Lieber 1992, 2000).

The Nutritional Status of Alcoholics

General observation suggests that many alcoholics do not consume a balanced diet; moreover, excessive alcohol consumption may interfere with these alcoholics' ability to absorb and use the nutrients they do consume. Accordingly, many alcoholics suffer from various degrees of both primary and secondary malnutrition. Primary malnutrition occurs when alcohol replaces other nutrients in the diet, resulting in overall reduced nutrient intake. Secondary malnutrition occurs when the drinker consumes adequate nutrients, but alcohol interferes with the absorption of those nutrients from the intestine so they are not available to the body.

The most severe malnutrition, which is accompanied by a significant reduction in muscle mass, generally is found in those alcoholics who are hospitalized for medical complications of alcoholism (e.g., alcohol-related liver disease or other organ damage). If these patients continue to drink, they will lose additional weight; conversely, if they abstain from drinking, they will gain weight. This pattern applies to patients with and without liver disease. People who drink heavily but do not require hospitalization for alcohol-related medical problems, in contrast, often are not malnourished or show less severe malnutrition (Feinman and Lieber 1998).

Alcohol's Effects on Digestion and Absorption of Essential Nutrients

Alcohol consumption, particularly at heavy drinking levels, not only influences the drinker's diet but also affects the metabolism of those nutrients that are consumed. Thus, even if the drinker ingests sufficient proteins, fats, vitamins, and minerals, deficiencies may develop if those nutrients are not adequately absorbed from the gastrointestinal tract into the blood, are not broken down properly, and/or are not used effectively by the body's cells. Two classes of nutrients for which such problems occur are proteins and vitamins.

A Person's Nutrition Affects Liver Function

Malnutrition, regardless of its causes, can lead to liver damage and impaired liver function. For example, children in underdeveloped countries whose diets do not contain enough protein can develop a disease called kwashiorkor. One symptom of this disorder is the accumulation of fat in the liver, a condition known as fatty liver. Studies performed during and after World War II indicated that severe malnutrition also could lead to liver injury in adults.

Because malnutrition also is common in alcoholics, clinicians initially thought that malnutrition, rather than alcohol itself, was responsible for alcohol-induced liver injury. Over the past 40 years, however, a more balanced view has evolved. Studies in humans, primates, and rodents have established that alcohol can cause liver damage even in well-nourished people (Lieber 1992). Moreover, controlled studies using hospitalized participants have demonstrated that even subjects receiving an enriched diet could develop fatty liver if the carbohydrates in the diet were replaced with alcohol. Finally, epidemiological analyses have found a close correlation between per capita alcohol consumption and the likelihood of cirrhosis, indicating that alcohol itself contributes to liver disease.

Management of Nutritional Deficiencies

Many drinkers who consume more than 30 percent of their total calories as alcohol ingest less than the recommended daily amounts of carbohydrates; proteins; fats; vitamins A, C, and B (especially thiamine); and minerals, such as calcium and iron. Deficiencies in these essential nutrients may exacerbate the effects of alcohol itself, resulting in serious disorders. To prevent these deficiencies, clinicians can provide alcoholics with a complete diet comparable to that of non-alcoholics. Even a complete, balanced diet, however, cannot prevent some of the organ damage that results from alcohol's direct toxic effects, including alcoholic liver disease.

Nevertheless, dietary supplements may prevent or ameliorate some of alcohol's harmful effects. For example, brain damage resulting from a lack of vitamin B_1 (thiamine), which can lead to conditions such as Wernicke-Korsakoff syndrome, can be reversed to some extent. Vitamin B_1 generally can be administered with a great margin of safety; therefore, all alcoholics undergoing treatment should be presumed to have a vitamin B_1 deficiency and should receive 50 mg of thiamine per day (either by injection if the patients are hospitalized or by mouth). Alcoholics also should receive supplements of vitamins B_2 (riboflavin) and B_6 (pyridoxine) at the dosages usually found in standard multivitamin preparations. Adequate folic acid levels can in most cases be achieved with a normal diet, unless there is evidence of a severe deficiency. Vitamin A should be given only to those alcoholics who have a well-documented deficiency, and who can stop or at least moderate their alcohol consumption, because of the potential harmful effects of vitamin A when combined with alcohol.

In addition to an improved diet to reverse nutritional deficiencies, alcoholics with moderate malnutrition also might benefit from treatment with anabolic steroids (Mendenhall et al. 1995). These compounds, which are derived from the male hormone testosterone, can be used in the short-term to promote overall body buildup and therefore may help the alcoholic recover from malnutrition.

Chapter 35

Physical Activity and Nutrition

Chapter Contents

Section 35.1

Physical Activity a Key Factor in Maintaining Health

"Physical Activity," from *Dietary Guidelines for Americans, 2005*, U.S. Department of Health and Human Services (HHS) and U.S. Department of Agriculture (USDA).

Americans tend to be relatively inactive. In 2002, 25 percent of adult Americans did not participate in any leisure time physical activities in the past month,[1] and in 2003, 38 percent of students in grades 9 to 12 viewed television three or more hours per day.[2] Regular physical activity and physical fitness make important contributions to one's health, sense of well-being, and maintenance of a healthy body weight. Physical activity is defined as any bodily movement produced by skeletal muscles resulting in energy expenditure. In contrast, physical fitness is a multi-component trait related to the ability to perform physical activity. Maintenance of good physical fitness enables one to meet the physical demands of work and leisure comfortably. People with higher levels of physical fitness are also at lower risk of developing chronic disease. Conversely, a sedentary lifestyle increases risk for overweight and obesity and many chronic diseases, including coronary artery disease, hypertension, type 2 diabetes, osteoporosis, and certain types of cancer. Overall, mortality rates from all causes of death are lower in physically active people than in sedentary people. Also, physical activity can aid in managing mild to moderate depression and anxiety.

Key Recommendations

Engage in regular physical activity and reduce sedentary activities to promote health, psychological well-being, and a healthy body weight.

- To reduce the risk of chronic disease in adulthood: Most days of the week, engage in at least 30 minutes of moderate-intensity physical activity, above usual activity at work or home.

- For most people, greater health benefits can be obtained by engaging in physical activity of more vigorous intensity or longer duration.

- To help manage body weight and prevent gradual, unhealthy body weight gain in adulthood: Engage in approximately 60 minutes of moderate to vigorous intensity activity on most days of the week while not exceeding caloric intake requirements.

- To sustain weight loss in adulthood: Participate in at least 60 to 90 minutes of daily moderate-intensity physical activity while not exceeding caloric intake requirements. Some people may need to consult with a healthcare provider before participating in this level of activity.

- Achieve physical fitness by including cardiovascular conditioning, stretching exercises for flexibility, and resistance exercises or calisthenics for muscle strength and endurance.

Key Recommendations for Specific Population Groups

- **Children and adolescents.** Engage in at least 60 minutes of physical activity on most, preferably all, days of the week.

- **Pregnant women.** In the absence of medical or obstetric complications, incorporate 30 minutes or more of moderate-intensity physical activity on most, if not all, days of the week. Avoid activities with a high risk of falling or abdominal trauma.

- **Breast-feeding women.** Be aware that neither acute nor regular exercise adversely affects the mother's ability to successfully breast-feed.

- **Older adults.** Participate in regular physical activity to reduce functional declines associated with aging and to achieve the other benefits of physical activity identified for all adults.

Most adults do not need to see their healthcare provider before starting a moderate-intensity physical activity program. However, men older than 40 years and women older than 50 years who plan a vigorous program or who have either chronic disease or risk factors for chronic disease should consult their physician to design a safe, effective program. It is also important during leisure time to limit sedentary behaviors, such as television watching and video viewing, and replace them with activities requiring more movement. Reducing these sedentary activities appears to be helpful in treating and preventing excessive weight gain among children and adolescents.

Different intensities and types of exercise confer different benefits. Vigorous physical activity (e.g., jogging or other aerobic exercise) provides greater benefits for physical fitness than does moderate physical activity and burns more calories per unit of time. Resistance exercise (such as weight training, using weight machines, and resistance band workouts) increases muscular strength and endurance and maintains or increases muscle mass. These benefits are seen in adolescents, adults, and older adults who perform resistance exercises on two or more days per week. Also, weight-bearing exercise has the potential to reduce the risk of osteoporosis by increasing peak bone mass during growth, maintaining peak bone mass during adulthood, and reducing the rate of bone loss during aging. In addition, regular exercise can help prevent falls, which is of particular importance for older adults.

The barrier often given for a failure to be physically active is lack of time. Setting aside 30 to 60 consecutive minutes each day for planned exercise is one way to obtain physical activity, but it is not the only way. Physical activity may include short sessions (e.g., 10 minutes at a time) of moderate-intensity activity. The accumulated total is what is important—both for health and for burning calories. Physical activity can be accumulated through three to six, 10 minute sessions over the course of a day.

Elevating the level of daily physical activity may also provide indirect nutritional benefits. A sedentary lifestyle limits the number of calories that can be consumed without gaining weight. The higher a person's physical activity level, the higher his or her energy requirement and the easier it is to plan a daily food intake pattern that meets recommended nutrient requirements.

Proper hydration is important when participating in physical activity. Two steps that help avoid dehydration during prolonged physical activity or when it is hot include: 1) consuming fluid regularly during the activity, and 2) drinking several glasses of water or other fluid after the physical activity is completed.

References

1. Behavioral Risk Factor Surveillance System, Surveillance for Certain Health Behaviors Among Selected Local Areas-United States, Behavioral Risk Factor Surveillance System, 2002, *Morbidity and Mortality Weekly Report* (MMWR), 53, No SS-05. http://www.cdc.gov/brfss.

2. Youth Risk Behavior Surveillance System, Youth Risk Behavior Surveillance-United States, 2003 *MMWR* 53(SS-2):1-29, 2004. http://www.cdc.gov/healthyyouth/yrbs.

Section 35.2

Guide to Eating for Sports

This information was provided by TeensHealth, one of the largest resources online for medically reviewed health information written for parents, kids, and teens. For more articles like this one, visit www.Teens Health.org, or www.KidsHealth.org. © 2002 The Nemours Center for Children's Health Media, a division of The Nemours Foundation.

Note: The information in this section is written for teens, but appropriate for all athletes.

You've prepared for the game in almost every way possible: you've trained hard with your teammates, heard inspirational speeches from your coach, washed your uniform, and gotten psyched up . . . but now what should you eat?

If this is something you hadn't thought of, you're not alone; many teen athletes don't really know how to combine food and fitness to reach their potential. And with all the different products available that can supposedly make an athlete perform even better, things can get pretty confusing.

The Funky Food Guide Pyramid

Fortunately, eating for sports isn't too complicated or difficult. It doesn't even require that you change your diet or buy any special foods or supplements.

One of the best ways to ensure you're in top form is to follow the Food Guide Pyramid. Sound simple? It is. By eating the recommended groups of foods in the suggested amounts, you are giving your body the nutrients it needs to succeed. You can find a copy of the Food Guide Pyramid on most boxes of cereal. (When following the Food Guide Pyramid, remember that some teen athletes may need more than the suggested daily servings of certain foods.) Eating regular meals and healthy snacks will keep you in top form.

The Food Guide Pyramid is a crucial part of eating for sports because it includes a huge variety of nutrients. You'll need a healthy combination of vitamins, minerals, protein, carbs, fats, and other nutrients from different foods to be at the top of your game.

That's why it's never a good idea to eat only one type of food when you're training for an event or game. You may have heard about people who swear by "carb loading" by eating only pasta before a big event, but this isn't the way to go if you're a teen. Carbohydrates are definitely an important source of fuel while you're active, but teens need different types of foods to do well in sports; eating from only one part of the pyramid will probably let your body down.

Although athletes do need a little more protein than less active teens, it's a myth that they need a huge daily intake of protein to build large, strong muscles. Amino acid supplements won't help either. Muscle growth comes from regular training and hard work.

We don't usually think of fats as being healthy, but athletes especially need to take in enough fat from their meals every day. When they are active and well-trained, our muscles quickly burn through carbs and need fats for long-lasting energy. When eaten in healthy foods—not sugary, high-fat snacks—fats are an extremely important source of direct energy for any athlete in training.

And don't forget iron and calcium. Most teens don't get enough of these two nutrients, and athletes' bodies require even more. All teens should make sure they get enough iron and calcium. The best sources of iron are lean red meats, grains that are iron-fortified, and green, leafy vegetables. For teens who play sports, calcium keeps the bones strong. Strong bones prevent stress fractures that can occur while working out or during a game. Foods from the milk group are the best sources of calcium.

Eat Extra Calories for Excellence

And while you're picking foods from the Food Guide Pyramid, it's very important that you are eating enough every day. Athletes should never skip meals.

Dieting is not a part of being an athlete, unless your doctor gives you instructions to do so. Most athletic teens need all the calories they normally consume to give them power and strength, and cutting calories can not only hinder performance, it can even be dangerous. This is especially true for teens who are wrestlers, swimmers, dancers, or gymnasts, because they are especially likely to be weight-conscious about their sport.

In addition, the growth spurts that teens undergo require some extra body fat, which translates to extra calories consumed. If anyone—a coach, a gym teacher, or another teammate—says that you should go (or have to go) on a diet, don't do anything until you talk to your doctor. If your doctor determines that a diet is necessary, he or she can work with you—or have you work with a dietitian—to get your program going.

What can happen if teens don't eat enough during heavy exercise and training? Lean body tissues, including the muscle mass necessary for peak performance, can break down. Simply put, you won't be as fast and as strong as you could be without taking in enough healthy calories every day. It can be difficult for your body to maintain its proper temperature, leading to illness and making you feel worn out—you'll be "hitting the wall" before your body can get fully warmed up. Your blood volume will drop, too, which means your tissues won't get the best oxygen, minerals, and nutrients they need. This hurts any active, growing teen, let alone an athletic teen in training.

Supplements, Sports Drinks, and You

Some athletes have the idea that while regular food is okay for building strength, supplements and sports foods and drinks must be used by athletes who want to win. Right? Wrong. It's easy to get tempted by the hundreds of sports bars, gels, supplements, protein powders, amino acid powders, and other products out there. Their commercials and packages make many promises about building athletes up, increasing their power and strength, and making them healthy, but the truth is that these products just aren't necessary, and usually aren't suitable for teens.

When an athlete drinks a mixture made with a protein product, her body has no idea that it's a sports supplement—it just treats it like plain, regular protein from food. In fact, most protein supplements offer the body no more protein than a cup (or 1/4 liter) of milk or one serving of meat, which is usually more tasty, anyway! In other words, these products don't provide you with any more energy that you would get from eating regular food from the Food Guide Pyramid. And regular food is a lot cheaper, too—sports bars and other supplements can deplete your savings because they tend to be very expensive.

Though none of these supplements do a whole lot of good, they won't really do you too much harm—except in the case of salt tablets. Athletes should never take salt tablets in an effort to compete better. These only serve to dehydrate you and could do potential damage to the lining of your stomach.

Ditch Dehydration

And speaking of dehydration, don't forget that food isn't the sole key to unlocking your power; water is just as important. When you are perspiring heavily during exercise and your body loses large amounts of water, it's easy to become overheated and not be able to perform to your full potential. In hot or humid weather, heat exhaustion can become a real hazard if you're not staying properly hydrated while you're exercising.

The best way to keep hydrated is to drink before, during, and after exercise (or a game or event). The amounts you should drink are as follows:

- 1 to 2 hours before exercising: 12 to 16 ounces of cold water (about 2 cups or ½ liter)

- 10 to 15 minutes before exercising: 12 to 16 ounces of cold water (about 2 cups or ½ liter)

- While exercising: 3 to 4 ounces of cold water every 15 minutes (about ½ cup or 1/10 liter)

- After exercising: 2 cups (about ½ liter) of cold water for every pound of weight loss through sweat (this means about 1 to 2 cups, or ¼ to ½ liter, for most teens; if it's a hot day you may feel thirsty enough to drink even more)

The main thing to remember about staying hydrated is to drink regardless of whether you feel thirsty. Thirst is a sign that your body has needed liquids for a while. And when deciding what to grab to quench your thirst, the best drink is cold water—it's the simplest thing for your body to absorb, it's usually easy to find, and it's free! If you like sports drinks, they are also okay, but like sports foods and supplements, they're not necessary for you to get what your body needs. They also tend to be pretty expensive. But if you like the taste and tend to drink more of a sports drink than you would of regular water, then it's fine.

If you want to drink water but want a tiny bit of taste, try mixing a splash of juice or a sports drink with the water in a water bottle. But be sure to avoid straight juice or soda because these contain carbohydrates that could give you a stomach ache while you're competing.

Also, the caffeine that's in many sodas can actually dehydrate you more, which defeats the purpose of drinking in the first place.

Edible Energy

When game day finally rolls around, most of your body's energy will come from the foods you've eaten in the last week, but you can enhance your performance even more by paying attention to the food you eat that day. Foods that are ideal for top performance contain carbohydrates for energy, a small to medium amount of protein, and very little fat.

- **Foods to eat 1 to 3 hours before the game or event:** fruit or vegetable juice or fruit (especially plums, melons, cherries, and peaches) with bread, a bagel, or an English muffin. (But if you like cream cheese or butter, now is a good time to skip it; the fat in these products could make you feel sick while you're competing.)

- **Foods to eat 3 or more hours before the game or event:** same as above, plus peanut butter, lean meat, low-fat cheese or yogurt, a baked potato, cereal with low-fat milk, or pasta with tomato sauce.

It's a good practice to avoid eating anything for the hour before you compete, because digestion requires energy—energy that you want to use to win! Also, eating too soon before certain types of events can cause food to slosh around in your stomach, which can leave you feeling sick and nauseated. It's also best to avoid candy bars or sodas before your event; these types of foods will give you quick energy, but it won't last long enough to see you through your event.

Part Five

Weight Control

Chapter 36

The Health Impact of Excessive Weight

Chapter Contents

Section 36.1

Defining Unhealthy Weight Ranges

"Defining Overweight and Obesity,"
Centers for Disease Control and Prevention (CDC),
Reviewed April 2005.

Overweight and obesity are both labels for ranges of weight that are greater than what is generally considered healthy for a given height. The terms also identify ranges of weight that have been shown to increase the likelihood of certain diseases and other health problems.

Definitions for Adults

For adults, overweight and obesity ranges are determined by using weight and height to calculate a number called the body mass index (BMI). BMI is used because, for most people, it correlates with their amount of body fat.

- An adult who has a BMI between 25 and 29.9 is considered overweight.

- An adult who has a BMI of 30 or higher is considered obese.

It is important to remember that although BMI correlates with the amount of body fat, BMI does not directly measure body fat. As a result, some people, such as athletes, may have a BMI that identifies them as overweight even though they do not have excess body fat.

Table 36.1. Example of Body Mass Index (BMI) for a 5'9" Adult

Height	Weight Range	BMI	Considered
5' 9"	124 lbs or less	Below 18.5	Underweight
	125 lbs to 168 lbs	18.5 to 24.9	Healthy weight
	169 lbs to 202 lbs	25.0 to 29.9	Overweight
	203 lbs or more	30 or higher	Obese

Other methods of estimating body fat and body fat distribution include measurements of skinfold thickness and waist circumference, calculation of waist-to-hip circumference ratios, and techniques such as ultrasound, computed tomography, and magnetic resonance imaging (MRI).

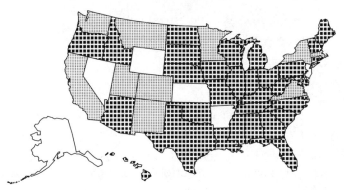

Obesity Trends* Among U.S. Adults
BRFSS, 1990
(*BMI ≥30, or ~ 30 lbs overweight for 5' 4" woman)

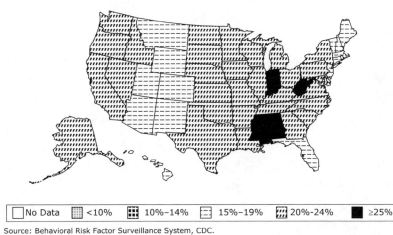

Obesity* Trends Among U.S. Adults
BRFSS, 2003
(*BMI ≥30, or about 30 lbs overweight for 5'4" person)

☐ No Data ▦ <10% ▦ 10%–14% ▤ 15%–19% ▨ 20%-24% ■ ≥25%

Source: Behavioral Risk Factor Surveillance System, CDC.

Figure 36.1. *Obesity Trends among U.S. Adults (Source: From "We Can!" National Institutes of Health, NIH Pub. No. 05-5273, June 2005).*

Definitions for Children and Teens

For children and teens, BMI ranges above a normal weight have different labels (at risk of overweight and overweight). Additionally, BMI ranges for children and teens are defined so that they take into account normal differences in body fat between boys and girls and differences in body fat at various ages.

Assessing Health Risks Associated with Overweight and Obesity

BMI is just one indicator of potential health risks associated with being overweight or obese. For assessing someone's likelihood of developing overweight- or obesity-related diseases, the National Heart, Lung, and Blood Institute guidelines recommend looking at two other predictors:

- The individual's waist circumference (because abdominal fat is a predictor of risk for obesity-related diseases).

- Other risk factors the individual has for diseases and conditions associated with obesity (for example, high blood pressure or physical inactivity).

Section 36.2

Factors Contributing to Obesity

"Overweight and Obesity: Contributing Factors,"
Centers for Disease Control and Prevention, Reviewed April 2005.

Overweight and Obesity: An Overview

The obesity epidemic covered on television and in the newspapers did not occur overnight. Obesity and overweight are chronic conditions. Overall there are a variety of factors that play a role in obesity. This makes it a complex health issue to address. This section will address how behavior, environment, and genetic factors may have an effect in causing people to be overweight and obese.

- Overweight and obesity result from an energy imbalance. This involves eating too many calories and not getting enough physical activity.

- Body weight is the result of genes, metabolism, behavior, environment, culture, and socioeconomic status.

- Behavior and environment play a large role causing people to be overweight and obese. These are the greatest areas for prevention and treatment actions.

Adapted from *U.S. Surgeon General's Call to Action to Prevent and Decrease Overweight and Obesity, 2001.*

Overweight and obesity are a result of energy imbalance over a long period of time. The cause of energy imbalance for each individual may be due to a combination of several factors. Individual behaviors, environmental factors, and genetics all contribute to the complexity of the obesity epidemic.

Energy imbalance: When the number of calories consumed is not equal to the number of calories used. Energy balance is like a scale. When calories consumed are greater than calories used weight gain results.

- **Weight Gain:** Calories consumed are greater than calories used

- **Weight Loss:** Calories consumed are less than calories used

- **No Weight Change:** Calories consumed equal the calories used

Genetics and the environment may increase the risk of personal weight gain. However, the choices a person makes in eating and physical activity also contribute to overweight and obesity. Behavior can increase a person's risk for gaining weight.

Calorie Consumption

In America, a changing environment has broadened food options and eating habits. Grocery stores stock their shelves with a greater selection of products. Pre-packaged foods, fast food restaurants, and soft drinks are also more accessible. While such foods are fast and convenient they also tend to be high in fat, sugar, and calories. Choosing many foods from these areas may contribute to an excessive calorie intake. Some foods are marketed as healthy, low fat, or fat-free, but may contain more calories than the fat containing food they are designed to replace. It is important to read food labels for nutritional information and to eat in moderation.

Portion size has also increased. People may be eating more during a meal or snack because of larger portion sizes. This results in increased calorie consumption. If the body does not burn off the extra calories consumed from larger portions, fast food, or soft drinks, weight gain can occur.

Choosing a variety of healthy foods in the correct portion sizes is helpful for achieving and maintaining a healthy weight. The *Dietary Guidelines for Americans* is a good resource to help people guide their dietary habits.

Calories Used

Our bodies need calories for daily functions such as breathing, digestion, and daily activities. Weight gain occurs when calories consumed exceed this need. Physical activity plays a key role in energy balance because it uses up calories consumed.

Physical activity is any bodily movement produced by skeletal muscles that results in an expenditure of energy with a range of activities such as the following:

- **Occupational work:** Carpentry, construction work, waiting tables, farming

- **Household chores:** Washing floors or windows, gardening, yard work

- **Leisure time activities:** Walking, skating, biking, swimming, playing Frisbee, dancing, structured sports, exercise, softball, tennis, football, aerobics

Regular physical activity is good for overall health. Physical activity decreases the risk for colon cancer, diabetes, and high blood pressure. It also helps to control weight, contributes to healthy bones, muscles, and joints; reduces falls among the elderly; and helps to relieve the pain of arthritis. Physical activity does not have to be strenuous to be beneficial. Moderate physical activity, such as 30 minutes of brisk walking five or more times a week, also has health benefits.

Despite all the benefits of being physically active, most Americans are sedentary. Technology has created many time and labor saving products. Some examples include cars, elevators, computers, dishwashers, and televisions. Cars are used to run short distance errands instead of people walking or riding a bicycle. As a result, these recent lifestyle changes have reduced the overall amount of energy expended in our daily lives. According to the *Behavioral Risk Factor Surveillance System*, in 2000 more than 26% of adults reported no leisure time physical activity.

The belief that physical activity is limited to exercise or sports, may keep people from being active. Another myth is that physical activity must be vigorous to achieve health benefits. Confidence in one's ability to be active will help people make choices to adopt a physically active lifestyle.

Environment

People may make decisions based on their environment or community. For example, a person may choose not to walk to the store or to work because of a lack of sidewalks. Communities, homes, and workplaces can all influence people's health decisions. Because of this influence, it is important to create environments in these locations that make it easier to engage in physical activity and to eat a healthy diet. The *Surgeon General's Call to Action to Prevent and Decrease Overweight and Obesity 2001* identified action steps for several locations that may help prevent and decrease obesity and overweight. Table 36.2 provides some examples of these steps.

Genetics

Science shows that genetics plays a role in obesity. Genes can directly cause obesity in disorders such as Bardet-Biedl syndrome and Prader-Willi syndrome. However, genes do not always predict future health. Genes and behavior may both be needed for a person to be overweight. In some cases, multiple genes may increase one's susceptibility for obesity and require outside factors; such as abundant food supply or little physical activity.

Other Factors

Diseases and Drugs

Some illnesses may lead to obesity or weight gain. These may include Cushing's disease, and polycystic ovary syndrome. Drugs such as steroids and some antidepressants may also cause weight gain. A doctor is the best source to tell you whether illnesses, medications, or psychological factors are contributing to weight gain or making weight loss hard.

Table 36.2. Action Steps to Prevent and Decrease Excess Weight

Location	Steps to Help Prevent and Decrease Overweight and Obesity
Home	Reduce time spent watching television and in other sedentary behaviors
	Build physical activity into regular routines
Schools	Ensure that the school breakfast and lunch programs meet nutrition standards
	Provide food options that are low in fat, calories, and added sugars
	Provide all children, from prekindergarten through grade 12, with quality daily physical education
Work	Create more opportunities for physical activity at work sites
Community	Promote healthier choices including at least 5 servings of fruits and vegetables a day, and reasonable portion sizes
	Encourage the food industry to provide reasonable food and beverage portion sizes
	Encourage food outlets to increase the availability of low-calorie, nutritious food items
	Create opportunities for physical activity in communities

Section 36.3

Health Risks of Excessive Weight

"Do You Know the Health Risks of Being Overweight?"
National Institute of Diabetes and Digestive and Kidney Diseases
(NIDDK), NIH Publication No. 04–4098, November 2004.

If you are overweight, you are more likely to develop certain health problems. You can improve your health by losing as little as 10 to 20 pounds. Weighing too much may increase your risk for developing many health problems. If you are overweight or obese on a body mass index (BMI) chart, you may be at risk for health problems such as the following:

- Type 2 diabetes
- Heart disease and stroke
- Cancer
- Sleep apnea
- Osteoarthritis
- Gallbladder disease
- Fatty liver disease.

Type 2 Diabetes

Type 2 diabetes used to be called adult-onset diabetes or noninsulin-dependent diabetes. It is the most common type of diabetes in the United States. Type 2 diabetes is a disease in which blood sugar levels are above normal. High blood sugar is a major cause of early death, heart disease, kidney disease, stroke, and blindness.

How is it linked to excessive weight?

More than 80 percent of people with type 2 diabetes are overweight. It is not known exactly why people who are overweight are more likely to suffer from this disease. It may be that being overweight causes cells to change, making them less effective at using sugar from the blood. This then puts stress on the cells that produce insulin (a hormone that carries sugar from the blood to cells) and makes them gradually fail.

What can weight loss do?

You can lower your risk for developing type 2 diabetes by losing weight and increasing the amount of physical activity you do. If you have type 2 diabetes, losing weight and becoming more physically active can help you control your blood sugar levels, and may allow your health care provider to reduce the amount of diabetes medication you take.

Heart Disease and Stroke

Heart disease means that the heart and circulation (blood flow) are not functioning normally. If you have heart disease, you may suffer from a heart attack, congestive heart failure, sudden cardiac death, angina (chest pain), or abnormal heart rhythm. During a stroke, blood and oxygen do not flow normally to the brain, possibly causing paralysis or death. Heart disease is the leading cause of death in the U.S., and stroke is the third leading cause.

How is it linked to being overweight?

People who are overweight are more likely to suffer from high blood pressure, high levels of triglycerides (blood fats) and LDL cholesterol (a fat-like substance often called the bad cholesterol), and low levels of HDL cholesterol (the good cholesterol). These are all risk factors for heart disease and stroke. In addition, people with more body fat have higher blood levels of substances that cause inflammation. Inflammation in blood vessels and throughout the body may raise heart disease risk.

What can weight loss do?

Losing 5 to 15 percent of your weight can lower your chances for developing heart disease or having a stroke. If you weigh 200 pounds, this means losing as little as 10 pounds. Weight loss may improve your blood pressure, triglyceride, and cholesterol levels; improve how your heart works and your blood flows; and decrease inflammation throughout your body.

Body Mass Index (BMI)

To use Table 36.3, find the appropriate height in the left-hand column labeled Height. Move across to a given weight. The number at

Table 36.3. Body Mass Index Table

BMI Height (Inches)	19	20	21	22	23	24	25	26	27	28	29	30	31	32	33	34	35	36	37	38	39	40
	Weight (Pounds)																					
58	91	96	100	105	110	115	119	124	129	134	138	143	148	153	158	162	167	172	177	181	186	191
59	94	99	104	109	114	119	124	128	133	138	143	148	153	158	163	168	173	178	183	188	193	198
60	97	102	107	112	118	123	128	133	138	143	148	153	158	163	168	174	179	184	189	194	199	204
61	100	106	111	116	122	127	132	137	143	148	153	158	164	169	174	180	185	190	195	201	206	211
62	104	109	115	120	126	131	136	142	147	153	158	164	169	175	180	186	191	196	202	207	213	218
63	107	113	118	124	130	135	141	146	152	158	163	169	175	180	186	191	197	203	208	214	220	225
64	110	116	122	128	134	140	145	151	157	163	169	174	180	186	192	197	204	209	215	221	227	232
65	114	120	126	132	138	144	150	156	162	168	174	180	186	192	198	204	210	216	222	228	234	240
66	118	124	130	136	142	148	155	161	167	173	179	186	192	198	204	210	216	223	229	235	241	247
67	121	127	134	140	146	153	159	166	172	178	185	191	198	204	211	217	223	230	236	242	249	255
68	125	131	138	144	151	158	164	171	177	184	190	197	203	210	216	223	230	236	243	249	256	262
69	128	135	142	149	155	162	169	176	182	189	196	203	209	216	223	230	236	243	250	257	263	270
70	132	139	146	153	160	167	174	181	188	195	202	209	216	222	229	236	243	250	257	264	271	278
71	136	143	150	157	165	172	179	186	193	200	208	215	222	229	236	243	250	257	265	272	279	286
72	140	147	154	162	169	177	184	191	199	206	213	221	228	235	242	250	258	265	272	279	287	294
73	144	151	159	166	174	182	189	197	204	212	219	227	235	242	250	257	265	272	280	288	295	302
74	148	155	163	171	179	186	194	202	210	218	225	233	241	249	256	264	272	280	287	295	303	311
75	152	160	168	176	184	192	200	208	216	224	232	240	248	256	264	272	279	287	295	303	311	319
76	156	164	172	180	189	197	205	213	221	230	238	246	254	263	271	279	287	295	304	312	320	328

the top of the column is the BMI at that height and weight. Pounds have been rounded off.

Cancer

Cancer occurs when cells in one part of the body, such as the colon, grow abnormally or out of control and possibly spread to other parts of the body, such as the liver. Cancer is the second leading cause of death in the United States.

How is it linked to overweight?

Being overweight may increase the risk of developing several types of cancer, including cancers of the colon, esophagus, and kidney. Overweight is also linked with uterine and postmenopausal breast cancer in women. Gaining weight during adult life increases the risk for several of these cancers. Being overweight also may increase the risk of dying from some cancers. It is not known exactly how being overweight increases cancer risk. It may be that fat cells make hormones that affect cell growth and lead to cancer. Also, eating or physical activity habits that may lead to being overweight may also contribute to cancer risk.

What can weight loss do?

Avoiding weight gain may prevent a rise in cancer risk. Weight loss, healthy eating, and physical activity habits may lower cancer risk.

Sleep Apnea

Sleep apnea is a condition in which a person stops breathing for short periods during the night. A person who has sleep apnea may suffer from daytime sleepiness, have difficulty concentrating, and even risk heart failure.

How is it linked to overweight?

The risk for sleep apnea is higher for people who are overweight. A person who is overweight may have more fat stored around his or her neck. This may make the airway smaller. A smaller airway can make breathing difficult, loud (snoring), or stop altogether. In addition, fat stored in the neck and throughout the body can produce substances that cause inflammation. Inflammation in the neck may be a risk factor for sleep apnea.

What can weight loss do?

Weight loss usually improves sleep apnea. Weight loss may help to decrease neck size and lessen inflammation.

Osteoarthritis

Osteoarthritis is a common joint disorder. With osteoarthritis, the joint bone and cartilage (tissue that protects joints) wear away. Osteoarthritis most often affects the joints of the knees, hips, and lower back.

How is it linked to overweight?

Extra weight may place extra pressure on joints and cartilage, causing them to wear away. In addition, people with more body fat may have higher blood levels of substances that cause inflammation. Inflammation at the joints may raise the risk for osteoarthritis.

What can weight loss do?

Weight loss can decrease stress on your knees, hips, and lower back, and lessen inflammation in your body. If you have osteoarthritis, losing weight may help improve your symptoms.

Gallbladder Disease

Gallstones are clusters of solid material that form in the gallbladder. They are made mostly of cholesterol and can sometimes cause abdominal or back pain.

How is it linked to overweight?

People who are overweight have a higher risk for developing gallbladder disease and gallstones. They may produce more cholesterol, a risk factor for gallstones. Also, people who are overweight may have an enlarged gallbladder, which may not work properly.

What can weight loss do?

Weight loss—especially fast weight loss (more than 3 pounds per week) or loss of a large amount of weight—can actually increase your chance of developing gallstones. Modest, slow weight loss of about ½ to 2 pounds a week is less likely to cause gallstones.

Fatty Liver Disease

Fatty liver disease occurs when fat builds up in the liver cells and causes injury and inflammation in the liver. It can sometimes lead to severe liver damage, cirrhosis (build-up of scar tissue that blocks proper blood flow in the liver), or even liver failure. Fatty liver disease is like alcoholic liver damage, but it is not caused by alcohol and can occur in people who drink little or no alcohol.

How is it linked to overweight?

People who have diabetes or pre-diabetes (when blood sugar levels are higher than normal, but not yet in the diabetic range) are more likely to have fatty liver disease than people without these conditions. People who are overweight are more likely to have diabetes. It is not known why some people who are overweight or diabetic get fatty liver and others do not.

What can weight loss do?

Losing weight can help you control your blood sugar levels. It can also reduce the build-up of fat in your liver and prevent further injury. People with fatty liver disease should avoid drinking alcohol.

Lower Your Health Risks

If you are overweight, losing as little as 5 percent of your body weight may lower your risk for several diseases, including heart disease and diabetes. If you weigh 200 pounds, this means losing 10 pounds. Slow and steady weight loss of ½ to 2 pounds per week, and not more than 3 pounds per week, is the safest way to lose weight.

To lose weight and keep it off over time, try to make long-term changes in your eating and physical activity habits. Choose healthy foods, such as vegetables, fruits, whole grains, and low-fat meat and dairy products more often, and eat just enough food to satisfy you. Try to do at least 30 minutes of moderate-intensity physical activity—like walking—on most days of the week, preferably every day. To lose weight, or to maintain weight loss, you may need to do more than 30 minutes of moderate physical activity daily.

Section 36.4

Helping Your Overweight Child

National Institute of Diabetes and Digestive and Kidney Diseases (NIDDK), NIH Publication No. 04–4096, July 2004.

Healthy eating and physical activity habits are key to your child's well-being. Eating too much and exercising too little can lead to excessive weight and related health problems that can follow children into their adult years. You can take an active role in helping your child—and your whole family—learn healthy eating and physical activity habits that can last for a lifetime.

Is my child overweight?

Because children grow at different rates at different times, it is not always easy to tell if a child is overweight. If you think that your child is overweight, talk to your health care provider. He or she can measure your child's height and weight and tell you if your child is in a healthy range.

How can I help my overweight child?

Involve the whole family in building healthy eating and physical activity habits. It benefits everyone and does not single out the child who is overweight.

Note: Do not put your child on a weight-loss diet unless your health care provider tells you to. If children do not eat enough, they may not grow and learn as well as they should.

Be Supportive

- Tell your child that he or she is loved, is special, and is important. Children's feelings about themselves often are based on their parents' feelings about them.

- Accept your child at any weight. Children will be more likely to accept and feel good about themselves when their parents accept them.

- Listen to your child's concerns about his or her weight. Overweight children probably know better than anyone else that they have a weight problem. They need support, understanding, and encouragement from parents.

Encourage Healthy Eating Habits

- Buy and serve more fruits and vegetables (fresh, frozen, or canned). Let your child choose them at the store.

- Buy fewer soft drinks and high fat, high calorie snack foods like chips, cookies, and candy. These snacks are okay once in a while, but keep healthy snack foods on hand and offer them to your child more often.

- Eat breakfast every day. Skipping breakfast can leave your child hungry, tired, and looking for less healthy foods later in the day.

- Plan healthy meals and eat together as a family. Eating together at meal times helps children learn to enjoy a variety of foods.

- Eat fast-food less often. When you visit a fast-food restaurant, try the healthier options offered.

- Offer your child water or low-fat milk more often than fruit juice. Fruit juice is a healthy choice, but is high in calories.

- Do not get discouraged if your child will not eat a new food the first time it is served. Some kids will need to have a new food served to them ten times or more before they will eat it.

- Try not to use food as a reward when encouraging kids to eat. Promising dessert to a child for eating vegetables, for example, sends the message that vegetables are less valuable than dessert. Kids learn to dislike foods they think are less valuable.

- Start with small servings and let your child ask for more if he or she is still hungry. It is up to you to provide your child with healthy meals and snacks, but your child should be allowed to choose how much food he or she will eat.

Here is a list of healthy snack foods for your child to try:

- Fresh fruit
- Fruit canned in juice or light syrup

- Small amounts of dried fruits such as raisins, apple rings, or apricots

- Fresh vegetables such as baby carrots, cucumber, zucchini, or tomatoes

- Reduced fat cheese or a small amount of peanut butter on whole-wheat crackers

- Low-fat yogurt with fruit

- Graham crackers, animal crackers, or low-fat vanilla wafers

Foods that are small, round, sticky, or hard to chew such as raisins, whole grapes, hard vegetables, hard chunks of cheese, nuts, seeds, and popcorn can cause choking in children under age 4. You can still prepare some of these foods for young children, for example, by cutting grapes into small pieces and cooking and cutting up vegetables. Always watch your toddler during meals and snacks.

Encourage Daily Physical Activity

Like adults, kids need daily physical activity. Here are some ways to help your child move every day:

- Set a good example. If your children see that you are physically active and have fun, they are more likely to be active and stay active throughout their lives.

- Encourage your child to join a sports team or class such as soccer, dance, basketball, or gymnastics at school or at your local community or recreation center.

- Be sensitive to your child's needs. If your child feels uncomfortable participating in activities like sports, help him or her find physical activities that are fun and not embarrassing.

- Be active together as a family. Assign active chores such as making the beds, washing the car, or vacuuming. Plan active outings such as a trip to the zoo or a walk through a local park.

Because his or her body is not ready yet, do not encourage your pre-adolescent child to participate in adult-style physical activity such as long jogs, using an exercise bike or treadmill, or lifting heavy weights. Fun physical activities are best for kids.

Kids need a total of about 60 minutes of physical activity a day, but this does not have to be all at one time. Short 10- or even 5-minute periods of activity throughout the day are just as good. If your children are not used to being active, encourage them to start with what they can do and build up to 60 minutes a day.

Discourage Inactive Pastimes

- Set limits on the amount of time your family spends watching television and videos, or playing video games.

- Help your child find fun things to do besides watching television, like acting out favorite books or stories, or doing a family art project. Your child may find that creative play is more interesting than television.

- Encourage your child to get up and move during commercials and discourage snacking when watching television.

Be a positive role model. Children watch adults and imitate what they see. Choose healthy foods and active pastimes for yourself. Your children will see that they can follow healthy habits that last a lifetime.

Find More Help

Your Health Care Provider

Ask your health care provider for brochures, booklets, or other information about healthy eating, physical activity, and weight control. He or she may be able to refer you to other health care professionals who work with overweight children, such as registered dietitians, psychologists, and exercise physiologists.

Weight-Control Program

You may want to think about a treatment program if:

- you have changed your family's eating and physical activity habits and your child has not reached a healthy weight.

- your health care provider has told you that your child's health or emotional well-being is at risk because of his or her weight.

The overall goal of a treatment program should be to help your whole family adopt healthy eating and physical activity habits that you can keep up for the rest of your lives. Here are some other things a weight-control program should do:

- Include a variety of health care professionals on staff: doctors, registered dietitians, psychiatrists or psychologists, and/or exercise physiologists.

- Evaluate your child's weight, growth, and health before enrolling in the program and watch these factors while enrolled.

- Adapt to the specific age and abilities of your child. Programs for 4-year-olds should be different from those for 12-year-olds.

- Help your family keep up healthy eating and physical activity behaviors after the program ends.

Additional Information

Weight-Control Information Network (WIN)
1 Win Way
Bethesda, MD 20892-3665
Toll-Free: 877-946-4627
Phone: 202-828-1025
Fax: 202-828-1028
Website: http://win.niddk.nih.gov
E-mail: win@info.niddk.nih.gov

Centers for Disease Control and Prevention
1600 Clifton Rd.
Atlanta, GA 30333
Toll-Free: 800-311-3435
Phone: 404-639-3534
Website: http://www.cdc.gov

Chapter 37

Choosing a Safe and Successful Weight Loss Program

Choosing a weight loss program may be a difficult task. You may not know what to look for in a weight loss program or what questions to ask. This chapter can help you make an informed decision about joining a program.

A Responsible and Safe Weight Loss Program

Experts agree that the best way to reach a healthy weight is to follow a sensible eating plan and engage in regular physical activity. Weight loss programs should encourage healthy behaviors that help you lose weight and that you can maintain over time. Safe and effective weight loss programs should include these components:

- Healthy eating plans that reduce calories, but do not rule out specific foods or food groups.

- Regular physical activity and/or exercise instruction.

- Tips on healthy behavior changes that also consider your cultural needs. Slow and steady weight loss of about ¾ to 2 pounds per week and not more than 3 pounds per week (weight loss may be faster at the start of a program).

National Institute of Diabetes and Digestive and Kidney Diseases (NIDDK), NIH Publication No. 03–3700, April 2003.

357

- Medical care if you are planning to lose weight by following a special formula diet, such as a very-low-calorie diet.

- A plan to keep the weight off after you have lost it.

Ask Questions

Gather as much information as you can before deciding to join a program. Providers of weight loss programs should be able to answer these questions:

- What does the weight loss program consist of?

- What are the staff qualifications?

- Does the product or program carry any risks?

- How much does the program cost?

- What results do participants typically have?

What does the weight loss program consist of?

- Does the program offer individual counseling and/or group classes?

- Do you have to follow a specific meal plan or keep food records?

- Do you have to purchase special food, drugs, or supplements?

- Does the program encourage you to be physically active, follow a specific physical activity plan, or provide exercise instruction?

- Does the program provide information on how to make positive and healthy behavior changes?

- Is the program sensitive to your lifestyle and cultural needs?

What are the staff qualifications?

- Who supervises the program?

- What type of weight management training, experience, education, and certifications does the staff have?

Does the product or program carry any risks?

- Are there risks related to following the program's eating or exercise plans?

- Are there risks related to using recommended drugs or supplements?

- Do participants talk with a medical professional?

- Does a medical professional oversee the program?

- Will the program providers work with your personal health care provider if you have a medical condition or are taking prescribed medications?

How much does the program cost?

- What is the total cost of the program?

- Are there recurring costs such as weekly attendance fees, costs of food and supplement purchases, etc.?

- Are there additional fees for a follow-up program or to re-enter the program for follow-up after you lose weight?

- Are there additional fees for medical tests?

What results do participants typically have?

- How much weight does an average participant lose, and how long have they kept off all, or part, of the lost weight?

- Can the program provide references?

If you are interested in locating a weight loss program in your area, ask your health care provider for a referral or contact your local hospital.

Additional Information

Weight-Control Information Network (WIN)
1 Win Way
Bethesda, MD 20892-3665
Toll-Free: 877-946-4627
Phone: 202-828-1025
Fax: 202-828-1028
Website: http://win.niddk.nih.gov
E-mail: win@info.niddk.nih.gov

Partnership for Healthy Weight Management
Website: http://www.consumer.gov/weightloss

Chapter 38

Weight Loss and Nutrition Myths

Diet Myths

Myth: **Fad diets work for permanent weight loss.**

Fact: Fad diets are not the best way to lose weight and keep it off. Fad diets often promise quick weight loss, or tell you to cut certain foods out of your diet. You may lose weight at first on one of these diets, but diets that strictly limit calories or food choices are hard to follow. Most people quickly get tired of them and regain any lost weight.

Fad diets may be unhealthy because they may not provide all of the nutrients your body needs. Also, losing weight at a very rapid rate (more than 3 pounds a week after the first couple weeks) may increase your risk for developing gallstones (clusters of solid material in the gallbladder that can be painful). Diets that provide less than 800 calories per day could result in heart rhythm abnormalities, which can be fatal.

Tip: Research suggests that losing ½ to 2 pounds a week by making healthy food choices, eating moderate portions, and building physical activity into your daily life is the best way to lose weight and keep it off. By adopting healthy eating and physical activity habits, you may

National Institute of Diabetes and Digestive and Kidney Diseases (NIDDK), NIH Publication No. 04–4561, March 2004.

also lower your risk for developing type 2 diabetes, heart disease, and high blood pressure.

Myth: **High-protein/low-carbohydrate diets are a healthy way to lose weight.**

Fact: The long-term health effects of a high-protein/low-carbohydrate diet are unknown. However, getting most of your daily calories from high-protein foods like meat, eggs, and cheese is not a balanced eating plan. You may be eating too much fat and cholesterol, which may raise heart disease risk. You may be eating too few fruits, vegetables, and whole grains, which may lead to constipation due to lack of dietary fiber. Following a high-protein/low-carbohydrate diet may also make you feel nauseous, tired, and weak.

Eating fewer than 130 grams of carbohydrate a day can lead to the buildup of ketones (partially broken-down fats) in your blood. A buildup of ketones in your blood (called ketosis) can cause your body to produce high levels of uric acid, which is a risk factor for gout (a painful swelling of the joints) and kidney stones. Ketosis may be especially risky for pregnant women and people with diabetes or kidney disease.

Tip: High-protein/low-carbohydrate diets are often low in calories because food choices are strictly limited, so they may cause short-term weight loss. But a reduced-calorie eating plan that includes recommended amounts of carbohydrate, protein, and fat will also allow you to lose weight. By following a balanced eating plan, you will not have to stop eating whole classes of foods, such as whole grains, fruits, and vegetables—and miss the key nutrients they contain. You may also find it easier to stick with a diet or eating plan that includes a greater variety of foods.

Myth: **Starches are fattening and should be limited when trying to lose weight.**

Fact: Many foods high in starch, like bread, rice, pasta, cereals, beans, fruits, and some vegetables (like potatoes and yams) are low in fat and calories. They become high in fat and calories when eaten in large portion sizes or when covered with high-fat toppings like butter, sour cream, or mayonnaise. Foods high in starch (also called complex carbohydrates) are an important source of energy for your body.

Tip: The *Dietary Guidelines for Americans* recommends eating 6 to 11 servings a day, depending on your calorie needs, from the bread, cereal, rice, and pasta group—even when trying to lose weight. Pay attention to your serving sizes—one serving is equal to 1 slice of bread, 1 ounce of ready-to-eat cereal, or ½ cup of pasta, rice, or cooked cereal. Try to avoid high-fat toppings and choose whole grains, like whole wheat bread, brown rice, oatmeal, and bran cereal. Choose other starchy foods that are high in dietary fiber too, like beans, peas, and vegetables.

Myth: **Certain foods, like grapefruit, celery, or cabbage soup, can burn fat and make you lose weight.**

Fact: No foods can burn fat. Some foods with caffeine may speed up your metabolism (the way your body uses energy or calories) for a short time, but they do not cause weight loss.

Tip: The best way to lose weight is to cut back on the number of calories you eat and be more physically active.

Myth: **Natural or herbal weight loss products are safe and effective.**

Fact: A weight loss product that claims to be natural or herbal is not necessarily safe. These products are not usually scientifically tested to prove that they are safe or that they work. For example, herbal products containing ephedra (now banned by the U.S. Government) have caused serious health problems and even death. Newer products that claim to be ephedra-free are not necessarily danger-free, because they may contain ingredients similar to ephedra.

Tip: Talk with your health care provider before using any weight loss product. Some natural or herbal weight loss products can be harmful.

Meal Myths

Myth: **"I can lose weight while eating whatever I want."**

Fact: To lose weight, you need to use more calories than you eat. It is possible to eat any kind of food you want and lose weight. You need to limit the number of calories you eat every day and/or increase your daily physical activity. Portion control is the key. Try eating smaller amounts of food and choosing foods that are low in calories.

Tip: When trying to lose weight, you can still eat your favorite foods—as long as you pay attention to the total number of calories that you eat.

Myth: **The terms low-fat and nonfat mean no calories.**

Fact: A low-fat or nonfat food is often lower in calories than the same size portion of the full-fat product. But many processed low-fat or nonfat foods have just as many calories as the full-fat version of the same food or even more calories. They may contain added sugar, flour, or starch thickeners to improve flavor and texture after fat is removed. These ingredients add calories.

Tip: Read the Nutrition Facts label on a food package to find out how many calories are in a serving. Check the serving size too it may be less than you are used to eating.

Myth: **Fast foods are always an unhealthy choice and you should not eat them when dieting.**

Fact: Fast foods can be part of a healthy weight loss program with a little bit of know-how.

Tip: Avoid supersized combo meals, or split one with a friend. Sip on water or nonfat milk instead of soda. Choose salads and grilled foods, like a grilled chicken breast sandwich or small hamburger. Try a fresco taco (with salsa instead of cheese or sauce) at taco stands. Fried foods, like french fries and fried chicken, are high in fat and calories, so order them only once in a while, order a small portion, or split an order with a friend. Also, use only small amounts of high-fat, high-calorie toppings, like regular mayonnaise, salad dressings, bacon, and cheese.

Myth: **Skipping meals is a good way to lose weight.**

Fact: Studies show that people who skip breakfast and eat fewer times during the day tend to be heavier than people who eat a healthy breakfast and eat four or five times a day. This may be because people who skip meals tend to feel hungrier later on, and eat more than they normally would. It may also be that eating many small meals throughout the day helps people control their appetites.

Tip: Eat small meals throughout the day that include a variety of healthy, low-fat, low-calorie foods.

Myth: **Eating after 8 p.m. causes weight gain.**

Fact: It does not matter what time of day you eat. It is what and how much you eat and how much physical activity you do during the whole day that determines whether you gain, lose, or maintain your weight. No matter when you eat, your body will store extra calories as fat.

Tip: If you want to have a snack before bedtime, think first about how many calories you have eaten that day. Try to avoid snacking in front of the television at night—it may be easier to overeat when you are distracted by the television.

Physical Activity Myth

Myth: **Lifting weights is not good to do if you want to lose weight, because it will make you bulk up.**

Fact: Lifting weights or doing strengthening activities like push-ups and crunches on a regular basis can actually help you maintain or lose weight. These activities can help you build muscle, and muscle burns more calories than body fat. So if you have more muscle, you burn more calories—even sitting still. Doing strengthening activities 2 or 3 days a week will not bulk you up. Only intense strength training, combined with a certain genetic background, can build very large muscles.

Tip: In addition to doing at least 30 minutes of moderate-intensity physical activity (like walking 2 miles in 30 minutes) on most days of the week, try to do strengthening activities 2 to 3 days a week. You can lift weights, use large rubber bands (resistance bands), do push-ups or sit-ups, or do household or garden tasks that make you lift or dig.

Food Myths

Myth: **Nuts are fattening and you should not eat them if you want to lose weight.**

Fact: In small amounts, nuts can be part of a healthy weight loss program. Nuts are high in calories and fat. However, most nuts contain healthy fats that do not clog arteries. Nuts are also good sources of protein, dietary fiber, and minerals including magnesium and copper.

Tip: Enjoy small portions of nuts. One-third cup of mixed nuts has about 270 calories.

Myth: **Eating red meat is bad for your health and makes it harder to lose weight.**

Fact: Eating lean meat in small amounts can be part of a healthy weight loss plan. Red meat, pork, chicken, and fish contain some cholesterol and saturated fat (the least healthy kind of fat). They also contain healthy nutrients like protein, iron, and zinc.

Tip: Choose cuts of meat that are lower in fat and trim all visible fat. Lower fat meats include pork tenderloin, and beef round steak, tenderloin, sirloin tip, flank steak, and extra lean ground beef. Also, pay attention to portion size. One serving is 2 to 3 ounces of cooked meat—about the size of a deck of cards.

Myth: **Dairy products are fattening and unhealthy.**

Fact: Low-fat and nonfat milk, yogurt, and cheese are just as nutritious as whole milk dairy products, but they are lower in fat and calories. Dairy products have many nutrients your body needs. They offer protein to build muscles and help organs work properly, and calcium to strengthen bones. Most milk and some yogurts are fortified with vitamin D to help your body use calcium.

Tip: The *Dietary Guidelines for Americans* recommend that people aged 9 to 18 and over age 50 have three servings of milk, yogurt, and cheese a day. Adults aged 19 to 49 need two servings a day, even when trying to lose weight. A serving is equal to 1 cup of milk or yogurt, 1½ ounces of natural cheese such as cheddar, or 2 ounces of processed cheese such as American. Choose low-fat or nonfat dairy products including milk, yogurt, cheese, and ice cream. If you cannot digest lactose (the sugar found in dairy products), choose low-lactose or lactose-free dairy products, or other foods and beverages that offer calcium and vitamin D including:

- **Calcium:** fortified fruit juice; soy-based beverage, or tofu made with calcium sulfate; canned salmon; dark leafy greens like collards or kale

- **Vitamin D:** fortified fruit juice; soy-based beverage; or cereal (getting some sunlight on your skin also gives you a small amount of vitamin D)

Myth: **Going vegetarian means you are sure to lose weight and be healthier.**

Fact: Research shows that people who follow a vegetarian eating plan, on average, eat fewer calories and less fat than non-vegetarians. They also tend to have lower body weights relative to their heights than non-vegetarians. Choosing a vegetarian eating plan with a low fat content may be helpful for weight loss. But vegetarians—like non-vegetarians—can make food choices that contribute to weight gain, like eating large amounts of high-fat, high-calorie foods or foods with little or no nutritional value. Vegetarian diets should be as carefully planned as non-vegetarian diets to make sure they are balanced. Nutrients that non-vegetarians normally get from animal products, but that are not always found in a vegetarian eating plan, are iron, calcium, vitamin D, vitamin B_{12}, zinc, and protein.

Tip: Choose a vegetarian eating plan that is low in fat and that provides all of the nutrients your body needs. Food and beverage sources of nutrients that may be lacking in a vegetarian diet include:

- **Iron:** cashews, spinach, lentils, garbanzo beans, fortified bread or cereal
- **Calcium:** dairy products, fortified soy-based beverages or fruit juices, tofu made with calcium sulfate, collard greens, kale, broccoli
- **Vitamin D:** fortified foods and beverages including milk, soy-based beverages, fruit juices, or cereal
- **Vitamin B_{12}:** eggs, dairy products, fortified cereal or soy-based beverages, tempeh, miso (tempeh and miso are foods made from soybeans)
- **Zinc:** whole grains (especially the germ and bran of the grain), nuts, tofu, leafy vegetables (spinach, cabbage, lettuce)
- **Protein:** eggs, dairy products, beans, peas, nuts, seeds, tofu, tempeh, soy-based burgers.

Additional Information

Weight-Control Information Network
1 Win Way
Bethesda, MD 20892-3665
Weight-Control Information Network (continued on next page)

Weight-Control Information Network

(continued)
Toll-Free: 877-946-4627
Phone: 202-828-1025
Fax: 202-828-1028
Website: http://win.niddk.nih.gov
E-mail: win@info.niddk.nih.gov

Federal Trade Commission

Website: http://www.ftc.gov/bcp/conline/features/wgtloss

American Dietetic Association

120 S. Riverside Plaza, Suite 2000
Chicago, IL 60606-6995
Toll-Free: 800-877-1600
Fax: 312-899-4899
Website: http://www.eatright.org/Public
E-mail: hotline@eatright.org

Chapter 39

Tips for Weight Loss and Maintenance

Have you decided to start eating healthier and become more physically active? Have you realized that healthy choices have a positive impact on not only yourself, but also those around you? If your goal is to lose weight or maintain your current healthy weight, here are some tips to help you achieve that goal. Remember, to maintain weight, you must balance calories with the energy you burn through physical activity. If you eat more than you expend, you gain weight. If you eat less (reduce calories) than you expend, you lose weight.

Make healthy choices a habit. This leads to a healthy lifestyle. Make a commitment to eat well, move more, and get support from family and friends. Even better, start eating healthier and being active together.

Remember to be realistic about your goals. If you try to reduce the calories, fat, saturated fat, and sugar in your diet, and at the same time promise to make a drastic change in your physical activity level, you may be setting yourself up for failure. Instead of trying to make many changes at once, set smaller, more realistic goals for yourself and add a new challenge each week.

Conduct an inventory of your meal/snack and physical activity patterns. Keep a food and activity journal. Write down not only

"Tipping the Scales in Your Favor," Centers for Disease Control and Prevention (CDC), April 2005.

what you ate, but where, when, and what you were feeling at the time. You will see what triggers your hunger and what satisfies your appetite. What foods do you routinely purchase? What snacks do you keep in the pantry?

Eat at least 5 servings of vegetables and fruits per day. If you are adding fruits and vegetables to your diet, try substituting them for higher calorie, less nutritious foods.

Eat foods that are high in fiber to help you feel full. Whole grain cereals, legumes (lentils and beans), vegetables, and fruits are good sources of fiber that may help you feel full with fewer calories.

Prepare and eat meals and snacks at home. This is a great way to save money, eat healthy, and spend time with your family. When preparing meals, choose low-fat/low-calorie versions of your favorite ingredients and learn how easy it is to substitute. For example:

- switch to 1% or nonfat milk and low-fat cheeses.

- use a cooking spray instead of oil or butter to decrease the amount of fat when you cook.

- prepare baked potatoes with low-fat blue cheese dressing or low-fat plain yogurt instead of butter or sour cream.

Use a scale and measuring cup to serve your food. Read food labels to determine serving sizes. One bowl of cereal may actually be two ¾-cup servings. A small frozen pizza may contain up to three servings (check the nutrition information label). This could add up to more calories than you think you are getting. Being aware of serving sizes may make it easier to avoid those extra calories.

Choose snacks that are nutritious and filling. A piece of fresh fruit, cut raw vegetables, or a container of low-fat yogurt are excellent (and portable) choices to tide you over until mealtimes. Take these snacks with you for a healthy alternative to chips, cookies, or candy.

Take your time. Eat only when you are hungry and enjoy the taste, texture, and smell of your meal as you eat it. Remember, it takes approximately 15 minutes for your stomach to signal your brain that you are full.

If you choose to eat out, remember these important suggestions: Watch your portions. Portion sizes at restaurants (including fast food) are usually more than one serving, which can result in overeating. Choose smaller portion sizes, order an appetizer and a leafy green salad with low-fat dressing, share an entree with a friend, or get a doggy bag and save half for another meal.

Forgive yourself. If you occasionally make mistakes, don't give up. Forgive yourself for making that choice and keep working on it. Eat an extra healthy lunch and dinner if you had a high-calorie, high-fat breakfast. Add more physical activity to your day.

Remember physical activity. Aim for at least 30 minutes (adults) or 60 minutes (children) of moderate-intensity physical activity five or more days of the week. If you are just starting to be physically active, remember that even small increases provide health benefits. Check with your physician first, and then start with a few minutes of activity a day and gradually increase, working your way up to 30 minutes. If you already get 30 minutes of moderate-intensity physical activity a day, you can gain even more health benefits by increasing the amount of time that you are physically active or by taking part in more vigorous-intensity activities.

Chapter 40

Popular Diets Reviewed

By the time you read this, there may already be a new best-selling diet book heading the list, but with some help from current or former American Dietetic Association (ADA) media spokespeople we have put together this information to give you the scoop on some current popular diets.

Dr. Phil's Ultimate Weight Solution

The Ultimate Weight Solution: The 7 Keys to Weight Loss Freedom by Phillip McGraw, PhD, Free Press, 2003.
Reviewed by: Lisa Dorfman, MS, RD, LMHC, Licensed Psychotherapist

Diet Summary: The theme of this program is that behavior modification and cognitive restructuring, along with a healthy diet and exercise, can lead to permanent weight management. Claiming an 80 percent success rate, the program's key points offer behavioral and nutritional advice ranging from portion control to supplement recommendations. Foods are divided into two categories: high response foods (good) and low response foods (bad).

While some of the book's advice is good (recycling behavior modification strategies that have been used in weight control programs for decades), several of the book's points contain erroneous or outdated nutrition and dietary recommendations. Additionally, the *Ultimate Weight Solution* includes seemingly simple advice for dealing with complicated emotional, eating, and family issues. Without proper supervision, managing these issues alone can lead to ultimate dietary disaster. Dr. Phil suggests enlisting a circle of support, including a nutritionist with technical expertise; however, this advice comes late in the book.

And for Adolescents

The Ultimate Weight Loss Solution for Teens: The 7 Keys to Weight Freedom by Jay McGraw, Free Press, 2003.

Written by Dr. Phil's son, this book is essentially a gentler version of the original *Ultimate Weight Solution*. While I do like the way it adapts the 7 Keys for kids with softer, hopeful language, this diet is still comprised of recycled behavior modification tips and unrealistically simple solutions to treating obesity and eating disorders.

The "New" Atkins Diet

Dr. Atkins' New Diet Revolution: Revised and Improved by Robert C. Atkins, M.D., Avon, 2001.
Reviewed by: Keith Ayoob, EdD, RD, FADA

Diet Summary: Arguably one of the most famous fad diets, the Atkins Diet program restricts carbohydrates and focuses on eating mostly protein with the use of vitamin and mineral supplements. According to the program, this will alter a body's metabolism so it will burn stored fat while building muscle mass. The "new" Atkins Diet is the same diet with a more liberal maintenance plan.

With the "new" Atkins diet, some of the sensationalism is gone and there is heavy promoting of low-carb bars and food products from Atkins Nutritionals, Inc. But the bottom line is still the same. Carbs are demonized and there are major restrictions on fruits and vegetables, whole grains, legumes, and low-fat dairy foods, which contradicts everything we know about health promotion and disease prevention.

The Zone Diet

The Zone: Revolutionary Life Plan to Put Your Body in Total Balance for Permanent Weight Loss by Barry Sears, M.D., Regan Books, 1995.
Reviewed by: Althea Zanecosky, MS, RD

Diet Summary: Promoting a "balanced nutritional approach," the Zone Diet is a complex eating plan that divides each meal into proportions of 40 percent carbohydrates, 30 percent proteins, and 30 percent fats. The Zone refers to the state in which the body is at its physical peak, presumably from following this diet.

While the Zone Diet is closer to what most dietetics professionals would recommend compared to other fad diets, there are still better nutrition and exercise programs that are less complicated and frustrating than constantly measuring proportions and counting calories.

South Beach Diet

The South Beach Diet: The Delicious, Doctor-Designed, Foolproof Plan for Fast and Healthy Weight Loss by Arthur Agaston, M.D., Rodale Press, 2003.
Reviewed by: Dawn Jackson, RD, LD

Diet Summary: Comprised of three phases, the South Beach Diet begins by banning carbohydrates such as fruit, bread, rice, potatoes, pasta, and baked goods and allowing normal-size portions of meat, poultry, shellfish, vegetables, eggs, and nuts. Dieters are told they will lose between 8 and 13 pounds in the first two weeks during the detoxification phase. The second phase reintroduces "good carbs" (as defined using an online glycemic index), and dieters expect to lose one to two pounds per week until the weight goal is reached. The third phase is the least restrictive, allowing the dieters to eat pretty much anything in moderation.

The theory behind the South Beach Diet is that the faster sugars and starches are digested, the more weight is gained. Instead, the diet will cause weight loss because it is a low-calorie plan with an average intake of about 1,400 to 1,500 calories per day. The diet's first phase promotes potentially dangerous accelerated weight loss; however, the second and third phases emphasize whole grains, lean proteins and dairy, unsaturated fats, fruits, and vegetables, in addition to consistent meal times, snacks, a healthy dessert, and plenty of water.

Raw Food Diets

The Raw Life: Becoming Natural in an Unnatural World by Paul Nison, 343 Publishing Company, 2000, and *Raw, the Uncooked Book* by Juliano Brotman and Erika Lenkert, Regan Books, 1999.
Reviewed by: Claudia M. González, MS, RD, LD/N

Diet Summary: Various versions of raw food diets exist, but they share the same basic principle: Cooked foods lose the natural vitamins, nutrients, and enzymes necessary to build a strong immune system. They recommend eating only fruits and vegetables picked ripe from the tree, garden, or vine (organic preferred); nuts, or seeds. Some raw food diets claim that it is not natural to eat sea vegetables, and others say that they are very important to include in the diet.

Raw food diets may be high in fiber and low in total fat, saturated fat, cholesterol, and calories, but they restrict so many important foods that it becomes a challenge to get all the nutrients the body needs. For example, avoiding all animal foods presents a challenge in getting enough vitamins B_{12} and D.

Sugar Busters

The New Sugar Busters! Cut Sugar to Trim Fat by H. Leighton Steward; Morrison C. Bethea, M.D.; Sam S. Andrews, M.D.; Luis A. Balart, M.D., Ballatine Books, 1998.
Reviewed by: Kathleen Zelman, MPH, RD, LD

Diet Summary: The basic tenet of *Sugar Busters* is that all sugars, including the sugar derived from complex carbohydrates and starches, are toxic because they produce excess insulin, which causes our bodies to store sugar as fat and make cholesterol. According to the book, foods with a high glycemic index produce a greater insulin response and fat storage. The book concludes with a list of acceptable foods and foods to avoid, a 14-day sample meal plan, and *Sugar Busters!* recipes. The diet is recommended as appropriate for children, pregnant women, people with diabetes, hypoglycemia sufferers and persons with a history of cardiovascular disease.

The carbohydrate/insulin response theory as a cause of weight gain has become popular in fad diets, but there is no evidence that excess insulin release causes obesity in people with normal pancreatic function. Obesity is more likely a result of a decline in physical activity and increase in calorie intake than increased sugar or carbohydrate consumption. While the authors mention that protein foods and fats should also be limited, some of the recipes suggest the contrary, such as the filet mignon recipe for four that includes four 10-ounce filets, a cup of blue cheese, and a half-pound of bacon.

Chapter 41

The Glycemic Index

The Skinny on the Glycemic Index

Although developed to help people with diabetes manage their food intake, the glycemic index (GI) has taken on new meaning as a weight loss strategy. In fact, several diet books tout the glycemic index as a foolproof way of identifying foods that raise blood sugar and insulin levels and therefore, can lead to weight gain.

But despite the hype, experts in nutrition and public health see very little practical use for the glycemic index and even the American Diabetes Association does not recommend this system for the prevention or treatment of diabetes. This is because of the many factors that affect the digestion of carbohydrates in the body. In fact, there is no clear evidence that avoiding foods high on the index is even beneficial.

The following describes what the glycemic index is and why the public health community does not recommend it in designing an eating plan.

The Glycemic Index and Its Limitations

Originally developed in 1981 as a laboratory tool to measure the rate at which carbohydrates are metabolized, the glycemic index is now being used by some as a measure of the degree to which a specific food raises a person's blood sugar, which in turn affects insulin

Reprinted with permission from http://www.essentialnutrition.org. © 2004 The Partnership for Essential Nutrition.

levels in the body. GI is calculated by measuring the effect of 50 grams of carbohydrates from various foods against a standard response from 50 grams of glucose. The higher the number, the greater the food's effect on blood sugar.

The reason for all the interest in the index is because it supports the theory of net carbs, which has facilitated the creation of the low-carb food industry and the launch of thousands of low-carb products. The theory is that high-GI foods cause a spike in the glucose level that prompts the body to release a flood of insulin. In turn, insulin drops blood sugar levels so that the person feels hungry again quickly and eats more. In contrast, low-GI foods are said to be digested more slowly and to release glucose more gradually.

But while many popular diet books make it sound as if the glycemic index is an accepted theory, in truth, there are very real problems with this system. First and foremost is the fact that the glycemic index deals with single foods eaten alone, not meals where foods are combined.

At the same time, this system does not take into account the serving size of commonly eaten foods, or the fact that there can be major differences even when comparing foods of the same type such as a relatively green banana compared with a ripe one. Another major limitation of the glycemic index is that it does not take into account the many factors that can alter the digestion and absorption of carbohydrates. These factors include the amount of fiber, fat, and protein in the food; how refined the ingredients are; whether the food was cooked; and what other foods are eaten at the same time.

Along with these limitations, there is no clear-cut evidence in the scientific literature that associates low-GI foods as either promoting satiety or reducing hunger. Moreover, nutritionists state that eliminating all foods that are high on the glycemic index is unhealthy, since many of these carbohydrates are rich in vitamins and minerals, phytochemicals, antioxidants, and dietary fiber that have been associated with a lower risk for certain cancers, diabetes, cardiovascular disease, and stroke, among other medical conditions. What is even more troubling is that many foods that have a low GI score, such as chocolate bars, are known to be high in fat and calories, while foods such as carrots with a high GI score are not.

The Implications for People with Diabetes

Because the glycemic index was developed to measure how fast blood sugar rises after a person eats foods containing carbohydrates, it is important to note that the premier organization focusing on the prevention and treatment of diabetes—the American Diabetes Association—does not recommend the use of this system. In its January 2002 nutrition recommendations, ADA stated that the available studies where glycemic index was controlled "do not provide convincing evidence of a benefit."[1] In addition, ADA's statement said that the research examining the index is very limited and involves only a small number of study groups. Therefore, ADA concluded, "the data reveal no clear trend in outcome benefits."

Rather, the ADA along with all the leading nutrition and public health groups recommend that for optimal health as well as weight loss, people should consume a diet that includes a variety of carbohydrate-containing foods, and especially fruits, vegetables, whole grains, and low-fat dairy products. Moreover, nutrition authorities are unanimous in stating that for weight loss, calories count, not the glycemic index. Although it may sound old-fashioned, the simple fact is that the key to successful weight loss is a combination of a reduced-calorie diet and increased physical activity—nothing more.

[1] Statement of the American Diabetes Association: Nutrition Recommendations for the Treatment and Prevention of Diabetes: January 2002 (*Diabetes Care* 2002;25:148-198).

Chapter 42

Weight Cycling

What Is Weight Cycling?

Weight cycling is the repeated loss and regain of body weight. When weight cycling is the result of dieting, it is often called yo-yo dieting. A weight cycle can range from small weight losses and gains (5–10 lbs. per cycle) to large changes in weight (50 lbs. or more per cycle).

Some research links weight cycling with certain health risks. To avoid potential risks, most experts recommend that obese adults adopt healthy eating and regular physical activity habits to achieve and maintain a healthier weight for life. Non-obese adults should try to maintain their weight through healthy eating and regular physical activity.

If I regain lost weight, won't losing it again be even harder?

A person who repeatedly loses and gains weight should not have more trouble trying to reach and maintain a healthy weight than a person attempting to lose weight for the first time. Most studies show that weight cycling does not affect one's metabolic rate—the rate at which the body burns fuel (food) for energy. Based on these findings, weight cycling should not affect the success of future weight-loss efforts. Metabolism does, however, slow down as a person ages. In addition, older people are often less physically active than when they

National Institute of Diabetes and Digestive and Kidney Diseases (NIDDK), NIH Publication No. 01–3901, updated March 2004.

were younger. Regardless of your age, making regular physical activity, as well as healthy eating habits, a part of your life will aid weight loss and improve health overall.

Will weight cycling leave me with more fat and less muscle than if I had not dieted at all?

Weight cycling has not been proven to increase the amount of fat tissue in people who lose and regain weight. Researchers have found that after a weight cycle, those who return to their original weights have the same amount of fat and lean tissue (muscle) as they did prior to weight cycling.

Some people are concerned that weight cycling can put more fat around their abdominal (stomach) area. People who tend to carry excess fat in the stomach area (apple-shaped), instead of in the hips, thighs, and buttocks (pear-shaped), are more likely to develop type 2 diabetes, heart disease, and high blood pressure. Studies have not found, however, that after a weight cycle, people have more fat around their stomachs than they did before weight cycling.

Is weight cycling harmful to my health?

Some studies suggest that weight cycling may increase the risk for certain health problems. These include high blood pressure, high cholesterol, and gallbladder disease. For adults who are not obese and do not have weight-related health problems, experts recommend maintaining a stable weight to avoid any potential health risks associated with weight cycling. Obese adults, however, should continue to try to achieve modest weight loss to improve overall health and reduce the risk of developing obesity-related diseases.

Losing and regaining weight may have a negative psychological effect if you let yourself become discouraged or depressed. Weight cycling should not be a reason to feel like a failure. Instead it is a reason to refocus on making long-term changes in your diet and level of physical activity to help you keep off the pounds you lose.

Is staying overweight healthier than weight cycling?

It is not known for certain whether weight cycling causes health problems. The diseases associated with being obese, however, are well known. These include the following:

- High blood pressure

- Heart disease
- Stroke
- Type 2 diabetes
- Certain types of cancer
- Arthritis
- Gallbladder disease

Not every adult who is overweight or obese has the same risk for disease. Whether you are a man or woman, the amount and location of your fat, and your family history of disease, all play a role in determining your disease risk. Experts agree, however, that even a modest weight loss of 10 percent of body weight over a period of six months or more can improve the health of an adult who is overweight or obese.

Conclusions

Further research on the effects of weight cycling is needed. In the meantime, if you are obese or are overweight and suffer from weight-related health problems, try to improve your health by achieving a modest weight loss. Although weight cycling may have some effect on disease risk, the serious health problems resulting from obesity are clearly understood. If you need to lose weight, you should be ready to commit to lifelong changes in your eating and physical activity behaviors.

If you are not obese or overweight with weight-related health problems, maintain your weight. Focus on adopting healthful eating habits and enjoying regular physical activity to manage weight and promote health for life.

Chapter 43

Dieting and Gallstones

If you are overweight or obese, you can lower your risk for type 2 diabetes, heart disease, stroke, and some forms of cancer by losing weight. People who are overweight are at greater risk for developing gallstones than people who are at a healthy weight. When choosing a weight loss program, be aware that the risk for developing gallstones increases with quick weight loss or a large weight loss. Gradual weight loss can lower the risk for obesity-related gallstones.

What are gallstones?

Gallstones are clusters of solid material that form in the gallbladder. They are made mostly of cholesterol. Gallstones may occur as one large stone or as many small ones. They vary in size and may be as large as a golf ball or as small as a grain of sand.

Experts estimate that 16 to 22 million people in the United States have gallstones—as many as one in every 12 Americans. Most people with gallstones do not know that they have them and experience no symptoms. Painless gallstones are called silent gallstones. Sometimes gallstones can cause abdominal or back pain. These are called symptomatic gallstones. In rare cases, gallstones can cause serious health problems. Symptomatic gallstones result in about 800,000 hospitalizations and more than 500,000 operations each year in the U.S.

Excerpted from "Dieting and Gallstones," National Institute of Diabetes and Digestive and Kidney Diseases (NIDDK), NIH Publication No. 02–3677, February 2002.

What are the symptoms of gallstones?

Some common symptoms of gallstones or gallstone attack include:

- severe pain in the upper abdomen that starts suddenly and lasts from 30 minutes to many hours;

- pain under the right shoulder or in the right shoulder blade;

- nausea or vomiting;

- indigestion after eating high-fat foods, such as fried foods or desserts.

Is obesity a risk factor for gallstones?

Obesity is a strong risk factor for gallstones, especially among women. People who are obese are more likely to have gallstones than people who are at a healthy weight. Researchers have found that people who are obese may produce high levels of cholesterol. This leads to the production of bile containing more cholesterol than it can dissolve. When this happens, gallstones can form. People who are obese may also have large gallbladders that do not empty normally or completely. Some studies have shown that men and women who carry fat around their midsections may be at a greater risk for developing gallstones than those who carry fat around their hips and thighs.

Is weight loss dieting a risk factor for gallstones?

Weight loss dieting increases the risk of developing gallstones. People who lose a large amount of weight quickly are at greater risk than those who lose weight more slowly. Rapid weight loss may also cause silent gallstones to become symptomatic. Studies have shown that people who lose more than 3 pounds per week may have a greater risk of developing gallstones than those who lose weight at slower rates.

A very low-calorie diet (VLCD) allows a person who is obese to quickly lose a large amount of weight. VLCDs usually provide about 800 calories or less per day in food or liquid form, and are followed for 12 to 16 weeks under the supervision of a health care provider. Studies have shown that 10 to 25 percent of people on a VLCD developed gallstones. These gallstones were usually silent—they did not produce any symptoms. About one-third of the dieters who developed gallstones, however, did have symptoms and some of these required gallbladder surgery.

Experts believe dieting may cause a shift in the balance of bile salts and cholesterol in the gallbladder. The cholesterol level is increased and the amount of bile salts is decreased. Following a diet too low in fat or going for long periods without eating (skipping breakfast, for example), a common practice among dieters, may also decrease gallbladder contractions. If the gallbladder does not contract often enough to empty out the bile, gallstones may form.

Is weight cycling a risk factor for gallstones?

Weight cycling, or losing and regaining weight repeatedly, may increase the risk of developing gallstones. People who weight cycle—especially with losses and gains of more than 10 pounds—have a higher risk for gallstones than people who lose weight and maintain their weight loss. In addition, the more weight a person loses and regains during a cycle, the greater the risk of developing gallstones.

Why weight cycling is a risk factor for gallstones is unclear. The rise in cholesterol levels during the weight loss phase of a weight cycle may be responsible.

Is surgery to treat obesity a risk factor for gallstones?

Gallstones are common among people who undergo gastrointestinal surgery to lose weight, also called bariatric surgery. Gastrointestinal surgery to reduce the size of the stomach or bypass parts of the digestive system is a weight loss method for people who have a body mass index (BMI) above 40. Experts estimate that one-third of patients who have bariatric surgery develop gallstones. The gallstones usually develop in the first few months after surgery and are symptomatic.

How can I safely lose weight and decrease the risk of gallstones?

You can take several measures to decrease the risk of developing gallstones during weight loss. Losing weight gradually, instead of losing a large amount of weight quickly, lowers your risk. Experts recommend losing 1 to 2 pounds per week. You can also decrease the risk of gallstones associated with weight cycling by aiming for a modest weight loss that you can maintain. Even a loss of 10 percent of body weight over a period of 6 months or more can improve the health of an adult who is overweight or obese.

Your food choices can also affect your gallstone risk. Experts recommend including some fat in your diet to stimulate gallbladder contracting and emptying. However, no more than 30 percent of your total calories should come from fat. Studies have also shown that diets high in fiber and calcium may reduce the risk of gallstone development. Finally, regular physical activity is related to a lower risk for gallstones.

Are the benefits of weight loss greater than the risk of getting gallstones?

Although weight loss increases the risk of developing gallstones, obesity poses an even greater risk. In addition to gallstones, obesity is linked to many serious health problems including the following:

- type 2 diabetes
- high blood pressure
- heart disease
- stroke
- certain types of cancer
- sleep apnea (when breathing stops for short periods during sleep)
- osteoarthritis (wearing away of the joints)
- gastroesophageal reflux disease (GERD)

For people who are obese, weight loss can lower the risk of developing these illnesses. Even a small weight loss of 10 to 20 pounds can improve health and lower disease risk. In addition, weight loss can bring other benefits such as better mood and positive self-image.

If you are thinking about starting an eating and physical activity plan to lose weight, talk with your health care provider first. Together, you can discuss various eating and exercise programs, your medical history, and the benefits and risks of losing weight including the risk of developing gallstones.

Additional Information

Weight-Control Information Network
1 Win Way
Bethesda, MD 20892-3665
Toll-Free: 877-946-4627
Phone: 202-828-1025
Fax: 202-828-1028
Website: http://win.niddk.nih.gov
E-mail: win@info.niddk.nih.gov

Part Six

Supplements

Chapter 44

What's in the Bottle? An Introduction to Dietary Supplements

Dietary supplements are a topic of great public interest. Whether you are in a store, using the Internet, or talking to people you know, you may hear about supplements and claims of benefits for health. How do you find out whether what's in the bottle is safe to take and whether science has proven that the product does what it claims? This chapter provides some answers.

What are dietary supplements?

Dietary supplements (also called nutritional supplements, or supplements for short) were defined in a law passed by Congress in 1994.[1, 2]

Dietary supplements:

- Are taken by mouth.

- Contain a dietary ingredient intended to supplement the diet. Examples of dietary ingredients include vitamins, minerals, herbs (as single herbs or mixtures), other botanicals, amino acids, and dietary substances such as enzymes and glandulars.

- Come in different forms, such as tablets, capsules, softgels, gelcaps, liquids, and powders.

Excerpted from "What's in the Bottle? An Introduction to Dietary Supplements," National Center for Complementary and Alternative Medicine, NCCAM Publication No. D191, September 2003, reviewed July 2004.

- Are not represented for use as a conventional food or as a sole item of a meal or the diet.

- Are labeled as being a dietary supplement.

Dietary supplements are sold in grocery, health food, drug, and discount stores, as well as through mail order catalogs, television programs, the Internet, and direct sales.

Is using supplements considered conventional medicine or complementary and alternative medicine (CAM)?

Some uses of dietary supplements have become part of conventional medicine. For example, scientists have found that the vitamin folic acid prevents certain birth defects, and a regimen of vitamins and zinc can slow the progression of the eye disease age-related macular degeneration.

On the other hand, some supplements are considered to be complementary and alternative medicine (CAM)—either the supplement itself or one or more of its uses. An example of a CAM supplement would be a herbal formula that claims to relieve arthritis pain, but has not been proven to do so through scientific studies. An example of a CAM use of a supplement would be taking 1,000 milligrams of vitamin C per day to prevent or treat a cold, as the use of large amounts of vitamin C for these purposes has not been proven.

Conventional medicine is medicine as practiced by holders of M.D. (medical doctor) or D.O. (doctor of osteopathy) degrees and by their allied health professionals, such as nurses, physical therapists, and dietitians. Other terms for conventional medicine include allopathy; Western, mainstream, orthodox, and regular medicine; and biomedicine.

Complementary and Alternative Medicine (CAM): Health care practices and products that are not presently considered to be part of conventional medicine are called CAM. Complementary medicine is used together with conventional medicine. Alternative medicine is used in place of conventional medicine. There is scientific evidence for the effectiveness of some CAM treatments. But for most, there are key questions yet to be answered through well-designed scientific studies, such as whether they are safe and work for the diseases or conditions for which they are used. The National Center for Complementary and Alternative Medicine (NCCAM), part of the National

Institutes of Health (NIH), is the Federal Government's lead agency for scientific research on CAM.

How can I get science-based information on a supplement?

There are several ways to get information on supplements that is based on the results of rigorous scientific testing, rather than on testimonials and other unscientific information.

- Ask your health care provider. Even if your provider does not happen to know about a particular supplement, he can access the latest medical guidance about its uses and risks.

- Dietitians and pharmacists also have helpful information.

- You can find out yourself whether there are any scientific research findings on the CAM supplement you are interested in. NCCAM and other Federal agencies have free publications, clearinghouses, and databases with this information.

If I am interested in using a supplement as CAM, how can I do so most safely?

Here are some points to keep in mind:

- It is important to talk to your health care provider (or providers, if you have more than one) about the supplement. This is for your safety and a complete treatment plan. It is especially important to talk to your provider if you:
  - are thinking about replacing your regular medical care with one or more supplements.
  - are taking any medications (whether prescription or over-the-counter). Some supplements have been found to interact with medications.
  - have a chronic medical condition.
  - are planning to have surgery. Certain supplements may increase the risk of bleeding or affect anesthetics and painkillers.
  - are pregnant or nursing a baby.
  - are thinking about giving a child a supplement. Many products being marketed for children have not been tested for their safety and effectiveness in children.[4]

- Do not take a higher dose of a supplement than what is listed on the label, unless your health care provider advises you to do so.

- If you experience any side effects that concern you, stop taking the supplement, and contact your provider. You can also report your experience to the U.S. Food and Drug Administration's (FDA) MedWatch program, which tracks consumer safety reports on supplements.

- For current information from the Federal Government on the safety of particular supplements, check the "Alerts and Advisories" section of the NCCAM website or the FDA website.

Can supplements and drugs interact?

- St. John's wort can increase the effects of prescription drugs used to treat depression. It can also interfere with drugs used to treat human immunodeficiency virus (HIV) infection, to treat cancer, for birth control, or to prevent the body from rejecting transplanted organs.

- Ginseng can increase the stimulant effects of caffeine (as in coffee, tea, and cola). It can also lower blood sugar levels, creating the possibility of problems when used with diabetes drugs.

- Ginkgo, taken with anticoagulant or antiplatelet drugs, can increase the risk of bleeding. It is also possible that ginkgo might interact with certain psychiatric drugs and with certain drugs that affect blood sugar levels.

I see the word natural on a lot of supplement labels. Does natural always mean safe?

There are many supplements, as well as many prescription drugs, that come from natural sources and are both useful and safe. However, natural does not always mean safe or without harmful effects. For example, consider mushrooms that grow in the wild—some are safe to eat, while others are poisonous.

The FDA issues warnings about supplements that pose risks to consumers, including those used for CAM therapies. The FDA found these products of concern because they:

- could damage health—in some cases severely.

- were contaminated—with other unlabeled herbs, pesticides, heavy metals, or prescription drugs.

- interacted dangerously with prescription drugs.

Here are examples of supplements that have carried FDA cautions about safety: [6, 7]

- Ephedra

- Kava

- Some dieter's teas

- L-tryptophan

- Herbal mixtures called PC SPES and SPES

- Aristolochic acid

- Comfrey

- St. John's wort

- GHB (gamma hydroxybutyric acid), GBL (gamma butyrolactone), and BD (1,4-butanediol)

- Certain products, marketed for sexual enhancement and claimed to be natural versions of the drug Viagra®, which were found to contain an unlabeled drug (sildenafil or tadalafil).

Does the federal government regulate supplements?

Yes, the federal government regulates supplements through the FDA. Currently, the FDA regulates supplements as foods rather than drugs. In general, the laws about putting foods (including supplements) on the market and keeping them on the market are less strict than the laws for drugs. The following list provides specific details about these differences:

- Research studies in people to prove a supplement's safety are not required before the supplement is marketed, unlike for drugs.

- The manufacturer does not have to prove that the supplement is effective, unlike for drugs. The manufacturer can say that the product addresses a nutrient deficiency, supports health, or reduces the risk of developing a health problem, if that is true. If the manufacturer does make a claim, it must be followed by the statement "This statement has not been evaluated by the Food and Drug Administration. This product is not intended to diagnose, treat, cure, or prevent any disease."

- The manufacturer does not have to prove supplement quality. Specifically:

  - The FDA does not analyze the content of dietary supplements.

  - At this time, supplement manufacturers must meet the requirements of the FDA's Good Manufacturing Practices (GMP) for foods. GMP describe conditions under which products must be prepared, packed, and stored. Food GMP do not always cover all issues of supplement quality. Some manufacturers voluntarily follow the FDA's GMP for drugs, which are stricter.

  - Some manufacturers use the term standardized to describe efforts to make their products consistent. However, U.S. law does not define standardization. Therefore, the use of this term (or similar terms such as verified or certified) does not guarantee product quality or consistency.

- If the FDA finds a supplement to be unsafe once it is on the market, only then can it take action against the manufacturer and/or distributor, such as by issuing a warning or requiring the product to be removed from the marketplace.

In March 2003, the FDA published proposed guidelines for supplements that would require manufacturers to avoid contaminating their products with other herbs, pesticides, heavy metals, or prescription drugs. The guidelines would also require supplement labels to be accurate.

The Federal Government also regulates supplement advertising, through the Federal Trade Commission. It requires that all information about supplements be truthful and not mislead consumers.

Does what's in the bottle always match what's on the label?

No. A supplement might:

- not contain the correct ingredient (plant species). For example, one study that analyzed 59 preparations of echinacea found that about half did not contain the species listed on the label.[8]

- contain higher or lower amounts of the active ingredient. For example, an NCCAM-funded study of ginseng products found that most contained less than half the amount of ginseng listed on their labels.[9]

- be contaminated.

Is NCCAM supporting research on supplements?

Yes, NCCAM is funding most of the nation's current research aimed at increasing scientific knowledge about supplements—including whether they work; if so, how they work; and how purer and more standardized products could be developed. Among the substances that researchers are studying are:

- yeast-fermented rice, to see if it can lower cholesterol levels in the blood.
- soy, to see if it slows the growth of tumors.
- ginger and turmeric, to see if they can reduce inflammation associated with arthritis and asthma.
- chromium, to better understand its biological effects and impact upon insulin in the body, possibly offering new pathways to treating type 2 diabetes.
- green tea, to find out if it can prevent heart disease.

NCCAM is also sponsoring or cosponsoring clinical trials on supplements, including:

- glucosamine hydrochloride and chondroitin sulfate, to find out if they relieve knee pain from osteoarthritis.
- black cohosh, to see if it reduces hot flashes and other symptoms of menopause.
- echinacea, to see if it shortens the length or lessens the severity of colds in children.
- garlic, to find out if it can lower moderately high cholesterol levels.
- ginkgo biloba, to determine whether it prevents or delays decline in cognitive (thinking) function in people aged 85 or older.
- ginger, to confirm whether it eases nausea and vomiting after cancer chemotherapy.

Definitions

Amino acid: Building block of proteins.

Botanical: (See herb) Botanical is a synonym for herb.

Clinical trials: Research studies in which a treatment or therapy is tested in people to see whether it is safe and effective.

Depression: An illness that involves the body, mood, and thoughts. The symptoms of depression often include feelings of sadness, hopelessness, or pessimism; and changes in sleep, appetite, and thinking.

Enzymes: Proteins that speed up chemical reactions in the body.

Glandulars: Dietary ingredients or supplements that are made from the glands of animals.

Heavy metals: A class of metals that, in chemical terms, have a density at least five times that of water. They are widely used in industry. A few examples of heavy metals that are toxic and have contaminated some dietary supplements are lead, arsenic, and mercury.

Herb: A plant or plant part that is used for its flavor, scent, and/or therapeutic properties.

Peer reviewed: Reviewed before publication by a group of experts in the same field.

Testimonials: Information provided by individuals who claim to have been helped or cured by a particular product. The information provided lacks the necessary elements to be evaluated in a rigorous and scientific manner and is not used in the scientific literature.

References

1. *Dietary Supplement Health and Education Act of 1994.* Food and Drug Administration Website. Accessed at www.fda.gov/opacom/laws/dshea.html on April 14, 2003.

2. *Dietary supplements: overview.* U.S. Food and Drug Administration, Center for Food Safety and Applied Nutrition Website. Accessed at www.cfsan.fda.gov/~dms/supplmnt.html on August 20, 2003.

3. Kaufman DW, Kelly JP, Rosenberg L, et al. Recent patterns of medication use in the ambulatory adult population of the United States: the Slone survey. *Journal of the American Medical Association.* 2002;287(3):337-344.

4. Federal Trade Commission. *Promotions for kids' dietary supplements leave sour taste.* Federal Trade Commission Website.

Accessed at www.ftc.gov/bcp/conline/features/kidsupp.pdf on May 2, 2003.

5. Natural Medicines Comprehensive Database. Natural Medicines Comprehensive Database Website. Accessed at naturaldatabase .com on August 20, 2003.

6. *MedWatch: the FDA safety information and adverse event reporting program.* U.S. Food and Drug Administration Website. Accessed at www.fda.gov/medwatch on August 20, 2003.

7. *Dietary supplements: warnings and safety information.* U.S. Food and Drug Administration, Center for Food Safety and Applied Nutrition Website. Accessed at www.cfsan.fda.gov/ ~dms/ds-warn.html on April 14, 2003.

8. Gilroy CM, Steiner JF, Byers T, et al. Echinacea and truth in labeling. *Archives of Internal Medicine.* 2003;163(6):699-704.

9. Harkey MR, Henderson GL, Gershwin ME, et al. Variability in commercial ginseng products: an analysis of 25 preparations. *American Journal of Clinical Nutrition.* 2001;73(6):1101-1106.

Additional Information

Center for Food Safety and Applied Nutrition (CFSAN)
5100 Paint Branch Parkway
College Park, MD 20740-3835
Toll-Free: 888-723-3366
Website: http://www.cfsan.fda.gov

Federal Trade Commission (FTC)
600 Pennsylvania Ave., N.W.
Washington DC 20580
Toll-Free: 877-382-4357
Website: http://www.ftc.gov

MedWatch
5600 Fishers Lane, HFD-410
Rockville, MD 20857
Toll-Free: 800-332-1088
Fax: 301-827-7241
Website: http://www.fda.gov/medwatch

NCCAM Clearinghouse

P.O. Box 7923
Gaithersburg, MD 20898-7923
Toll-Free: 888-644-6226
International: 301-519-3153
Toll-Free TTY: 866-464-3615
Toll-Free Fax: 866-464-3616
Fax-on-Demand service: 888-644-6226
Website: http://nccam.nih.gov
E-mail: info@nccam.nih.gov

Office of Dietary Supplements (ODS)

Room 3B01, MSC 7517
6100 Executive Blvd.
Bethesda, MD 20892-7515
Phone: 301-435-2920
Fax: 301-480-1845
Website: http://dietary-supplements.info.nih.gov
E-mail: ods@nih.gov

U.S. Food and Drug Administration (FDA)

5600 Fishers Lane
Rockville, MD 20857
Toll-Free: 888-463-6335
Website: http://www.fda.gov

Chapter 45

Ensuring the Safety of Dietary Supplements

When taken appropriately, some dietary supplements have clear benefits. Folic acid lowers the risk of some birth defects. Calcium supplements can strengthen bones and help prevent osteoporosis. But some dietary supplements pose health risks. They may be improperly manufactured or handled, or their ingredients may cause harmful effects on the body.

Under the Dietary Supplement Health and Education Act of 1994 (DSHEA), dietary supplements are regulated like foods. Unlike new drugs, dietary supplements do not generally have to go through review by the Food and Drug Administration for safety and effectiveness or be approved before they can be marketed. But manufacturers must provide pre-market notice and evidence of safety for any supplements they plan to sell that contain dietary ingredients that were not on the market before DSHEA was passed.

The FDA evaluates the safety of dietary supplements after they are on the market primarily through research and adverse event monitoring. Those who market and make dietary supplements are responsible for ensuring that any claims are substantiated with adequate evidence, and they cannot claim that the dietary supplements will treat or cure any disease.

FDA Consumer, July-August 2004, U.S. Food and Drug Administration (FDA).

Monitoring Industry

The dietary supplement industry has changed a lot in the last decade. When DSHEA was passed, there were about 4,000 dietary supplements on the market. Now there are about 29,000 on the market, with another 1,000 new products introduced each year, according to a recent Institute of Medicine report that was sponsored by the FDA. "We have seen a huge growth in the industry over the last 10 years, including the introduction of products that seem far removed from the vitamins and minerals of the pre-DSHEA days," says Dr. Lester M. Crawford, Acting FDA Commissioner. "Unlike most foods, some dietary supplements are pharmacologically active." When a substance is pharmacologically active, it can cause changes in the body. Such a substance could be toxic on its own or cause dangerous interactions with over-the-counter or prescription drugs.

Ephedra, which was often marketed for weight control and improved energy, was linked to cardiovascular problems, such as increased blood pressure and irregular heart rhythm. In the first formal action to stop the sale of a dietary supplement since DSHEA was passed, the FDA banned ephedra in 2003. "This is an example of how we can get a dietary supplement off the market if we have solid scientific proof that it does more harm than good," Crawford says.

Manufacturers and retailers can make claims about the impact of dietary supplements on the structure or function of the body, but these claims must be truthful. An example of such a claim is "calcium builds strong bones." The FDA plans to issue guidance for what data substantiates these types of claims. The agency has worked closely with the Federal Trade Commission to aggressively enforce the law against dietary supplements that are labeled with fraudulent health claims. In April 2004, the FDA sent warning letters to 16 firms, asking them to stop making false claims for weight loss.

From November 2003 to April 2004, the FDA inspected 180 domestic dietary supplement manufacturers, sent 119 warning letters to dietary supplement distributors, refused entry to 1,171 foreign shipments of dietary supplements, and seized or supervised the voluntary destruction of almost $18 million worth of mislabeled or adulterated dietary supplement products.

In March 2004, the FDA requested that 23 companies stop distributing dietary supplements containing androstenedione, also known as andro. Widely marketed to athletes and body builders, androstenedione has been touted as a way to increase muscle growth and reduce fat. However, it acts like a steroid in the body and increases the risk of serious diseases. For example, women who use these products may be at increased risk for breast cancer and endometrial cancer. Children who use these products are at risk of early onset of puberty and of premature cessation of bone growth.

Additionally, the FDA is developing regulations for industry on good manufacturing practices (GMP) for dietary supplements. When finalized, the rule will set standards for the manufacturing and handling of dietary supplements to ensure that consumers are provided with high-quality dietary supplements.

"The GMP regulation is the linchpin for properly regulating dietary supplements," Crawford says. "It gives FDA benchmarks for regulating dietary supplements and it gives clear instructions to the industry on how to manufacture products that meet rigorous quality standards."

Continuing Research

Crawford says that these initiatives are an important part of the agency's science-based approach to regulating dietary supplements. The FDA continues to collaborate with federal research partners at the National Institutes of Health and other organizations to gather evidence about the safety and effectiveness of dietary supplements. "In evaluating dietary supplements, we look at scientific information from a range of sources," Crawford says, "including published research, evidence-based reports, and data about the pharmacology or toxicology of a compound." Crawford notes that the agency has particular interest in gathering safety data about certain dietary supplements suspected to pose human health risks, including:

- an ephedra substitute called *Citrus aurantium*, also known as bitter orange, which may present health risks similar to ephedra;

- usnic acid, marketed for weight loss and linked to liver damage;

- kava, a botanical ingredient that has caused liver failure; and

- pyrrolizidine alkaloids, which are found in some plants and have been shown to have toxic effects that can cause liver damage.

The FDA recommends that consumers talk with a health care provider before using a dietary supplement. People who think they have been harmed by a dietary supplement should contact their health providers, and also report it to:

MedWatch
5600 Fishers Lane, HFD-410
Rockville, MD 20857
Toll-Free: 800-332-1088
Fax: 301-827-7241
Website: http://www.fda.gov/medwatch

—by Michelle Meadows

Chapter 46

Supplements May Cause Adverse Health Effects

Partners in Health—Working with Your Health Care Providers

With the abundance of conflicting information available about dietary supplements, it is more important than ever to talk with your doctor and other health care providers (dietitian, nurse, pharmacist, etc.) to help you sort the reliable information from the questionable.

Dietary Supplements—More Than Vitamins

Today's dietary supplements are not only vitamins and minerals. They also include other less familiar substances, such as herbals, botanicals, amino acids, and enzymes. Dietary supplements come in a variety of forms, such as tablets, capsules, powders, energy bars, or drinks.

If you do not consume a variety of foods, as recommended in the Food Guide Pyramid and *Dietary Guidelines for Americans*, some supplements may help ensure that you get adequate amounts of essential nutrients or help promote optimal health and performance. However, dietary supplements are not intended to treat, diagnose, mitigate, prevent, or cure diseases; therefore, manufacturers may not

Excerpts from "What Dietary Supplements Are You Taking?" Center for Food Safety and Applied Nutrition (CFSAN), U.S. Food and Drug Administration (FDA), December 2004.

make such claims. In some cases, dietary supplements may have unwanted effects, especially if taken before surgery or with other dietary supplements or medicines, or if you have certain health conditions.

Unlike drugs, but like conventional foods, dietary supplements are not approved by the Food and Drug Administration (FDA) for safety and effectiveness. It is the responsibility of dietary supplement manufacturers/distributors to ensure that their products are safe and that their label claims are accurate and truthful. Once a product enters the marketplace, FDA has the authority to take action against any dietary supplement product that presents a significant or unreasonable risk of illness or injury.

Scientific evidence supporting the benefits of some dietary supplements (e.g., vitamins and minerals) is well established for certain health conditions, but others need further study. Whatever your choice, supplements should not replace prescribed medications or the variety of foods important to a healthful diet.

Potential Risks of Using Dietary Supplements

Although certain products may be helpful to some people, there may be circumstances when these products can pose unexpected risks. Many supplements contain active ingredients that can have strong effects in the body. Taking a combination of supplements, using these products together with medicine, or substituting them in place of prescribed medicines could lead to harmful, even life-threatening results. Also, some supplements can have unwanted effects before, during, and after surgery. It is important to let your doctor and other health professionals know about the vitamins, minerals, botanicals, and other products you are taking, especially before surgery.

Here a few examples of dietary supplements believed to interact with specific drugs:

- **Calcium** and heart medicine (e.g., Digoxin), thiazide diuretics (Thiazide), and aluminum and magnesium-containing antacids.

- **Magnesium** and thiazide and loop diuretics (e.g., Lasix®, etc.), some cancer drugs (e.g., Cisplatin, etc.), and magnesium-containing antacids.

- **Vitamin K** and a blood thinner (e.g., Coumadin). St. John's Wort and selective serotonin reuptake inhibitor (SSRI) drugs (i.e., anti-depressant drugs and birth control pills).

What Should I Know before Using Dietary Supplements?

Be savvy! Follow these tips before buying a dietary supplement:

- **Safety First.** Some supplement ingredients, including nutrients and plant components, can be toxic based on their activity in your body. Do not substitute a dietary supplement for a prescription medicine or therapy.

- **Think twice about chasing the latest headline.** Sound health advice is generally based on research over time, not a single study touted by the media. Be wary of results claiming a quick fix that depart from scientific research and established dietary guidance.

- **Learn to Spot False Claims.** If something sounds too good to be true, it probably is. Some examples of false claims on product labels:

  - Quick and effective cure-all

  - Can treat or cure disease

  - Totally safe, all natural, and has definitely no side effects

  - Limited availability, no-risk, money-back guarantees, or requires advance payment

- **More may not be better.** Some products can be harmful when consumed in high amounts, for a long time, or in combination with certain other substances.

- **The term natural doesn't always mean safe.** Do not assume that this term ensures wholesomeness or safety. For some supplements, natural ingredients may interact with medicines, be dangerous for people with certain health conditions, or be harmful in high doses. For example, tea made from peppermint leaves is generally considered safe to drink, but peppermint oil (extracted from the leaves) is much more concentrated and can be toxic if used incorrectly.

- **Is the product worth the money?** Resist the pressure to buy a product or treatment on the spot. Some supplement products may be expensive or may not provide the benefit you expect. For example, excessive amounts of water-soluble vitamins, like vitamin C and B vitamins, are not used by the body and are eliminated in the urine.

Bottom Line

- Do not self diagnose any health condition. Work with your health care providers to determine how best to achieve optimal health.

- Check with your health care providers before taking a supplement, especially when combining or substituting them with other foods or medicine.

- Some supplements can help you meet your daily requirements for certain nutrients, but others may cause health problems.

- Dietary supplements are not intended to treat, diagnose, mitigate, prevent, or cure disease, or to replace the variety of foods important to a healthful diet.

Because many products are marketed as dietary supplements, it is important to remember that supplements include vitamins and minerals, as well as botanicals and other substances.

FDA MedWatch

If you suspect that you have had a serious reaction to a dietary supplement, you and your doctor should report it to:

MedWatch
5600 Fishers Lane, HFD-410
Rockville, MD 20857
Toll-Free: 800-332-1088
Fax: 301-827-7241
Website: http://www.fda.gov/medwatch

Chapter 47

Supplements for People over 50

Bill's retired and lives alone. Often he's just not hungry or is too tired to fix a whole meal. Does he need a multivitamin or one of those dietary supplements he sees in ads everywhere? He wonders if they work—will one help his arthritis, or another give him more energy? And, are they safe?

Dietary supplements used to make you think only of vitamins and minerals. But, today this big business makes and sells many different types of dietary supplements that have vitamins, minerals, fiber, amino acids, herbs, or hormones in them. Supplements come in the form of pills, capsules, powders, gel tabs, extracts, or liquids. Sometimes you find them added to drinks or energy bars. They might be used to add nutrients to your diet or to prevent health problems. You don't even need a prescription from your doctor to buy dietary supplements.

Do I need a dietary supplement?

Ads for supplements seem to promise to make you feel better, keep you from getting sick, or even help you live longer. Often there is little, if any, scientific support for these claims. In fact, some supplements can hurt you. Others are a waste of money because they don't give you any health benefits.

"Dietary Supplements: More Is Not Always Better," National Institute on Aging (NIA), August 2002.

So, should you take a supplement? You might want to talk to your doctor or a registered dietitian to answer that question. A friend or neighbor, or someone on a commercial shouldn't be suggesting a supplement for you.

Are these supplements safe?

Are you thinking about using dietary supplements? Remember that these over-the-counter substances are not like the penicillin or blood pressure medicine your doctor might prescribe for you. The U.S. Food and Drug Administration (FDA) has to check prescription drugs to make sure they are safe and do what they promise before they are sold. The same is true for over-the-counter drugs like cold and pain medicines. It is not the FDA's job to check dietary supplements in the same way. That means they are not reviewed by the FDA before being sold, but it is the FDA's job to take action against unsafe products on the market. Only if enough people report problems with a dietary supplement, can the FDA study these possible problems and take action.

Besides the FDA, many federal government agencies and private groups are interested in dietary supplements. The National Institutes of Health (NIH) is the federal focal point for medical research in the United States. NIH supports research studies looking at the safety and helpfulness of some of the ingredients found in many supplements.

Business and consumer groups are also interested in dietary supplements. So are private professional groups such as the National Academy of Sciences (NAS). The NAS develops guidelines saying how much of each vitamin and mineral people need.

What about vitamins and minerals?

Vitamins and minerals are nutrients found naturally in food. We need them to stay healthy. The benefits and side effects of many vitamins and minerals have been studied. The best way to get vitamins and minerals is through the food you eat, not any supplements you might take. Try to eat the number of servings of food recommended by the U.S. Department of Agriculture's Food Guide Pyramid each day. Pick foods that are lower in fat and added sugars. If you can't eat enough, then ask your doctor if you should be taking a multivitamin and mineral supplement. And, remember these tips:

- The supplement does not need to be a senior formula.

- It should not have large or mega-doses of vitamins and minerals.

- Generally store or generic brands are fine.

How much should you take? The NAS has developed recommendations for vitamins and minerals. Check the label on your supplement bottle. It shows the level of vitamins and minerals in a serving compared with the suggested daily intake. For example, a vitamin A intake of 100% DV (Daily Value) means the supplement is giving you the full amount of vitamin A you need each day. This is in addition to what you are getting from your food.

Some people might think that if a little is good, a lot must be better. But, that does not necessarily apply to vitamins and minerals. Depending on the supplement, your age, and your health, taking more than 100% DV could be harmful to your health. Also, if your body cannot use the entire supplement you take, you have wasted money. Finally, large doses of some vitamins and minerals can also keep your prescription medications from working as they should.

Anything special for people over 50?

Even if you eat a good variety of foods, if you are over 50, you might need certain supplements. Talk to your doctor or a registered dietitian. Depending on your needs, he or she might suggest you get the following amounts from food and, if needed, supplements:

- **Vitamin B$_{12}$**—2.4 mcg (micrograms) of B$_{12}$ each day. Some foods, such as cereals, are fortified with this vitamin. But, up to one-third of older people can no longer absorb natural vitamin B$_{12}$ from their food. They need this vitamin to keep their blood and nerves healthy.

- **Calcium**—1200 mg (milligrams), but not more than 2500 mg a day. As you age, you need more of this and vitamin D to keep bones strong and to keep the bone you have. Bone loss can lead to fractures, mainly of the hip, spine, or wrist, in both older women and men.

- **Vitamin D**—400 IU (international units) for people age 51 to 70 and 600 IU for those over 70, but not more than 2000 IU each day.

- **Iron**—extra iron for women past menopause who are using hormone replacement therapy (men and other postmenopausal women need 8 mg of iron). Iron helps keep red blood cells healthy. Postmenopausal women who use hormone replacement therapy may still experience a monthly period. They need extra iron to make up for that loss of blood.

- **Vitamin B$_6$**—1.7 mg for men and 1.5 mg for women. This vitamin is needed for forming red blood cells and to keep you healthy.

What are antioxidants?

You may have heard about the possible benefits of antioxidants, natural substances found in food. Right now, there is no proof that large doses of antioxidants will prevent chronic diseases such as heart disease, diabetes, or cataracts. Eating fruits and vegetables (at least five servings a day) rather than taking a supplement is the best way to get antioxidants. Vegetable oil and nuts are also good sources of some antioxidants. Non-dairy calcium sources are especially good for people who cannot use dairy products.

Sources of calcium include:

- dairy products like milk and cheese and foods made with them,
- canned fish with soft bones like salmon and sardines,
- dark green leafy vegetables,
- calcium-fortified products such as orange juice, and
- breads and cereals made with calcium-fortified flour.

What about herbal supplements?

You may have heard of ginkgo biloba, ginseng, Echinacea, or black cohosh. These are examples of herbal supplements. They are dietary supplements that come from certain plants. It is easy to think they are safe because they come from plants. And, although herbal supplements are not approved as drugs, some are being studied as possible treatments for illness. But, it is still too soon to tell. Remember some strong poisons like hemlock and prescription medicines such as cancer drugs come from plants as well. You need to be careful.

When you use any dietary supplement, including herbals, for a health problem, you are using that supplement as a drug. Because their ingredients may have an effect on your body, they can interfere with medications you may already be taking. Some herbal supplements can also cause serious side effects such as high blood pressure, nausea, diarrhea, constipation, fainting, headaches, seizures, heart attack, or stroke.

What's best for me?

If you are thinking about using dietary supplements for any reason, remember these guidelines:

- Talk to your doctor or a registered dietitian. Just because something worked for your neighbor, does not mean the same will be true for you.

- Use only the supplement your doctor or dietitian and you decide on—do not buy combinations that have things you do not want or need.

- If your doctor does not suggest a dietary supplement, but you decide to use one anyway, tell your doctor. Then he or she can keep an eye on your health and adjust your other medications if needed.

- Learn as much as you can about the supplement you are thinking about, but be aware of the source of the information. Could the writer or group profit from the sale of a particular supplement?

- Buy brands you know from companies you, your doctor, your dietitian, or your pharmacist know are reputable.

Remember that many of the claims made about supplements are not based on enough scientific proof. If you have questions about a supplement, contact the firm and ask if it has information on the safety and/or effectiveness of the ingredients in its product.

What else can I do?

Stick to a healthy diet, exercise, keep your mind active, don't smoke, and see your doctor regularly.

Additional Information

Center for Food Safety and Applied Nutrition
Food and Drug Administration
5100 Paint Branch Parkway
College Park, MD 20740-3835
Toll-Free: 888-723-3366
Website: http://www.cfsan.fda.gov

Food and Nutrition Information Center

Department of Agriculture
10301 Baltimore Ave.
Beltsville, MD 20705-2351
Phone: 301-504-5719
TTY: 301-504-6856
Fax: 301-504-6409
Website: http://www.nal.usda.gov/fnic
E-mail: fnic@nal.usda.gov

National Institute on Aging (NIA)

Building 31, Room 5C27
31 Center Drive, MSC 2292
Bethesda, MD 20892
Toll-Free: 800-222-2225
Toll-Free TTY: 800-222-4225
Phone: 301-496-1752
Fax: 301-496-1072
Website: http://www.nia.nih.gov

Office of Dietary Supplements

National Institutes of Health
Room 3B01, MSC 7517
6100 Executive Blvd.
Bethesda, MD 20892-7515
Phone: 301-435-2920
Fax: 301-480-1845
Website: http://dietary-supplements.info.nih.gov
E-mail: ods@nih.gov

Chapter 48

Supplements for Heart Disease and Cholesterol Control: Some Work, Others Are Worthless

What Works?

Some 1,400 Americans will die of heart disease today. That's about how many died yesterday and how many will die tomorrow.

With a toll that high, it doesn't make sense to waste precious time and money on worthless supplements. But that's just what millions of people do. Little do they know that some supplements really can lower your LDL (bad) cholesterol or triglycerides. Or that others really can raise your HDL (good) cholesterol. Or that still others may even slash your odds of dying of cardiac arrest.

So the next time the vitamin-store clerk tells you that vitamin E or garlic or guggulipids or tocotrienols are just what the doctor ordered for your heart, say no thanks. Then pick up the following:

Fish Oil

"Studies show that eating fish, especially higher-fat fish, at least twice a week cuts the risk of dying from a heart attack by a quarter to a half, even in people who don't already have heart disease," says William Harris of the University of Missouri–Kansas City School of Medicine.

What about fish oil supplements? Researchers haven't tested them on healthy people, but they have looked at people who have survived a heart attack. In a large Italian study, 2,800 heart attack survivors were given a daily dose of fish oil that contained 850 milligrams of omega-3 fats. Over the next 3½ years, they suffered 20 percent fewer deaths from heart disease than 2,800 survivors who weren't taking fish oil.[a]

The only problem: the study didn't compare the fish oil takers to placebo takers, so it's impossible to say whether it was the fish oil—or just the fact that people were taking a pill—that led to the decline. Still, the evidence is promising.

"The risk of dying from a heart attack in the Italian study began to drop within the first three months of taking the fish oil," notes Harris.

Fish oil may act quickly by preventing sudden death heart attacks. According to the American Heart Association (AHA), 250,000 Americans die each year of cardiac arrest before reaching a hospital. In most cases, sudden death occurs following an arrhythmia—when the heartbeat becomes chaotic.

The two omega-3 fatty acids in fish oil, eicosapentaenoic acid (EPA) and docosahexaenoic acid (DHA), seem to have a unique ability to stabilize arrhythmias. "They become part of the heart's muscle cells and can stop a sudden heart arrhythmia from becoming fatal," says Harris.

The AHA advises heart disease patients who don't eat fish regularly to talk with their doctors about taking a daily supplement with one gram (1,000 mg) of omega-3 fats. While larger amounts—two to four grams a day—can reduce blood triglyceride levels (which may lower heart disease risk even further), three grams a day or more causes internal bleeding in a small number of people. To figure out how many fish oil capsules to take, add up the amount of EPA and DHA per capsule or per serving in the information that's listed on the label. ([a] *Lancet* 354: 447, 1999.)

Psyllium

The soluble fiber psyllium, which is the main ingredient in the bulk-forming laxative Metamucil, is proven to lower LDL. In 197 men and women with high cholesterol who took two teaspoons of Metamucil (about seven grams) before breakfast and before lunch every day for six months, LDL dropped seven percent more than in 55 similar people who took four teaspoons of a placebo every day.[b] The psyllium takers were no more likely to complain of diarrhea or constipation than the placebo takers. The Food and Drug Administration allows manufacturers to claim that consuming at least seven grams a day of soluble fiber from psyllium may help reduce the risk of heart disease. ([b] *American Journal of Clinical Nutrition* 71: 1433, 2000.)

Niacin (Vitamin B₃)

Niacin (Vitamin B$_3$)

At very high doses, it really acts as a drug, not a vitamin. But whatever you call it, niacin is the most potent pill you can take to raise your HDL (good) cholesterol. Megadoses (500 milligrams to 1,000 milligrams a day) can boost HDL by 15 to 35 percent and can lower triglycerides by 20 to 50 percent. (The government's recommended daily intake for niacin as a vitamin is 20 mg.)

"But using niacin effectively is complicated," says John Pieper, dean of the University of New Mexico College of Pharmacy in Albuquerque. "So you need to work with a physician who knows what he or she is doing."

Many people can't tolerate its side effects. "The most troublesome and common one," says Pieper, "is a painful facial flushing that feels like someone is sticking pins into your skin." That can sometimes be prevented by starting with a low dose, taking aspirin or ibuprofen 30 minutes before the niacin, and taking the niacin with meals.

"Sustained-release niacin, which is absorbed much more slowly, doesn't produce as much flushing, but it can cause reversible liver damage in some people," cautions Pieper. A new extended-release niacin, available by prescription as Niaspan, produces less flushing and less liver toxicity than the other forms of niacin, says Pieper.

The take-home message: If you have high triglycerides or low HDL, niacin works. But don't take high doses of any form of niacin without a doctor's supervision.

Phytosterols

"Plant sterols are more effective in lowering LDL than all the currently available dietary supplements," says endocrinologist Ronald Ostlund of Washington University in St. Louis. "By interfering with the absorption of cholesterol from the intestinal tract, they can reduce LDL by about 10 percent." (Statin drugs like Lipitor and Pravachol lower LDL by 20 to 40 percent, depending on the drug and the dosage.)

Small amounts of plant sterols (they're also called phytosterols) occur naturally in pine trees and foods like soybeans, nuts, grains, and oils. Manufacturers concentrate them to create supplements or margarine-like "cholesterol-lowering" spreads like Benecol, Take Control, and Smart Balance Omega Plus. Minute Maid has introduced "Heart Wise," a phytosterol-fortified orange juice.

The evidence is so clear that the Food and Drug Administration (FDA) allows foods that contain at least 400 milligrams of phytosterols per serving to claim that they can help prevent heart disease (though you need at least 800 mg a day to get the benefits, says the FDA). And the National Cholesterol Education Program (NCEP) now recommends two grams (2,000 mg) of plant sterols every day as a way to lower LDL if changes in diet aren't sufficient.

"If your cholesterol is high, plant sterols may not lower it enough," says Ostlund. "But if you're on statins, taking plant sterols will lower your cholesterol even more because they work in different ways."

Aspirin

It may be an over-the-counter medicine, not a dietary supplement, but odds are you've got a bottle of aspirin sitting next to your vitamins. And odds are you take it—or have heard that you should take it—every day to lower your risk of having a heart attack. Should you? It depends on who you are.

"Taking aspirin regularly has been proven to reduce the risk of having a second heart attack by 34 percent and a second stroke by 22 percent in both men and women," says researcher Charles Hennekens of the University of Miami School of Medicine, who led some of the landmark studies on aspirin and heart disease. "And aspirin can lower the risk of dying from a heart attack by 23 percent if it's taken during the attack and afterwards."

Should you take it regularly if you've never had a heart attack or stroke? Not necessarily. Aspirin is a double-edged sword. While it can prevent the clots that block arteries and cause heart attacks and strokes, it can also cause bleeding in the intestinal tract and, rarely, in the brain.

"The American Heart Association has concluded that if your risk of having a first heart attack is 10 percent or more over the next ten years, then the benefits of aspirin outweigh the risks, whether you're a man or woman," says Hennekens. Doctors determine ten-year risk using data from the Framingham Heart Study. "But the final decision should be made by the health-care provider, not the patient," cautions Hennekens. "The doctor can weigh aspirin's benefits and side effects against the patient's overall risk."

How much aspirin works? "For prevention, 75 milligrams a day is as good as 325," says Hennekens. "You see more side effects when you exceed 325 milligrams a day." (A full-strength aspirin has 325 mg. A baby aspirin has 81 mg, as do products like Bayer Low Strength Aspirin Regimen.)

"If you're having a heart attack," Hennekens adds, "you should take a regular 325-milligram aspirin." That dose seems to inhibit clotting within minutes, while a baby aspirin may take days.

Folic Acid and B₁₂

Folic Acid and B$_{12}$

People who have higher levels of homocysteine in their blood have a higher risk of dying of heart disease. Whether lowering homocysteine reduces that risk is still an open question. But the ability of the B-vitamin folic acid to lower homocysteine isn't.

A daily dose of 500 micrograms of folic acid lowers homocysteine levels by 25 percent, according to the pooled results of 12 studies.[c] (That's close enough to the 400 micrograms that are in most multivitamins.) Combining folic acid with 20 micrograms of vitamin B_{12} lowers homocysteine by an additional seven percent. ([c] *British Medical Journal* 316: 894, 1998.)

Don't Bet Your Heart on These

If stores could only sell supplements that worked, you'd have a hard time finding any of these heart disease fighters.

Antioxidants

Talk about underachievers. Despite promising early evidence in animals and people, high doses of beta-carotene and vitamin E have repeatedly failed to prevent heart attacks and death from heart disease.

Taking 50 IU to 800 IU of vitamin E a day didn't cut the risk of dying from heart disease in seven major studies that followed more than 81,000 men and women for up to six years.[1] And there's so little evidence for vitamin C that no one's been willing to fund a major heart disease trial.

While vitamin E doesn't help, at least it doesn't hurt. Not so beta-carotene. In eight studies that monitored a total of 138,000 men and women for two to twelve years, those who were given high doses of beta-carotene—15 mg to 50 mg (25,000 IU to 83,000 IU)—every day were 10 percent more likely to die from heart disease than similar people who took a placebo.[1]

"The use of vitamin supplements containing that much beta-carotene should be actively discouraged," cautions Marc Penn of the Cleveland Clinic Foundation, who was on the team that examined the eight studies. (There's no need to cut back on sweet potatoes and other foods that contain beta-carotene.)

If you take Lipitor, Pravachol, or other statin drugs plus large doses of the B-vitamin niacin to control your cholesterol, there's another reason to avoid high doses of antioxidants: they may interfere with the drugs. In a three-year trial of 160 patients with heart disease, three percent of those who were given statins plus niacin to raise their HDL (good) cholesterol and lower their triglycerides suffered a heart attack, stroke, or other cardiovascular event.[2] The rate jumped to 14 percent in patients who combined the statins and niacin with large daily doses of antioxidants—800 IU of vitamin E, 1,000 mg of vitamin C, and 100 micrograms of selenium.

"Antioxidant vitamins should rarely, if ever, be recommended for cardiovascular protection," concludes the study's lead author, B. Greg Brown of the University of Washington School of Medicine in Seattle.

Garlic

It's "cholesterol's natural enemy," say the makers of Garlique. Yet according to a U.S. government-sponsored review of the evidence, garlic's effect on cholesterol levels is unclear. While garlic supplements seem to produce a slight drop in LDL for the first three months, the decline disappears after six months.[3] In fact, the better the design and execution of garlic studies, the less likely they were to detect any benefit, concluded a review by British alternative-medicine scientists in 2000.[4]

In Germany, where much of the early enthusiasm for garlic's cholesterol-busting potential originated, the government no longer allows companies to claim that garlic can lower cholesterol.

Guggul

The first good test of this tree-resin extract outside its native India backfired last year. Researchers at the University of Pennsylvania gave 67 men and women with high cholesterol one or two grams a day of a standardized guggul extract called guggulipid. (The manufacturer, Sabinsa Corporation of Piscataway, New Jersey, funded the study.)

Instead of lowering LDL, Sabinsa's guggulipid actually raised it by five percent.[5] And six of the guggul takers (but none of the placebo takers) developed unpleasant rashes that went away only after they stopped taking the supplement.

Tocotrienols

In early studies by researchers with a financial interest in the outcome, these vitamin E-like compounds, found in rice and other plant foods, seemed to lower LDL in people with high cholesterol. But three larger and longer trials by independent scientists have come up empty. In the most recent one, the tocotrienol formulation used in Evolve, once the leading national brand, had no impact on LDL.[6]

"Tocotrienols don't seem to affect cholesterol levels in people," says Andre Theriault of the University of Hawaii in Honolulu. "Cholesterol is made by the liver and tocotrienols can inhibit that process in test tubes, but it appears that not enough tocotrienols get into the liver when people consume them as supplements."

Isoflavones

Isoflavones are estrogen-like compounds that are found in soybeans, clover, and some other plants. Eating at least 25 grams of soy protein a day can lower cholesterol, but "there's no definitive experimental evidence to establish that this is due to the isoflavones in soy," says Thomas Clarkson of the Wake Forest University School of Medicine in Winston-Salem, North Carolina.

In fact, isoflavones extracted from soybeans or from red clover have failed in most attempts to lower LDL. According to a recent analysis that pooled the results of 10 studies, the drop in LDL from eating soy protein was unrelated to the amount of isoflavones in the protein.[7]

Red Yeast Rice

For centuries, people in China have used powdered rice that has been fermented by red yeast to make wine, preserve food, and improve blood circulation. In a 1999 UCLA study that was funded by the company, the Cholestin brand of red yeast rice lowered LDL by an impressive 22 percent in 83 people with high cholesterol levels.[8]

But in 2001, the Food and Drug Administration persuaded a federal district court to ban Cholestin because the supplement contained the same active ingredients found in the prescription statin drug Mevacor. Cholestin's manufacturer, Nu Skin of Provo, Utah, replaced the red yeast rice with a plant extract called policosanol.

A lab analysis of eight other brands of red yeast rice found that none contained the same mix of cholesterol-lowering ingredients as the original Cholestin.[9]

The bottom line: the only red yeast rice known to lower cholesterol is no longer for sale.

Policosanol

Policosanol (or polycosanol) extracted from sugarcane lowered LDL by 17 to 31 percent in 19 trials involving more than 1,900 people. But 16 of the studies were carried out by just one group of researchers in Havana, Cuba. (The other three were small trials done in Mexico, Argentina, and Chile.) Policosanol has never been tested in good studies in the U.S., Canada, Europe, or Japan.

What's more, the policosanol used in most U.S. supplements (including the reformulated Cholestin—see "Red Yeast Rice") is extracted from beeswax, not sugarcane. Beeswax policosanol hasn't been tested on cholesterol levels.

References

1. *Lancet* 361: 2017, 2003.

2. *New England Journal of Medicine* 345: 1583, 2001.

3. www.ahrq.gov/clinic/epcsums/garlicsum.htm.

4. *Annals of Internal Medicine* 133: 420, 2000.

5. *Journal of the American Medical Association* 290: 765, 2003.

6. *American Journal of Clinical Nutrition* 76: 1237, 2002.

7. *European Journal of Clinical Nutrition* 57: 940, 2003.

8. *American Journal of Clinical Nutrition* 69: 231, 1999.

9. *Journal of Alternative and Complementary Medicine* 7: 133, 2001.

Chapter 49

Sports Supplement Dangers

Anabolic Steroid Abuse

One of the main reasons people give for abusing steroids is to improve their performance in sports. Among competitive bodybuilders, steroid abuse has been estimated to be very high. Among other athletes, the incidence of abuse probably varies depending on the specific sport.

Another reason people give for taking steroids is to increase their muscle size and/or reduce their body fat. This group includes some people who have a behavioral syndrome (muscle dysmorphia) in which a person has a distorted image of his or her body. Men with this condition think that they look small and weak, even if they are large and muscular. Similarly, women with the syndrome think that they look fat and flabby, even though they are actually lean and muscular.

While conditions such as muscle dysmorphia, a history of physical or sexual abuse, or a history of engaging in high-risk behaviors may increase the risk of initiating or continuing steroid abuse, researchers

This chapter includes text from "Research Report Series: Anabolic Steroid Abuse," National Institute on Drug Abuse (NIDA), February 4, 2005; and excerpts from "NIDA InfoFacts: Rohypnol and GHB," NIDA, revised March 2005. Also, "Sales of Supplements Containing Ephedrine Alkaloids (Ephedra) Prohibited," U.S. Food and Drug Administration (FDA), February 4, 2004; and an excerpt from "Dietary Supplements Containing Ephedrine Alkaloids: Final Rule Summary," FDA, 2004.

agree that most steroid abusers are psychologically normal when they start abusing the drugs.

How are anabolic steroids used?

Some anabolic steroids are taken orally, others are injected intramuscularly, and still others are provided in gels or creams that are rubbed on the skin. Doses taken by abusers can be 10 to 100 times higher than the doses used for medical conditions.

Steroid abusers typically stack the drugs, meaning that they take two or more different anabolic steroids, mixing oral and/or injectable types, and sometimes even including compounds that are designed for veterinary use. Abusers think that the different steroids interact to produce an effect on muscle size that is greater than the effects of each drug individually, a theory that has not been tested scientifically.

Often, steroid abusers also pyramid their doses in cycles of 6 to 12 weeks. At the beginning of a cycle, the person starts with low doses of the drugs being stacked and then slowly increases the doses. In the second half of the cycle, the doses are slowly decreased to zero. This is sometimes followed by a second cycle in which the person continues to train but without drugs. Abusers believe that pyramiding allows the body time to adjust to the high doses and the drug-free cycle allows the body's hormonal system time to recuperate. As with stacking, the perceived benefits of pyramiding and cycling have not been substantiated scientifically.

What are the health consequences of steroid abuse?

Anabolic steroid abuse has been associated with a wide range of adverse side effects ranging from some that are physically unattractive such as acne and breast development in men, to others that are life-threatening such as heart attacks and liver cancer. Most are reversible if the abuser stops taking the drugs, but some are permanent.

Hormonal System: Steroid abuse disrupts the normal production of hormones in the body, causing both reversible and irreversible changes. Changes that can be reversed include reduced sperm production and shrinking of the testicles (testicular atrophy). Irreversible changes include male-pattern baldness and breast development (gynecomastia). In one study of male bodybuilders, more than half had testicular atrophy, and more than half had gynecomastia. Gynecomastia is thought to occur due to the disruption of normal hormone balance. In the female body, anabolic steroids cause masculinization.

Breast size and body fat decrease, the skin becomes coarse, the clitoris enlarges, and the voice deepens. Women may experience excessive growth of body hair but lose scalp hair. With continued administration of steroids, some of these effects are irreversible.

Musculoskeletal System: Rising levels of testosterone and other sex hormones normally trigger the growth spurt that occurs during puberty and adolescence. Subsequently, when these hormones reach certain levels, they signal the bones to stop growing, locking a person into his or her maximum height.

When a child or adolescent takes anabolic steroids, the resulting artificially high sex hormone levels can signal the bones to stop growing sooner than they normally would have done.

Cardiovascular System: Steroid abuse has been associated with cardiovascular diseases (CVD), including heart attacks and strokes, even in athletes younger than 30. Steroids contribute to the development of CVD, partly by changing the levels of lipoproteins that carry cholesterol in the blood. Steroids, particularly the oral types, increase the level of low-density lipoprotein (LDL) and decrease the level of high-density lipoprotein (HDL). High LDL and low HDL levels increase the risk of atherosclerosis, a condition in which fatty substances are deposited inside arteries and disrupt blood flow. If blood is prevented from reaching the heart, the result can be a heart attack. If blood is prevented from reaching the brain, the result can be a stroke. Steroids also increase the risk that blood clots will form in blood vessels, potentially disrupting blood flow and damaging the heart muscle so that it does not pump blood effectively.

Liver: Steroid abuse has been associated with liver tumors and a rare condition called peliosis hepatis, in which blood-filled cysts form in the liver. Both the tumors and the cysts sometimes rupture, causing internal bleeding.

Skin: Steroid abuse can cause acne, cysts, and oily hair and skin.

Infection: Many abusers who inject anabolic steroids use nonsterile injection techniques or share contaminated needles with other abusers. In addition, some steroid preparations are manufactured illegally under non-sterile conditions. These factors put abusers at risk for acquiring life-threatening viral infections, such as human immunodeficiency virus (HIV) and hepatitis B and C. Abusers also can develop infective endocarditis, a bacterial illness that causes a potentially fatal inflammation of the inner lining of the heart. Bacterial infections also can cause pain and abscess formation at injection sites.

Gamma Hydroxybutyrate (GHB)

GHB is predominantly a central nervous system depressant. Because it is often colorless, tasteless, and odorless, it can be added to beverages and ingested unknowingly.

This substance emerged a few years ago as a drug-assisted assault drug, also known as date rape drug or drug rape. Because of concern about its abuse, Congress passed the "Drug-Induced Rape Prevention and Punishment Act of 1996" in October 1996. This legislation increased Federal penalties for use of any controlled substance to aid in sexual assault.

Since about 1990, GHB (gamma hydroxybutyrate) has been abused in the U.S. for its euphoric, sedative, and anabolic (body building) effects. It is a central nervous system depressant that was widely available over-the-counter in health food stores during the 1980s and until 1992. It was purchased largely by body builders to aid in fat reduction and muscle building. Street names include liquid ecstasy, soap, easy lay, vita-G, and Georgia home boy.

Coma and seizures can occur following abuse of GHB. Combining use with other drugs such as alcohol can result in nausea and breathing difficulties. GHB may also produce withdrawal effects, including insomnia, anxiety, tremors, and sweating. GHB and two of its precursors, gamma butyrolactone (GBL) and 1,4 butanediol (BD) have been involved in poisonings, overdoses, date rapes, and deaths.

What is the extent of use?

According to the *2004 Monitoring the Future*[1] (MTF) survey, NIDA's annual survey of drug use among the Nation's high school students, annual use of GHB among 8th graders and 12th graders remained relatively stable from 2003 to 2004, but 10th graders reported a significant decrease according to MTF findings. In 2004, 0.7 percent of 8th graders, 0.8 percent of 10th graders, and 2.0 percent of 12th graders reported annual use. (Annual use refers to use at least once during the year preceding an individual's response to the survey.)

Hospital emergency department (ED) episodes involving GHB rose from 56 in 1994 to 4,969 in 2000, then declined in 2002 to 3,330. Among ED mentions involving club drugs, however, only ecstasy is cited more frequently than GHB.[2]

[1] These data are from the *2004 Monitoring the Future* survey, funded by the National Institute on Drug Abuse, National Institutes of Health, DHHS, and conducted annually by the University of Michigan's Institute for Social Research. The survey has tracked 12th graders' illicit drug use and related attitudes since 1975; in 1991, 8th and 10th graders were added to the study. The latest data are online at http://www.drugabuse.gov.

[2] Emergency department data are from the annual *Drug Abuse Warning Network*, funded by the Substance Abuse and Mental Health Services Administration, DHHS. The survey provides information about emergency department visits that are induced by or related to the use of an illicit drug or the nonmedical use of a legal drug. The latest annual data are available at 800-729-6686 or online at http://www.samhsa.gov.

Sales of Supplements Containing Ephedrine Alkaloids (Ephedra) Prohibited

On April 12, 2004, an FDA final rule went into effect prohibiting the sale of dietary supplements containing ephedrine alkaloids (ephedra).

Ephedra, also called Ma huang, is a naturally occurring substance derived from plants. Its principal active ingredient is ephedrine, which when chemically synthesized is regulated as a drug. In recent years, ephedra products have been extensively promoted to aid weight loss, enhance sports performance, and increase energy. But FDA has determined that ephedra presents an unreasonable risk of illness or injury. It has been linked to significant adverse health effects, including heart attack and stroke.

Final Rule Summary Conclusion: Multiple studies demonstrate that dietary supplements containing ephedrine alkaloids, like other sympathomimetics, raise blood pressure and increase heart rate. These products expose users to several risks, including the consequences of a sustained increase in blood pressure (e.g., serious illnesses or injuries including stroke and heart attack that can result in death). There is also a risk of increased morbidity and mortality from worsened heart failure and pro-arrhythmic effects. Although the pro-arrhythmic effects of these products typically occur only in susceptible individuals, the long-term risks from elevated blood pressure can occur even in nonsusceptible, healthy individuals.

427

These risks are not outweighed by the known or reasonable likely benefits of dietary supplements containing ephedrine alkaloids. These products do not provide a meaningful health benefit. The best clinical evidence for a benefit is for weight loss, but even there, the evidence supports only a modest short-term weight loss insufficient to positively affect cardiovascular risk factors or health conditions associated with being overweight or obese. Other possible benefits, such as enhanced athletic performance, enhanced energy, or a feeling of alertness, lack scientific support and/or they would provide only temporary benefits that are trivial in comparison to the risks.

Additional Information

National Institute on Drug Abuse (NIDA)
National Institutes of Health
6001 Executive Blvd., Room 5213
Bethesda, MD 20892-9561
Phone: 301-443-1124
Website: http://www.drugabuse.gov
E-mail: information@nida.nih.gov

National Clearinghouse for Drug and Alcohol Information (NCDAI)
Toll-Free: 800-729-6686
Toll-Free TDD: 800-487-4889
Website: http://ncadi.samhsa.gov

U.S. Food and Drug Administration (FDA)
5600 Fishers Lane
Rockville, MD 20857
Toll-Free: 888-463-6335
Website: http://www.fda.gov

Part Seven

Nutrition for People with Specific Medical Concerns

Chapter 50

Artificial Hydration and Nutrition

When do people need artificial hydration and nutrition?

If a patient isn't able to swallow because of a medical problem, he or she can be given fluids and nutrition in ways other than by mouth. This is referred to as artificial hydration and nutrition. This is sometimes done when someone is recovering from a temporary problem. It may also be done when someone has an advanced, life-threatening illness and is dying.

What is involved in artificial nutrition and hydration?

An intravenous (IV) catheter (a thin plastic tube that slides in over a needle) may be placed in the vein under the patient's skin. Fluids and sometimes nutrition are given through the catheter.

Another method of artificial nutrition and hydration is through a plastic tube called a nasogastric tube (also called an NG tube). This tube is put through the nose, down the throat, and into the stomach.

It can only be left in for a short time, usually 1 to 4 weeks. If the tube has to be in longer, a different kind of feeding tube may be used. It's placed into the wall of the stomach (also called a PEG [percutaneous endoscopic gastrotomy] tube or g-tube).

What happens if artificial hydration or nutrition are not given?

Persons who don't receive any food or fluids will eventually fall into a deep sleep (coma) and usually die in 1 to 3 weeks.

What are the benefits?

A person with a temporary illness who can't swallow may be hungry and thirsty. A feeding tube may help. Sometimes a person may become confused because of dehydration. Dehydration is when the body doesn't get enough fluids. Giving a patient fluid through a tube reduces dehydration and may lessen his or her confusion. Giving fluids and nutrition helps the patient as he or she is recovering.

For a patient with an advanced life-threatening illness who is dying, artificial hydration and nutrition may not provide many benefits. Artificial hydration and nutrition in these patients may make the patient live a little longer, but not always.

What are the risks?

There's always a risk when someone is fed through a tube. Liquid might enter the lungs. This can cause coughing and pneumonia. Feeding tubes may feel uncomfortable. They can become plugged, causing pain, nausea, and vomiting. Feeding tubes may also cause infections. Sometimes, patients may need to be physically restrained or sedated to keep them from pulling out the feeding tube.

How do we decide whether to use artificial hydration and nutrition?

The patient and his or her family should talk with the doctor about the patient's medical condition, and the risks and benefits of giving artificial hydration and nutrition. Each situation is different. Your doctor can help you make the decision that is right for the patient and family.

Making the Decision: Tube Feeding—Frequently Asked Questions

What is a feeding tube?

Feeding tubes may provide nutrition to people who have difficulty swallowing or unable to eat for medical reasons. A feeding tube is device which transports liquid nutrition to your stomach. A feeding tube can be inserted into the stomach (G-tubes), through the nose and into the stomach (NG-tubes), or through the nose and into the small intestine (NJ tubes). The NG and NJ tubes are considered to be temporary and the G tube is considered more permanent, but it can be removed.

In some circumstances, a person with a feeding tube can continue eating. Here, the feeding tube is providing additional nutrition because of poor intake by the patient. However, the majority of feeding tubes are inserted because the patient has difficulty swallowing, and they are unable to continue eating without the risk of swallowing food into the lungs.

The decision to use or not use a feeding tube must be made carefully. Discuss it with your physician, your family, and other persons important to you. It is the patient's right to use or not use a feeding tube. For the persons with severe dementia, a physician must rely on previously stated preferences in an advanced directive, or rely on a family member to provide information on the patient's wishes. A decision to use or not use a feeding tube must be made by weighing the risks and benefits.

Does tube feeding prevent aspiration pneumonia?

Aspiration pneumonia is caused by food going into the lungs rather than the stomach. Aspiration pneumonia is common in persons with advance dementia and often indicates that persons are dying. Surprisingly, there is no evidence that tube feedings prevent aspiration pneumonias. Even if tube fed, a person is always producing saliva. Tube feeding does not correct the swallowing problem with dementia, and the patient is still at risk of aspiration pneumonia. Research has found that despite feeding tubes, dementia patients still have a high risk of aspiration pneumonia.

Does tube feeding prolong a person's life?

Data suggests that tube feeding is beneficial if the patient has a reversible illness, which is usually not the case in patients who have

433

advanced dementia. If a person is actively dying, their body no longer absorbs nutrients and cannot utilize the nutrients for the work of the body. Therefore, tube feeding at the end stages of dementia may not be beneficial in prolonging a person's life. Vigorous hand feeding for some persons can prevent the use of a feeding tube. Stopping, or not starting, a feeding tube in someone who cannot be hand fed will result in death. In making a decision regarding the use of a feeding tube, ask for a swallowing evaluation by a specialist. There are no easy answers. You should discuss it with your physician and family.

Does tube feeding increase quality of life and reduce suffering?

Tube feedings can cause discomfort, the need for physical restraints to prevent the tube from being pulled out, and increased risk infection. Terminally ill patients rarely experience hunger or thirst. Of those who do, relief is achieved with small amounts of food and fluids, or by ice chips and lip lubrication. In addition, tube-fed patients with advanced dementia may miss the human contact that comes with assisted oral feeding.

Are there alternatives to tube feeding?

Getting an appropriate evaluation is the key. Discontinuing medications may reduce eating difficulties. Some drugs, such as sedatives, tranquilizers, and anti-cholinergics, may cause difficulty swallowing.

Interventions such as medication adjustments, use of assistive devices, changing the type of food, proper feeding technique, and dental care may prevent the use of a feeding tube. Useful techniques include: the use of finger foods and preferred foods; strong flavors; hot or cold rather than tepid food; and gravy, juices, and enrichers such as cream. Other helpful techniques are reminders to swallow and swallow multiple times per bolus (bolus size of less than 1 teaspoon); gentle coughs after each swallow; liquid supplements; and facilitation techniques such as vibration, gentle brushing, and icing of the cheeks and neck may help. Getting a feeding specialist, usually a speech therapist, is an important first step.

Where do I turn for help?

Support can come from your family and professionals who can offer guidance and assist with this kind of decision-making including your physician, nurse, social worker, speech therapist, chaplain, or dietitian. Support from clergy often helps guide a family through this decision. In addition, some hospitals and nursing homes have ethics committees who can assist with decision-making on alternative feeding. The best advice is for persons to state preferences concerning the use of a feeding tube in a written advance directive.

Chapter 51

Cancer: Nutrition Care

Overview of Nutrition in Cancer Care

Cancer and Cancer Treatments May Cause Nutrition-Related Side Effects

The diet is an important part of cancer treatment. Eating the right kinds of foods before, during, and after treatment can help the patient feel better and stay stronger. To ensure proper nutrition, a person has to eat and drink enough of the foods that contain key nutrients (vitamins, minerals, protein, carbohydrates, fat, and water). For many patients, however, some side effects of cancer and cancer treatments make it difficult to eat well. Symptoms that interfere with eating include anorexia, nausea, vomiting, diarrhea, constipation, mouth sores, trouble with swallowing, and pain. Appetite, taste, smell, and the ability to eat enough food or absorb the nutrients from food may be affected. Malnutrition (lack of key nutrients) can result, causing the patient to be weak, tired, and unable to resist infections or withstand cancer therapies. Eating too little protein and calories is the most common nutrition problem facing many cancer patients. Protein and calories are important for healing, fighting infection, and providing energy.

Excerpts from PDQ® Cancer Information Summary. National Cancer Institute; Bethesda, MD. Nutrition in Cancer Care (PDQ®): Supportive Care–Patient. Updated 05/2005. Available at http://cancer.gov. Accessed August 29, 2005.

Anorexia and Cachexia Are Common Causes of Malnutrition in Cancer Patients

Anorexia (the loss of appetite or desire to eat) is a common symptom in people with cancer. Anorexia may occur early in the disease or later, when the tumor grows and spreads. Some patients may have anorexia when they are diagnosed with cancer. Almost all patients who have widespread cancer will develop anorexia. Anorexia is the most common cause of malnutrition in cancer patients. Cachexia is a wasting syndrome that causes weakness and a loss of weight, fat, and muscle. It commonly occurs in patients with tumors of the lung, pancreas, and upper gastrointestinal tract and less often in patients with breast cancer or lower gastrointestinal cancer. Anorexia and cachexia often occur together. Weight loss can be caused by eating fewer calories, using more calories, or a combination of the two. Cachexia can occur in people who are eating enough, but who cannot absorb the nutrients. Cachexia is not related to the tumor size, type, or extent. Cancer cachexia is not the same as starvation. A healthy person's body can adjust to starvation by slowing down its use of nutrients, but in cancer patients, the body does not make this adjustment.

Good Eating Habits during Cancer Care Help the Patient Cope

Nutrition therapy can help cancer patients get the nutrients needed to maintain body weight and strength, prevent body tissue from breaking down, rebuild tissue, and fight infection. Eating guidelines for cancer patients can be very different from the usual suggestions for healthful eating. Nutrition recommendations for cancer patients are designed to help the patient cope with the effects of the cancer and its treatment. Some cancer treatments are more effective if the patient is well nourished and getting enough calories and protein in the diet. People who eat well during cancer treatment may even be able to handle higher doses of certain treatments. Being well-nourished has been linked to a better prognosis (chance of recovery).

Nutrition Therapy Overview

Nutrition Screening and Assessment

- Finding and treating nutrition problems early may improve the patient's prognosis.

- Screening and assessment are done before beginning anticancer therapy, and assessment continues throughout treatment.

- Ongoing assessment is completed by a healthcare team with expertise in nutritional management.

Goals of Nutrition Therapy

The goals of nutrition therapy for cancer patients in active treatment and recovery are designed to restore nutrient shortages, maintain nutritional health, and prevent complications. The goals of nutrition therapy for patients in active treatment and recovery are to do the following:

- Prevent or correct malnutrition
- Prevent wasting of muscle, bone, blood, organs, and other lean body mass
- Help the patient tolerate treatment
- Reduce nutrition-related side effects and complications
- Maintain strength and energy
- Protect ability to fight infection
- Help recovery and healing
- Maintain or improve quality of life

Good nutrition continues to be important for patients who are in remission or whose cancer has been cured.

The goals of nutrition therapy for patients who have advanced cancer are designed to improve the quality of life including the following:

- Reduce side effects
- Reduce risk of infection
- Maintain strength and energy
- Improve quality of life

Methods of Nutrition Care

Nutrition support provides nutrition to patients who cannot eat normally. Eating by mouth is the preferred method and should be used whenever possible, but some patients may not be able to take any or enough food by mouth due to complications from cancer or cancer treatment. A patient may be fed using enteral nutrition (through a tube inserted into the stomach or intestine), or parenteral nutrition (infused into the bloodstream directly). Enteral nutrition keeps the stomach and intestines working normally and has fewer complications than parenteral nutrition. Nutrients are used more easily by the body in enteral feeding.

Patients with certain conditions are most appropriate for treatment with nutrition support. Nutrition support may be helpful for patients who have one or more of the following characteristics:

- Low body weight
- Inability to absorb nutrients
- Holes or draining abscesses in the esophagus or stomach
- Inability to eat or drink by mouth for more than 5 days
- Moderate or high nutritional risk
- Ability, along with the caregiver, to handle tube feedings at home

Enteral Nutrition

Enteral nutrition is also called tube feeding. Enteral nutrition is food (in liquid form) given to the patient through a tube that is inserted into the stomach or the small intestine.

If the tube is placed in the stomach, food may be given through the tube continuously or in batches several times a day. If the tube is placed in the small intestine, the food is delivered continuously. Different formulas are available. Some provide complete nutrition and others provide certain nutrients. Formulas that meet the patient's specific needs are selected. Formulas are available for patients who have other health conditions, such as diabetes.

Enteral nutrition is sometimes used when the patient is able to eat small amounts by mouth, but cannot obtain enough food that way. The patient may continue to eat or drink as able, and the tube feeding provides the balance of calories and nutrients that are needed.

Enteral nutrition may be appropriate for patients whose gastrointestinal tract is still working. Enteral nutrition continues to use the stomach and/or intestines to digest food. Enteral nutrition may be used for patients who have cancer of the head, neck, or digestive system and whose treatment with chemotherapy and radiation therapy causes side effects that limit eating or drinking.

Enteral nutrition is not appropriate for the following patients:

- Patients whose stomach and intestines are not working or have been removed

- Patients who have a blockage in the bowel

- Patients who have severe nausea, vomiting, and/or diarrhea

- Patients whose platelet count is low. Platelets are blood cells that help prevent bleeding by causing blood clots to form

- Patients who have low levels of all blood cells (white blood cells, red blood cells, and platelets)

Enteral nutrition may continue after a patient leaves the hospital. If enteral nutrition is to be part of the patient's care after leaving the hospital, the patient and caregiver will be trained in use of the tube and pump, and in care of the patient. The home must be clean and the patient must be monitored often by the nutrition support team.

Parenteral Nutrition

Parenteral nutrition provides the patient with nutrients delivered into the blood stream. Parenteral nutrition is used when the patient cannot take food by mouth or by enteral feeding. Parenteral feeding bypasses the normal digestive system. Nutrients are delivered to the patient directly into the blood, through a catheter (thin tube) inserted into a vein. Patients with the following problems may benefit from parenteral nutrition:

- Stomach and intestines that are not working or have been removed

- Severe nausea, diarrhea, or vomiting

- Severe sores in the mouth or esophagus

- A fistula (hole) in the stomach or esophagus

- Loss of body weight and muscle with enteral nutrition

Trained medical staff should manage the use of parenteral nutrition. The techniques and formulas involved in parenteral nutrition support are precise and require management by trained medical staff or a nutrition support team. However, parenteral nutrition support may continue after a patient leaves the hospital. If parenteral nutrition is to be part of the patient's care after leaving the hospital, the patient and caregiver will be trained in the procedures and in care of the patient. The home must be clean and the patient must be monitored often by the nutrition support team.

Experienced medical staff should manage the patient's removal from parenteral nutrition support. Going off parenteral nutrition support needs to be done gradually and under medical supervision. The parenteral feedings are reduced by small amounts over time as the patient is changed to enteral or oral feeding.

Nutrition Suggestions for Symptom Relief

When side effects of cancer or cancer treatment interfere with normal eating, adjustments can be made to ensure the patient continues to get the necessary nutrition. Medications may be given to stimulate the appetite. Eating foods that are high in calories, protein, vitamins, and minerals is usually advised. Meal planning, however, should be individualized to meet the patient's nutritional needs and tastes in food.

Anorexia

Anorexia (lack of appetite) is one of the most common problems for cancer patients. The following suggestions may help cancer patients manage anorexia:

- Eat small high-protein and high-calorie meals every 1–2 hours instead of 3 larger meals.

- Have help with preparing meals.

- Add extra calories and protein to food (such as butter, skim milk powder, honey, or brown sugar).

- Take liquid supplements (special drinks containing nutrients), soups, milk, juices, shakes, and smoothies when eating solid food is a problem.

- Eat snacks that contain plenty of calories and protein.

- Prepare and store small portions of favorite foods so they are ready to eat when hungry.

- Eat breakfasts that contain one-third of the calories and protein needed for the day.

- Eat foods with odors that are appealing. Strong odors can be avoided by using boiling bags, cooking outdoors on the grill, using a kitchen fan when cooking, serving cold food instead of hot (since odors are in the rising steam), and taking off any food covers to release the odors before entering a patient's room. Small portable fans can be used to blow food odors away from patients. Cooking odors can be avoided by ordering take-out food.

- Try new foods. Be creative with desserts. Experiment with recipes, flavorings, spices, types, and consistencies of food. Food likes and dislikes may change from day to day.

The following high-calorie, high-protein foods are recommended:

- Cheese and crackers
- Muffins
- Puddings
- Nutritional supplements
- Milkshakes
- Yogurt
- Ice cream
- Powdered milk added to foods such as pudding, milkshakes, or any recipe using milk
- Finger foods (handy for snacking) such as deviled eggs, cream cheese or peanut butter on crackers or celery, or deviled ham on crackers

Taste Changes

Changes in how foods taste may be caused by radiation treatment, dental problems, or medicines. Cancer patients often complain of changes in their sense of taste when undergoing chemotherapy, in particular a bitter taste sensation. A sudden dislike for certain foods may occur. This may result in food avoidance, weight loss, and anorexia, which can greatly reduce the patients' quality of life. Some or all of the sense of taste may return, but it may be a year after treatment ends before the sense of taste is normal again. Drinking plenty of fluids, changing the types of foods eaten, and adding spices or flavorings to food may help.

The following suggestions may help cancer patients manage changes in taste:

- Rinse mouth with water before eating.

- Try citrus fruits (oranges, tangerines, lemons, grapefruit) unless mouth sores are present.

- Eat small meals and healthy snacks several times a day.

- Eat meals when hungry rather than at set mealtimes.

- Use plastic utensils if foods taste metallic.

- Try favorite foods.

- Eat with family and friends.

- Have others prepare meals.

- Try new foods when feeling best.

- Substitute poultry, fish, eggs, and cheese for red meat.

- Find non-meat, high-protein recipes in a vegetarian or Chinese cookbook.

- Use sugar-free lemon drops, gum, or mints if there is a metallic or bitter taste in the mouth.

- Add spices and sauces to foods.

- Eat meat with something sweet, such as cranberry sauce, jelly, or applesauce.

- Taking zinc sulfate tablets during radiation therapy to the head and neck may speed the return of normal taste after treatment.

Dry Mouth

Dry mouth is often caused by radiation therapy to the head and neck. Some medicines may also cause dry mouth. Dry mouth may affect speech, taste, ability to swallow, and the use of dentures or braces. There is also an increased risk of cavities and gum disease because less saliva is produced to wash the teeth and gums. The main treatment for dry mouth is drinking plenty of liquids, about ½ ounce per pound of body weight per day.

Other suggestions to manage dry mouth include the following:

- Eat moist foods with extra sauces, gravies, butter, or margarine.

- Suck on hard candy or chew gum.
- Eat frozen desserts (such as frozen grapes and ice pops) or ice chips.
- Clean teeth (including dentures) and rinse mouth at least four times per day (after each meal and before bedtime).
- Keep water handy at all times to moisten the mouth.
- Avoid liquids and foods that contain a lot of sugar.
- Avoid mouth rinses containing alcohol.
- Drink fruit nectar instead of juice.
- Use a straw to drink liquids.

Mouth Sores and Infections

Mouth sores can result from chemotherapy and radiation therapy. These treatments target rapidly-growing cells because cancer cells grow rapidly. Normal cells inside the mouth may be damaged by these cancer treatments because they also grow rapidly. Mouth sores may become infected and bleed, making eating difficult. By choosing certain foods and taking good care of their mouths, patients can usually make eating easier. Suggestions to help manage mouth sores and infections include the following:

- Eat soft foods that are easy to chew and swallow, such as the following:
  - Soft fruits, including bananas, applesauce, and watermelon
  - Peach, pear, and apricot nectars
  - Cottage cheese
  - Mashed potatoes
  - Macaroni and cheese
  - Custards; puddings
  - Gelatin
  - Milkshakes
  - Scrambled eggs
  - Oatmeal or other cooked cereals
- Use the blender to process vegetables (such as potatoes, peas, and carrots) and meats until smooth.

- Avoid rough, coarse, or dry foods, including raw vegetables, granola, toast, and crackers.

- Avoid foods that are spicy or salty. Avoid foods that are acidic, such as vinegar, pickles, and olives.

- Avoid citrus fruits and juices, including orange, grapefruit, and tangerine.

- Cook foods until soft and tender.

- Cut foods into small pieces.

- Use a straw to drink liquids.

- Eat foods cold or at room temperature. Hot and warm foods can irritate a tender mouth.

- Clean teeth (including dentures) and rinse mouth at least four times per day (after each meal and before bedtime).

- Add gravy, broth, or sauces to food.

- Drink high-calorie, high-protein drinks in addition to meals.

- Numb the mouth with ice chips or flavored ice pops.

Using a mouth rinse that contains glutamine may reduce the number of mouth sores. Glutamine is a substance found in plant and animal proteins.

Nausea

Nausea caused by cancer treatment can affect the amount and kinds of food eaten. The following suggestions may help cancer patients manage nausea:

- Eat before cancer treatments.

- Avoid foods that are likely to cause nausea. For some patients, this includes spicy foods, greasy foods, and foods that have strong odors.

- Eat small meals several times a day.

- Slowly sip fluids throughout the day.

- Eat dry foods such as crackers, breadsticks, or toast throughout the day.

- Sit up or lie with the upper body raised for one hour after eating.

- Eat bland, soft, easy-to-digest foods rather than heavy meals.

- Avoid eating in a room that has cooking odors or that is overly warm. Keep the living space at a comfortable temperature and with plenty of fresh air.

- Rinse out the mouth before and after eating.

- Suck on hard candies such as peppermints or lemon drops if the mouth has a bad taste.

Diarrhea

Diarrhea may be caused by cancer treatments, surgery on the stomach or intestines, or by emotional stress. Long-term diarrhea may lead to dehydration (lack of water in the body) and/or low levels of salt and potassium, important minerals needed by the body. The following suggestions may help cancer patients manage diarrhea:

- Eat broth, soups, sports drinks, bananas, and canned fruits to help replace salt and potassium lost by diarrhea.

- Avoid greasy foods, hot or cold liquids, and caffeine.

- Avoid high-fiber foods—especially dried beans and cruciferous vegetables (such as broccoli, cauliflower, and cabbage).

- Drink plenty of fluids through the day. Room temperature liquids may cause fewer problems than hot or cold liquids.

- Limit milk to 2 cups, or eliminate milk and milk products until the source of the problem is found.

- Limit gas-forming foods and beverages such as peas, lentils, cruciferous vegetables, chewing gum, and soda.

- Limit sugar-free candies or gum made with sorbitol (sugar alcohol).

- Drink at least one cup of liquid after each loose bowel movement.

Taking oral glutamine may help keep the intestines healthy when taking the anticancer drug fluorouracil.

Low White Blood Cell Count

Cancer patients may have a low white blood cell count for a variety of reasons, some of which include radiation therapy, chemotherapy, or the cancer itself. Patients who have a low white blood cell count are at an increased risk of infection. The following suggestions may help cancer patients prevent infections when white blood cell counts are low:

- Check dates on food and do not buy or use the food if it is out of date.
- Do not buy or use food in cans that are swollen, dented, or damaged.
- Thaw foods in the refrigerator or microwave. Never thaw foods at room temperature. Cook foods immediately after thawing.
- Refrigerate all leftovers within 2 hours of cooking and eat them within 24 hours.
- Keep hot foods hot, and cold foods cold.
- Avoid old, moldy, or damaged fruits and vegetables.
- Avoid unwrapped tofu sold in open bins or containers.
- Cook all meat, poultry, and fish thoroughly. Avoid raw eggs or raw fish.
- Buy foods packed as single servings to avoid leftovers.
- Avoid salad bars and buffets when eating out.
- Avoid large groups of people and people who have infections.
- Wash hands often to prevent the spread of bacteria.

Hot Flashes

Hot flashes occur in most women with breast cancer and men with prostate cancer. When caused by natural or treatment-related menopause, hot flashes can be relieved with estrogen replacement. Many women, however, (including women with breast cancer), are not able to take estrogen replacement. Eating soy foods, which contain an estrogen-like substance, is sometimes suggested to relieve hot flashes in patients who cannot take estrogen replacement, but no benefit has been proven.

Fluid Intake

The body needs plenty of water to replace the fluids lost every day. Long-term diarrhea, nausea, vomiting, and pain may prevent the patient from drinking and eating enough to get the water needed by the body. One of the first signs of dehydration (lack of water in the body) is extreme tiredness. The following suggestions may help cancer patients prevent dehydration:

- Drink 8 to 12 cups of liquids a day. This can be water, juice, milk, or foods that contain a large amount of liquid such as puddings, ice cream, ice pops, flavored ices, and gelatins.

- Take a water bottle whenever leaving home. It is important to drink even if not thirsty, as thirst is not a good sign of fluid needs.

- Limit drinks that contain caffeine, such as sodas, coffee, and tea (both hot and cold).

- Drink most liquids after and/or between meals.

- Use medicines that help relieve nausea and vomiting.

Constipation

Constipation is defined as fewer than 3 bowel movements per week. It is a very common problem for cancer patients and may result from lack of water or fiber in the diet; lack of physical activity; anticancer therapies such as chemotherapy; and medications. Prevention of constipation is a part of cancer care. The following suggestions may help cancer patients prevent constipation:

- Eat more fiber-containing foods on a regular basis. The recommended fiber intake is 25 to 35 grams per day. Increase fiber gradually and drink plenty of fluids at the same time to keep the fiber moving through the intestines.

- Drink 8 to 10 cups of fluid each day. Water, prune juice, warm juices, lemonade, and tea without caffeine can be very helpful.

- Take walks and exercise regularly. Proper footwear is important.

If constipation does occur, the following suggestions for diet, exercise, and medication may help correct it:

- Continue to eat high-fiber foods and drink plenty of fluids. Try adding wheat bran to the diet; begin with 2 heaping tablespoons each day for 3 days, then increase by 1 tablespoon each day until constipation is relieved. Do not exceed 6 tablespoons per day.

- Maintain physical activity.

- Include over-the-counter constipation treatments, if necessary. This refers to bulk-forming products (such as Citrucel, Metamucil, Fiberall, FiberCon, and Fiber-Lax); stimulants (such as Dulcolax tablets or suppositories and Senokot); stool softeners (such as Colace, Surfak, and Dialose); and osmotics (such as milk of magnesia). Cottonseed and aerosol enemas can also help relieve the problem. Lubricants such as mineral oil are not recommended because they may prevent the body's use of important nutrients.

Other Nutrition Issues

Advanced Cancer

Nutrition-related side effects may occur or become worse as cancer becomes more advanced. The usual treatment for these problems in patients with advanced cancer is palliative care to reduce the symptoms and improve the quality of life. Palliative care includes nutrition therapy and/or drug therapy. Eating less solid food is common in advanced cancer. Patients usually prefer soft foods and clear liquids. Those who have problems swallowing may do better with thick liquids than with thin liquids.

When cancer is advanced, food should be viewed as a source of enjoyment. Eating should not just be about calories, protein, and other nutrient needs. Dietary restriction is not usually necessary, as intake of prohibited foods (such as sweets for a patient with diabetes) is not enough to be of concern. Some patients, however, may need certain diet restrictions. For example, patients who have pancreatic cancer, uterine cancer, ovarian cancer, or another cancer affecting the abdominal area may need a soft diet (no raw fruits or vegetables, no nuts, no skins, no seeds) to prevent a blockage in the bowel. Diet restrictions should be considered in terms of quality of life and the patient's wishes.

The benefits and risks of nutrition support vary for each patient. Decisions about using nutrition support should be made with the following considerations:

- Will quality of life be improved?

- Do the possible benefits outweigh the risks and costs?

- Is there an advanced directive? An advanced directive is a written instruction about the provision of health care or power of attorney in the event an individual can no longer make his or her wishes known.

- What are the wishes and needs of the family?

Cancer patients and their caregivers have the right to make informed decisions. The healthcare team, with guidance from a registered dietitian, should inform patients and their caregivers about the benefits and risks of using nutrition support in advanced disease. In most cases, the risks outweigh the benefits. However, for someone who still has good quality of life, but also physical barriers to achieving adequate food and water by mouth, enteral feedings may be appropriate. Parenteral support is not usually appropriate.

Weight Loss and Drug-Nutrient Interactions

Weight loss that results from cancer and its treatment may cause a number of symptoms and side effects. Early treatment of anorexia with nutrition therapy and drugs can help the patient maintain a healthy weight.

Cancer patients may be treated with a number of drugs throughout their care. Some foods or nutritional supplements do not mix safely with certain drugs. The combination of these foods and drugs may reduce or change the effectiveness of anticancer therapy or cause life-threatening side effects. The combination of some herbs with certain foods and drugs may reduce or change the effectiveness of anticancer therapy or cause life-threatening side effects.

Always discuss questions about nutrition and medications with your health care providers.

Additional Information

American Institute for Cancer Research
1759 R Street N.W.
Washington, DC 20009
Toll-Free: 800-843-8114
Phone: 202-328-7744
Fax: 202-328-7226
Website: http://www.aicr.org
E-mail: aicrweb@aicr.org

National Cancer Institute (NCI)
Toll-Free: 800-4-CANCER (800-422-6237)
Toll-Free TTY: 800-332-8615
Website: http://www.cancer.gov
E-mail: cancergovstaff@mail.nih.gov.

Chapter 52

Celiac Disease

Celiac disease is a digestive disease that damages the small intestine and interferes with absorption of nutrients from food. People who have celiac disease cannot tolerate a protein called gluten, which is found in wheat, rye, and barley. When people with celiac disease eat foods containing gluten, their immune system responds by damaging the small intestine. Specifically, tiny finger-like protrusions, called villi, on the lining of the small intestine are lost. Nutrients from food are absorbed into the bloodstream through these villi. Without villi, a person becomes malnourished—regardless of the quantity of food eaten.

Because the body's own immune system causes the damage, celiac disease is considered an autoimmune disorder. However, it is also classified as a disease of malabsorption because nutrients are not absorbed. Celiac disease is also known as celiac sprue, nontropical sprue, and gluten-sensitive enteropathy.

Celiac disease is a genetic disease, meaning that it runs in families. Sometimes the disease is triggered—or becomes active for the

This chapter includes excerpts from "Celiac Disease," National Institute of Diabetes and Digestive and Kidney Diseases (NIDDK), NIH Publication No. 04–4269, February 2004. Also, text under the heading, "Gluten-Free Diet Examples," is from "Celiac Disease and the Gluten-free Diet: An Overview," by Marion Zarkadas, MSc, RD and Shelley Case, BSc, Rd. *Topics in Clinical Nutrition* 2005 April–June: 20 (2): 127–138. © 2005 Lippincott Williams and Wilkins. Reprinted with permission.

first time—after surgery, pregnancy, childbirth, viral infection, or severe emotional stress.

Treatment for Celiac Disease

The only treatment for celiac disease is to follow a gluten-free diet—that is, to avoid all foods that contain gluten. For most people, following this diet will stop symptoms, heal existing intestinal damage, and prevent further damage. Improvements begin within days of starting the diet, and the small intestine is usually completely healed—meaning the villi are intact and working—in 3 to 6 months. (It may take up to 2 years for older adults.)

The gluten-free diet is a lifetime requirement. Eating any gluten, no matter how small an amount, can damage the intestine. This is true for anyone with the disease, including people who do not have noticeable symptoms. Depending on a person's age at diagnosis, some problems, such as delayed growth and tooth discoloration, may not improve.

A small percentage of people with celiac disease do not improve on the gluten-free diet. These people often have severely damaged intestines that cannot heal even after they eliminate gluten from their diet. Because their intestines are not absorbing enough nutrients, they may need to receive intravenous nutrition supplements. Drug treatments are being evaluated for unresponsive celiac disease. These patients may need to be evaluated for complications of the disease.

The Gluten-Free Diet

A gluten-free diet means avoiding all foods that contain wheat (including spelt, triticale, and kamut), rye, and barley—in other words,

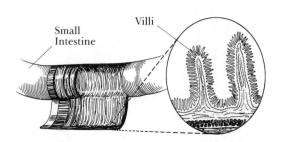

Figure 52.1. Villi on the lining of the small intestine help absorb nutrients.

most grain, pasta, cereal, and many processed foods. Despite these restrictions, people with celiac disease can eat a well-balanced diet with a variety of foods, including bread and pasta. For example, instead of wheat flour, people can use potato, rice, soy, or bean flour. Or, they can buy gluten-free bread, pasta, and other products from special food companies. Plain meat, fish, rice, fruits, and vegetables do not contain gluten, so people with celiac disease can eat as much of these foods as they like.

Whether people with celiac disease should avoid oats is controversial because some people have been able to eat oats without having a reaction. Scientists are doing studies to find out whether people with celiac disease can tolerate oats. Until the studies are complete, people with celiac disease should follow their physician or dietitian's advice about eating oats. A dietitian is a health care professional who specializes in food and nutrition.

The gluten-free diet is complicated. It requires a completely new approach to eating that affects a person's entire life. People with celiac disease have to be extremely careful about what they buy for lunch at school or work, eat at cocktail parties, or grab from the refrigerator for a midnight snack. Eating out can be a challenge as the person with celiac disease learns to scrutinize the menu for foods with gluten, and question the waiter or chef about possible hidden sources of gluten. Hidden sources of gluten include additives, preservatives, and stabilizers found in processed food, medicines, and mouthwash. If ingredients are not itemized, you may want to check with the manufacturer of the product. With practice, screening for gluten becomes second nature.

A dietitian can help people learn about their new diet. Also, support groups are particularly helpful for newly diagnosed people and their families as they learn to adjust to a new way of life.

Prevalence of Celiac Disease

Celiac disease is the most common genetic disease in Europe. In Italy about 1 in 250 people and in Ireland about 1 in 300 people have celiac disease. Recent studies have shown that it may be more common in Africa, South America, and Asia than previously believed.

Until recently, celiac disease was thought to be uncommon in the United States. However, studies have shown that celiac disease occurs in an estimated 1 in 133 Americans. Among people who have a first-degree relative diagnosed with celiac, as many as 1 in 22 people may have the disease. A recent study in which random blood samples from the Red Cross were tested for celiac disease suggests that as many as 1 in every 250 Americans may have it. Celiac disease could be under-diagnosed in the United States for a number of reasons:

- Celiac symptoms can be attributed to other problems.
- Many doctors are not knowledgeable about the disease.
- Only a handful of U.S. laboratories are experienced and skilled in testing for celiac disease.

More research is needed to find out the true prevalence of celiac disease among Americans.

Gluten-Free Diet Examples

Flours, Cereal, and Starches Allowed on a Gluten-Free Diet

- Arrowroot
- Amaranth
- Buckwheat
- Corn
- Flax
- Indian rice grass (Montina™)
- Legume flours (bean, chickpea/garbanzo, lentil, pea)
- Millet
- Nut flours (almond, hazelnut, pecan)
- Potato flour
- Potato starch
- Quinoa
- Rice (black, brown, glutinous/sweet, white, wild)
- Rice bran
- Rice polish
- Sago
- Sorghum
- Soy
- Sweet potato flour
- Tapioca (cassava/manioc)
- Teff

Table 52.1. Examples of Foods That Are Allowed on a Gluten-Free Diet and Foods to Question

Food Group	Foods allowed on a gluten-free diet	Foods to question
Grain products	Breads and baked goods, cereals, and pastas made with allowed cereals, flours, and starches	Rice and corn cereals (often have barley or malt added), buckwheat pasta
Fruits and vegetables	All fresh, frozen, and canned, with no gluten-containing sauces	Fruit pie fillings, dried fruits, french fries in restaurants
Meat and alternates	Meats: plain fresh, frozen, canned (no gluten fillers or thickened gravy) Eggs: fresh or frozen Legumes: lentils, chick peas, beans, peas, fresh, canned, and dried (no gluten-containing sauces) seeds and nuts—plain	Processed meats, for example, ham, luncheon meats such as bologna, salami, meat loaf, meat patties, sausages, pate, wieners, imitation fish Dry roasted nuts Baked beans
Milk and milk products	Plain milk products, including milk, cream, yogurt, butter-milk, cheese, most ice creams, processed and plain cheeses	Milk drinks, flavored yogurt, frozen yogurt, sour cream, cheese sauces and spreads
Miscellaneous	Fats and oils: all fats and oils and some salad dressings Soups: all made with allowed ingredients Desserts: gelatin, sherbet, custard, some rice pudding, whipped toppings, baked goods, all made with allowed ingredients Beverages: regular tea, coffee, cocoa, soft drinks, distilled alcoholic beverages Sweets: honey, jam, jelly, marmalade, maple syrup, sugar, candy made with allowed ingredients Condiments: plain pickles, relish, olives, ketchup, plain mustard, spices, vinegar (except malt vinegar), gluten-free soy sauce Snacks: plain popcorn, nuts, and soy nuts	Salad dressings (may contain wheat four or modified food starch) Canned soup, soup mixes, bases, bouillon cubes Milk puddings, custard powder, pudding mixes Flavored, herbal, and instant tea; coffee substitutes, chocolate drinks and mixes Chocolate bars Seasoning mixes Flavored potato chips, corn and taco chips

457

Additional Information

American Celiac Society
57 Crystal Ave.
West Orange, NJ 07052
Phone: 504-737-3293
Fax: 973-669-8808
E-mail:
amerceliacsoc@onebox.com

American Dietetic Association
120 S. Riverside Plaza
Suite 2000
Chicago, IL 60606-6995
Toll-Free: 800-877-1600
Fax: 312-89904899
Website: http://
www.eatright.org/Public
E-mail: hotline@eatright.org

Celiac Disease Foundation
13251 Ventura Blvd., #1
Studio City, CA 91604
Phone: 818-990-2354
Fax: 818-990-2379
Website: http://www.celiac.org
E-mail: cdf@celiac.org

Celiac Sprue Association/ USA Inc.
P.O. Box 31700
Omaha, NE 68131-0700
Toll-Free: 877-CSA-4CSA (272-4272)
Phone: 402-558-0600
Fax: 402-558-1347
Website: http://
www.csaceliacs.org
E-mail: celiacs@csaceliacs.org

Gluten Intolerance Group (GIG) of North America
15110 10th Ave. S.W., Suite A
Seattle, WA 98166
Phone: 206-246-6652
Fax: 206-246-6531
Website: http://www.gluten.net
E-mail: info@gluten.net

National Institute of Diabetes and Digestive and Kidney Diseases (NIDDK)
Information Clearinghouse
5 Information Way
Bethesda, MD 20892-3560
Toll-Free: 800-860-8747
Phone: 301-654-3810
Website: http://
www.niddk.nih.gov

Chapter 53

Cystic Fibrosis Nutrition: Changes through Life

Good nutrition is crucial for people with cystic fibrosis (CF). It begins at birth and continues through life. A balanced, high-calorie diet with salt, fat, and protein give the body what it needs to grow normally and live well. Normal weight and height help build strong lungs and preserve lung function. Good nutrition also helps to build and keep a strong immune system to fight infections. Fewer infections and stronger lungs mean a longer, healthier life.

Getting Off to a Good Start

Good nutrition starts with teaching infants and children good eating skills. Children learn by watching others. Parents should give the right types of foods. Parents should also eat meals and snacks with their children so they can see how to eat a balanced diet and enjoy meal times.

Children should be allowed to decide how much food to eat. This teaches them how to listen to the body's cues about hunger and fullness. Do not force feed a child. Mealtime is a time to relax and enjoy being together. Turn the television and telephone ringer off and make it free time to eat and enjoy.

Malabsorption and Pancreatic Enzyme Replacement

Most people with CF have a pancreas that does not work as well as it should. This is called pancreatic insufficiency. Pancreatic insufficiency causes maldigestion and malabsorption of food (especially fat). Pancreatic enzymes taken before each meal and snack help prevent maldigestion and malabsorption. Infants should take enzymes with every feeding. If a child cannot swallow an enzyme capsule, the capsule can be opened up and the beads inside put in a small amount of acidic food like baby food fruit. Talk to your CF dietitian or care provider about problems with enzymes.

Symptoms of maldigestion or malabsorption may include:

- poor weight gain despite a good (sometimes ravenous) appetite;
- frequent, loose and/or large bowel movements;
- foul-smelling bowel movements;
- mucus or oil in the bowel movement;
- excessive gas and/or stomach pain; and/or
- distention or bloating.

If any of these symptoms occur for more than three days, call your CF dietitian or care provider. The enzyme dose may need to be changed or a medicine to control stomach acid may need to be added to help the enzymes work better. Do not change the enzyme dose without talking to the CF dietitian or care provider.

Poor Growth or Poor Weight Gain

Normal height and weight and good nutrition are vital in the care of CF. People with CF may need to eat 20–50% more calories than people without CF. This can be hard to do. Even if people with CF eat often and well, they still may not get enough calories to grow normally.

Here are some ways to increase calories in the diet:

- Eat high-calorie/high-fat foods (ask your CF dietitian or care provider for ideas).
- Eat meals and snacks often.
- Supplement meals and snacks with homemade milkshakes and smoothies or store-bought nutrition supplements.

Tube Feedings

Some people still do not gain weight or grow normally even after adding extra calories. Your CF dietitian or care provider may suggest tube feedings. Tube feedings may give the extra calories needed to grow taller or gain weight. They are often given at night during sleep, but also may be given during the day. Tube feedings are a supplement to eating, not a substitute.

Tube feedings can be given through:

- the mouth (orogastric tube or OG);

- the nose (nasogastric tube or NG);

- the stomach (gastrostomy or GT); or

- the intestine (jejunostomy or JT).

Cystic Fibrosis-Related Diabetes (CFRD)

Diabetes related to CF occurs in 10–20% of people with CF. It usually begins in the teen or young adult years. CFRD is different from type 1 or type 2 diabetes. People with CF should have their blood glucose (blood sugar) checked yearly to test for CFRD. If CFRD is found, it is vital to get care from a doctor specializing in diabetes (an endocrinologist) and a CF dietitian and care provider. Right now, the best treatment for CFRD is insulin and checking glucose often.

If a person has CFRD, it is vital to learn good diabetes care. Good diabetes care leads to good diabetes control and fewer problems. A person with CF who has poor diabetes control may get sick more often, take longer to heal, and have trouble gaining or keeping weight. Poor diabetes control may lead to blindness, kidney disease, and poor blood flow.

Osteoporosis

People with CF are at risk for poor bone health. This increases their risk for osteoporosis and broken bones later in life. Getting enough calcium and vitamin D in the diet builds bone mass in children and teens and helps keep adult bones healthy. Weight-bearing exercise (walking, jogging, jumping rope, dancing, weight lifting, etc.) is also very important in building and keeping healthy bones. A DEXA (dual energy x-ray absorptiometry) scan—a type of x-ray—screens for bone health. Your CF dietitian or care provider can answer questions about preventing osteoporosis.

CF and Pregnancy

Women with CF can have healthy pregnancies. Severity of lung disease, presence of diabetes, and nutrition status before pregnancy seem to affect outcomes the most. Women whose pulmonary function tests show moderate to severe lung disease have a higher risk of having a preterm infant and reduced lung function than women with milder lung disease. It is vital for all women of childbearing age to take extra folic acid to help prevent birth defects of the spine in their babies.

A woman with CF should discuss with her CF dietitian or care provider which vitamin supplements are best to take before she gets pregnant. Once pregnant, she will need extra calories each day to gain enough weight. Good weight gain will help her and her baby to be healthy. The woman with CF also should be tested every trimester for pregnancy-related diabetes. If she decides to breast-feed, she will still need extra calories each day to keep healthy and her milk supply enough for the baby to grow. Good nutrition is crucial during pregnancy and breast-feeding for the mother and baby.

In CF, nutrition is the key to good health through life. You must to eat well to grow normally, maintain lung function, and fight infections.

Additional Information

Cystic Fibrosis Foundation
6931 Arlington Rd.
Bethesda, MD 20814
Toll-Free: 800-FIGHT CF (344-4823)
Phone: 301-951-4422
Fax: 301-951-6378
Website: http://www.cff.org
E-mail: info@cff.org

Chapter 54

Diabetes: What You Need to Know about Eating

Whether you have type 1 or type 2 diabetes, what, when, and how much you eat all affect your blood glucose. Blood glucose is the main sugar found in the blood and the body's main source of energy.

If you have diabetes (or impaired glucose tolerance), your blood glucose can go too high if you eat too much. If your blood glucose goes too high, you can get sick. Your blood glucose can also go too high or drop too low if you do not take the right amount of diabetes medicine.

If your blood glucose stays high too much of the time, you can get heart, eye, foot, kidney, and other problems. You can also have problems if your blood glucose gets too low (hypoglycemia). Keeping your blood glucose at a healthy level will prevent or slow down diabetes problems. Ask your doctor or diabetes teacher what a healthy blood glucose level is for you.

Blood Glucose Levels

What should my blood glucose levels be?

For most people, target blood glucose levels are 90 to 130 before meals, and less than 180 one to two hours after the start of a meal. Talk with your health care provider about your blood glucose target levels. Ask your doctor how often you should check your blood glucose.

Excerpted from "What I Need to Know about Eating and Diabetes," National Institute of Diabetes and Digestive and Kidney Diseases (NIDDK), NIH Publication No. 03–5043, July 2003.

The results from your blood glucose checks will tell you if your diabetes care plan is working. Also, ask your doctor for an A1c test at least twice a year. Your A1c number gives your average blood glucose for the past 3 months.

How can I keep my blood glucose at a healthy level?

- Eat about the same amount of food each day.
- Eat your meals and snacks at about the same times each day.
- Do not skip meals or snacks.
- Take your medicines at the same times each day.
- Exercise at about the same times each day.

Why should I eat about the same amount at the same times each day?

Your blood glucose goes up after you eat. If you eat a big lunch one day and a small lunch the next day, your blood glucose levels will change too much. Keep your blood glucose at a healthy level by eating about the same amount of carbohydrate foods at about the same times each day. Carbohydrate foods, also called carbs, provide glucose for energy. Starches, fruits, milk, starchy vegetables such as corn, and sweets are all carbohydrate foods. Talk with your doctor or diabetes teacher about how many meals and snacks to eat each day.

Your Diabetes Medicines

What you eat and when affects how your diabetes medicines work. Talk with your doctor or diabetes teacher about the best times to take your diabetes medicines based on your meal plan.

Your Exercise Plan

What you eat, and when, depends on how much you exercise. Exercise is an important part of staying healthy and controlling your blood glucose. Physical activity should be safe and enjoyable, so talk with your doctor about what types of exercise are right for you. Whatever kind of exercise you do, here are some special things that people with diabetes need to remember:

- Take care of your feet. Make sure your shoes fit properly and your socks stay clean and dry. Check your feet for redness or sores after exercising. Call your doctor if you have sores that do not heal.

- Drink about 2 cups of water before you exercise, about every 20 minutes during exercise, and after you finish, even if you do not feel thirsty.

- Warm up and cool down for 5 to 10 minutes before and after exercising. For example, walk slowly at first, then walk faster. Finish up by walking slowly again.

- Test your blood glucose before and after exercising. Do not exercise if your fasting blood glucose level is above 300. Eat a small snack if your blood glucose is below 100.

- Know the signs of low blood glucose (hypoglycemia) and how to treat it.

Hypoglycemia (Low Blood Sugar)

You should know the signs of hypoglycemia (low blood sugar) such as feeling weak or dizzy, sweating more, noticing sudden changes in your heartbeat, or feeling hungry. If you experience these symptoms, stop exercising and test your blood glucose. If it is 70 or less, eat one of the following right away:

- 2 or 3 glucose tablets
- ½ cup (4 ounces) of any fruit juice
- ½ cup (4 ounces) of a regular (not diet) soft drink
- 1 cup (8 ounces) of milk
- 5 or 6 pieces of hard candy
- 1 or 2 teaspoons of sugar or honey

After 15 minutes, test your blood glucose again to find out whether it has returned to a healthier level. Once blood glucose is stable, if it will be at least an hour before your next meal, it is a good idea to eat a snack.

To be safe when you exercise, carry something to treat hypoglycemia, such as glucose tablets or hard candy. Another good idea is to wear a medical identification bracelet or necklace (in case of emergency). Teach your exercise partners the signs of hypoglycemia and what to do about it.

What Should I Eat Each Day?

Talk with your diabetes teacher to make a meal plan that fits the way you usually eat, your daily routine, and your diabetes medicines. Then make your own plan. Have about 1,600 to 2,000 calories a day if you are:

- a large woman who wants to lose weight;
- a small man at a healthy weight;
- a medium man who does not exercise much;
- a medium to large man who wants to lose weight.

Have about 2,000 to 2,400 calories a day if you are:

- a medium to large man who does a lot of exercise or has a physically active job;
- a large man at a healthy weight;
- a large woman who exercises a lot or has a physically active job.

Starches

Starches are bread, grains, cereal, pasta, or starchy vegetables like corn and potatoes. They give your body energy, vitamins, minerals, and fiber. Whole grain starches are healthier because they have more vitamins, minerals, and fiber.

Eat some starches at each meal. People might tell you not to eat starches, but that is not correct. Eating starches is healthy for everyone, including people with diabetes. A serving of starch is: one slice of bread, one small potato, ½ cup cooked cereal, ¾ cup dry cereal flakes, or one small tortilla.

Healthy Ways to Eat Starches

- Buy whole grain breads and cereals.
- Eat fewer fried and high-fat starches such as regular tortilla chips and potato chips, french fries, pastries, or biscuits. Try pretzels, fat-free popcorn, baked tortilla or potato chips, baked potatoes, or low-fat muffins.
- Use low-fat or fat-free yogurt or fat-free sour cream instead of regular sour cream on a baked potato.

- Use mustard instead of mayonnaise on a sandwich.
- Use the low-fat or fat-free substitutes such as low-fat mayonnaise or light margarine on bread, rolls, or toast.
- Eat cereal with fat-free (skim) or low-fat (1%) milk.

Vegetables

Vegetables give you vitamins, minerals, and fiber, with very few calories. A serving of vegetables is: ½ cup cooked vegetables, 1 cup salad, ½ cup vegetable juice, or 1 cup tomato sauce.

Healthy Ways to Eat Vegetables

- Eat raw and cooked vegetables with little or no fat, sauces, or dressings.
- Try low-fat or fat-free salad dressing on raw vegetables or salads.
- Steam vegetables using a small amount of water or low-fat broth.
- Mix in some chopped onion or garlic.
- Use a little vinegar or some lemon or lime juice.
- Add a small piece of lean ham or smoked turkey instead of fat to vegetables when cooking.
- Sprinkle with herbs and spices. These flavorings add almost no fat or calories.
- If you do use a small amount of fat, use canola oil, olive oil, or soft margarines (liquid or tub types) instead of fat from meat, butter, or shortening.

Fruit

Fruit gives you energy, vitamins, minerals, and fiber. One serving of fruit is: one small apple, ½ cup juice, or ½ grapefruit.

What are healthy ways to eat fruit?

- Eat fruits raw or cooked, as juice with no sugar added, canned in their own juice, or dried.
- Buy smaller pieces of fruit.

- Eat pieces of fruit rather than drinking fruit juice. Pieces of fruit are more filling.

- Drink fruit juice in small amounts.

- Save high-sugar and high-fat fruit desserts such as peach cobbler or cherry pie for special occasions.

Milk and Yogurt

Milk and yogurt give you energy, protein, fat, calcium, vitamin A, and other vitamins and minerals. One serving is: 1 cup fat-free or low-fat yogurt, or 1 cup skim or 1% milk.

What are healthy ways to have milk and yogurt?

- Drink fat-free (skim or nonfat) or low-fat (1%) milk.

- Eat low-fat or fat-free fruit yogurt sweetened with a low-calorie sweetener.

- Use low-fat plain yogurt as a substitute for sour cream.

Meat and Meat Substitutes

The meat and meat substitutes group includes meat, poultry, eggs, cheese, fish, and tofu. Eat small amounts of some of these foods each day. Meat and meat substitutes help your body build tissue and muscles. They also give your body energy and vitamins and minerals. One serving equals: 2–3 ounces of cooked lean meat, chicken, or fish, one egg, 4 ounces (½ cup) of tofu, or 2 tablespoons of peanut butter. Two to three ounces of cooked meat is about the size of a deck of cards.

What are healthy ways to eat meat or meat substitutes?

- Buy cuts of beef, pork, ham, and lamb that have only a little fat on them. Trim off extra fat.

- Eat chicken or turkey without the skin.

- Cook meat or meat substitutes in low-fat ways: broil, grill, stir-fry, roast, steam, or stew.

- To add more flavor, use vinegars, lemon juice, soy or teriyaki sauce, salsa, ketchup, barbecue sauce, and herbs and spices.

- Cook eggs with a small amount of fat or use cooking spray.

- Limit the amounts of nuts, peanut butter, and fried chicken that you eat. They are high in fat.
- Choose low-fat or fat-free cheese.

Fats and Sweets

Limit the amounts of fats and sweets you eat. They have calories, but not much nutrition. Some contain saturated fats and cholesterol that increase your risk of heart disease. Limiting these foods will help you lose weight and keep your blood glucose and blood fats under control. One serving of sweets is: one 3 inch cookie, one plain cake doughnut, 4 chocolate kisses, or one tablespoon maple syrup. One serving of fat is: one strip of bacon or one teaspoon of oil.

How can I satisfy my sweet tooth?

It is okay to have sweets once in a while. Try having sugar-free popsicles, diet soda, fat-free ice cream or frozen yogurt, or sugar-free hot cocoa mix. Here are some additional tips:

- Share desserts in restaurants.
- Order small or child-size servings of ice cream or frozen yogurt.
- Divide homemade desserts into small servings and wrap each individually. Freeze extra servings.
- Do not keep dishes of candy in the house or at work.

Remember, fat-free and low-sugar foods still have calories. Talk with your diabetes teacher about how to fit sweets into your meal plan.

Alcohol

Alcohol has calories but no nutrients. If you drink alcohol on an empty stomach, it can make your blood glucose level too low. Alcohol also can raise your blood fats. If you want to drink alcohol, talk with your doctor or diabetes teacher about how it fits into your meal plan.

Measuring Your Food

To make sure your food servings are the right size, use the following tools:

- measuring cups

- measuring spoons
- a food scale

Also, the Nutrition Facts label on food packages tells you how much of that food is in one serving. Weigh or measure foods to make sure you eat the right amounts. These tips will help you choose the right serving sizes.

- Measure a serving size of dry cereal, hot cereal, pasta, or rice and pour it into a bowl or plate. The next time you eat that food, use the same bowl or plate and fill it to the same level.

- For one serving of milk, measure 1 cup and pour it into a glass. See how high it fills the glass. Always drink milk out of that size glass.

- Meat weighs more before it is cooked. For example, 4 ounces of raw meat will weigh about 3 ounces after cooking. For meat with a bone, like a pork chop or chicken leg, cook 5 ounces raw to get 3 ounces cooked.

- One serving of meat or meat substitute is about the size and thickness of the palm of your hand or a deck of cards.

- A small fist is equal to about ½ cup of fruit, vegetables, or starches like rice.

- A small fist is equal to 1 small piece of fresh fruit.

- A thumb is equal to about 1 ounce of meat or cheese.

- The tip of a thumb is equal to about 1 teaspoon.

When You Are Sick

It is important to take care of your diabetes even when you are ill. Here are some tips on what to do:

- Even if you cannot keep food down, keep taking your diabetes medicine.

- Drink at least one cup (8 ounces) of water or other calorie-free, caffeine-free liquid every hour while you are awake.

- If you cannot eat your usual food, try drinking juice or eating crackers, popsicles, or soup.

- If you cannot eat at all, drink clear liquids such as ginger ale. Eat or drink something with sugar in it if you have trouble keeping food down, because you still need calories. If you do not have enough calories, you increase your risk of hypoglycemia (low blood sugar).

- Make sure that you check your blood glucose. Your blood glucose level may be high even if you are not eating.

- Call your doctor right away if you throw up more than once or have diarrhea for more than 6 hours.

Points to Remember

- What, when, and how much you eat all affect your blood glucose level.

- You can keep your blood glucose at a healthy level if you follow these guidelines:
  - Eat about the same amount of food each day.
  - Eat at about the same times each day.
  - Take your medicines at the same times each day.
  - Exercise at the same times each day.

- Every day, choose foods from these food groups: starches, vegetables, fruit, meat and meat substitutes, and milk and yogurt. How much of each depends on how many calories you need a day.

- Limit the amounts of fats and sweets you eat each day.

Additional Information

American Association of Diabetes Educators
100 W. Monroe, Suite 400
Chicago, IL 60603
Toll-Free: 800-832-6874
Fax: 312-424-2427
Website: http://www.aadenet.org
E-mail: aade@aadenet.org

American Diabetes Association
1701 N. Beauregard St.
Alexandria, VA 22311
Toll-Free: 800-342-2383
Website: http://www.diabetes.org
E-mail: askADA@diabetes.org

National Diabetes Information Clearinghouse
1 Information Way
Bethesda, MD 20892-3560
Toll-Free: 800-860-8747
Fax: 703-738-4929
Website: http://diabetes.niddk.nih.gov
E-mail: ndic@info.niddk.nih.gov

Chapter 55

Eating Disorders Treatments

Facts about Eating Disorders

Eating is controlled by many factors, including appetite; food availability; family, peer, and cultural practices; and, attempts at voluntary control. Dieting to a body weight leaner than needed for health is highly promoted by current fashion trends, sales campaigns for special foods, and in some activities and professions. Eating disorders involve serious disturbances in eating behavior, such as extreme and unhealthy reduction of food intake or severe overeating, as well as feelings of distress or extreme concern about body shape or weight. Researchers are investigating how and why initially voluntary behaviors, such as eating smaller or larger amounts of food than usual, at some point move beyond control in some people and develop into an eating disorder. Studies on the basic biology of appetite control and its alteration by prolonged overeating or starvation have uncovered enormous complexity, but in the long run have the potential to lead to new pharmacologic treatments for eating disorders.

Eating disorders are not due to a failure of will or behavior; rather, they are real, treatable, medical illnesses in which certain maladaptive

This chapter includes an excerpt from "Eating Disorders: Facts about Eating Disorders and the Search for Solutions," National Institute of Mental Health (NIMH), NIH Publication No. 01–4901, 2001; and "About Eating Disorders: Treatment," reprinted with permission from the Academy for Eating Disorders, http://www.aedweb.org. © 2005 Academy for Eating Disorders. All rights reserved.

patterns of eating take on a life of their own. The main types of eating disorders are anorexia nervosa and bulimia nervosa. A third type, binge eating disorder, has been suggested, but has not yet been approved as a formal psychiatric diagnosis. Eating disorders frequently develop during adolescence or early adulthood, but some reports indicate their onset can occur during childhood or later in adulthood.

Eating disorders frequently co-occur with other psychiatric disorders such as depression, substance abuse, and anxiety disorders. In addition, people who suffer from eating disorders can experience a wide range of physical health complications, including serious heart conditions and kidney failure which may lead to death. Therefore, recognition of eating disorders as real and treatable diseases is critically important.

Females are much more likely than males to develop an eating disorder. Only an estimated 5 to 15 percent of people with anorexia or bulimia and an estimated 35 percent of those with binge eating disorder are male.

Treatment

Patients with eating disorders typically require a treatment team consisting of a primary care physician, dietitian, and a mental health professional knowledgeable about eating disorders. The multidisciplinary membership of the Academy for Eating Disorders reflects the consensus view that treatment must often involve clinicians from different health disciplines including psychologists, psychotherapists, physicians, dietitians, and nurses.

Research on the treatment of eating disorders is exploring how different treatments can be helpful for different types of eating disorders. The American Psychiatric Association has published a set of practice guidelines for the treatment of patients with eating disorders (American Psychiatric Association, Practice Guidelines for Eating Disorders, *American Journal of Psychiatry*, 2000).

There is general agreement that good treatment often requires a spectrum of treatment options. These options can range from basic educational interventions designed to teach nutritional and symptom management techniques to long-term residential treatment (living away from home in treatment centers).

Most individuals with eating disorders are treated on an outpatient basis after a comprehensive evaluation. Individuals with medical complications due to severe weight loss or due to the effects of binge eating and purging may require hospitalization. Other individuals, for whom outpatient therapy has not been effective, may benefit from day hospital treatment, hospitalization, or residential placement.

Treatment is usually conducted in the least restrictive setting that can provide adequate safety for the individual. Many patients with eating disorders also have depression, anxiety disorders, drug and/or alcohol use disorders and other psychiatric problems requiring treatment along with the eating disorder.

Initial Assessment

The initial assessment of individuals with eating disorders involves a thorough review of the patient's history, current symptoms, physical status, weight control measures, and other psychiatric issues or disorders such as depression, anxiety, substance abuse, or personality issues. Consultation with a physician and a registered dietitian is often recommended. The initial assessment is the first step in establishing a diagnosis and treatment plan.

Outpatient Treatment

Outpatient treatment for an eating disorder often involves a coordinated team effort between the patient, a psychotherapist, a physician, and a dietitian (yet, many patients are treated by their pediatrician or physician with or without a mental health professional's involvement).

Similarly, many patients are seen and helped by generalist mental health clinicians without specialist involvement. Not all individuals, then, will receive a multidisciplinary approach, but the qualified clinician should have access to all of these resources.

Psychotherapy

There are several different types of outpatient psychotherapies with demonstrated effectiveness in patients with eating disorders. These include cognitive-behavioral therapy, interpersonal psychotherapy, family therapy, and behavioral therapy. Some of these therapies may be relatively short-term (i.e., four-months), but other psychotherapies may last years.

It is very difficult to predict who will respond to short-term treatments versus longer term treatments. Other therapies which some clinicians and patients have found to be useful include feminist therapies, psychodynamic psychotherapies, and various types of group therapy.

Psychopharmacology

Psychiatric medications have a demonstrated role in the treatment of patients with eating disorders. Most of the research to date has involved antidepressant medications such as fluoxetine (for example Prozac®), although some clinicians and patients have found that other types of medications may also be effective.

Nutritional Counseling

Regular contact with a registered dietitian can be an effective source of support and information for patients who are regaining weight, or who are trying to normalize their eating behavior. Dietitians may help patients to gain a fundamental understanding of adequate nutrition, and may also conduct dietary counseling, which is a more specific process designed to help patients change the nature of their eating behavior.

Medical Treatment

Patients with eating disorders are subject to a variety of physical and medical concerns. Adequate medical monitoring is a cornerstone of effective outpatient treatment. Individuals with anorexia nervosa may be followed quite closely (i.e., weekly or more) because of the significant medical problems that this disorder poses for patients. Individuals with bulimia nervosa should be seen regularly, but may not require the intensive medical monitoring often seen in anorexia nervosa. Individuals with binge eating disorder may need medical treatment for a variety of complications of obesity, such as diabetes and hypertension.

Day Hospital Care

Patients for whom outpatient treatment is ineffective may benefit from the increased structure provided by a day hospital treatment program. Generally, these programs are scheduled from three to eight hours a day and provide several structured eating sessions per day, along with various other therapies, including cognitive behavioral therapy, body image therapies, family therapy, and numerous other interventions. Day hospital care allows the patient to live at home when they are not in treatment, and often continue to work or attend school.

Inpatient Treatment

Inpatient treatment provides a structured and contained environment in which the patient with an eating disorder has access to clinical support 24-hours a day. Many programs are now affiliated with a day hospital program so that patients can "step-up" and "step-down" to the appropriate level of care depending on their clinical needs.

Although eating disorder patients can sometimes be treated on general psychiatric units with individuals experiencing other psychiatric disorders, such an approach often poses problems with monitoring and containing eating disorder symptoms. Therefore, most inpatient programs for eating disordered individuals only treat patients with anorexia nervosa, bulimia nervosa, binge eating disorder, or variants of these disorders.

Residential Care

Residential programs provide a longer term treatment option for patients who require longer term treatment. This treatment option generally is reserved for individuals who have been hospitalized on several occasions, but have not been able to reach a significant degree of medical or psychological stability.

Chapter 56

Food Allergies

Food allergy affects up to 6 to 8 percent of children under the age of three and 2 percent of adults. If you have an unpleasant reaction to something you have eaten, you might wonder if you have a food allergy. One out of three people either believe they have a food allergy or modify their or their family's diet. Thus, while food allergy is commonly suspected, health care providers diagnose it less frequently than most people believe.

Food allergy is an abnormal response to a food triggered by the body's immune system. Allergic reactions to food can cause serious illness and, in some cases, death. Therefore, if you have a food allergy, it is extremely important for you to work with your health care provider to find out what food(s) causes your allergic reaction.

Sometimes, a reaction to food is not an allergy at all, but another type of reaction called food intolerance. Food intolerance is more common than food allergy. The immune system does not cause the symptoms of a food intolerance, though these symptoms can look and feel like those of a food allergy.

Allergic Reactions

An immediate allergic reaction involves two actions of the immune system.

Excerpted from "Food Allergy: An Overview," National Institute of Allergy and Infectious Diseases (NIAID), NIH Publication No. 04-5518, July 2004.

- The immune system produces immunoglobulin E (IgE), a type of protein that works against a specific food. This protein is called a food-specific antibody, and it circulates through the blood.

- The food-specific IgE then attaches to mast cells, cells found in all body tissues. They are more often found in areas of the body that are typical sites of allergic reactions. Those sites include the nose, throat, lungs, skin, and gastrointestinal (GI) tract.

Generally, your immune system will form IgE against a food if you come from a family in which allergies are common—not necessarily food allergies, but perhaps other allergic diseases such as hay fever or asthma. If you have two allergic parents, you are more likely to develop food allergy than someone with one allergic parent.

If your immune system is inclined to form IgE to certain foods, you must be exposed to the food before you can have an allergic reaction.

- As this food is digested, it triggers certain cells in your body to produce a food-specific IgE in large amounts. The food-specific IgE is then released and attaches to the surfaces of mast cells.

- The next time you eat that food, it interacts with food-specific IgE on the surface of the mast cells and triggers the cells to release chemicals such as histamine.

- Depending upon the tissue in which they are released, these chemicals will cause you to have various symptoms of food allergy.

Food allergens are proteins within the food that enter your bloodstream after the food is digested. From there, they go to target organs, such as your skin or nose, and cause allergic reactions. An allergic reaction to food can take place within a few minutes to an hour. The process of eating and digesting food affects the timing and the location of a reaction.

- If you are allergic to a particular food, you may first feel itching in your mouth as you start to eat the food.

- After the food is digested in your stomach, you may have gastrointestinal (GI) symptoms such as vomiting, diarrhea, or pain.

- When the food allergens enter and travel through your bloodstream, they may cause your blood pressure to drop.

- As the allergens reach your skin, they can cause hives or eczema.

- When the allergens reach your lungs, they may cause asthma.

Cross-Reactivity

If you have a life-threatening reaction to a certain food, your health care provider will show you how to avoid similar foods that might trigger this reaction. For example, if you have a history of allergy to shrimp, testing will usually show that you are not only allergic to shrimp, but also to crab, lobster, and crayfish. This is called cross-reactivity.

Another interesting example of cross-reactivity occurs in people who are highly sensitive to ragweed. During ragweed pollen season, they sometimes find that when they try to eat melons, particularly cantaloupe, they experience itching in their mouths and simply cannot eat the melon. Similarly, people who have severe birch pollen allergy also may react to apple peels. This is called the oral allergy syndrome.

Common Food Allergies

In adults, the foods that most often cause allergic reactions include the following:

- Shellfish such as shrimp, crayfish, lobster, and crab
- Peanuts
- Tree nuts such as walnuts
- Fish
- Eggs

The most common foods that cause problems in children are the following:

- Eggs
- Milk
- Peanuts

Tree nuts and peanuts are the leading causes of deadly food allergy reactions called anaphylaxis.

Adults usually keep their allergies for life, but children sometimes outgrow them. Children are more likely to outgrow allergies to milk or soy than allergies to peanuts or shrimp. The foods to which adults or children usually react are those foods they eat often. In Japan, for example, rice allergy is more frequent. In Scandinavia, codfish allergy is more common.

Food Allergy or Food Intolerance?

If you go to your health care provider and say, "I think I have a food allergy," your provider has to consider other possibilities that may cause symptoms and could be confused with food allergy such as food intolerance. To find out the difference between food allergy and food intolerance, your provider will go through a list of possible causes for your symptoms. This is called a differential diagnosis. This type of diagnosis helps confirm that you do indeed have a food allergy rather than food intolerance or other illness.

Types of Food Intolerance

Food poisoning. One possible cause of symptoms like those of food allergy is foods contaminated with microbes such as bacteria, and bacterial products such as toxins. Contaminated meat and dairy products sometimes cause symptoms, including GI discomfort, that resemble a food allergy when it is really a type of food poisoning.

Histamine toxicity. There are substances, such as histamine present in certain foods, that cause a reaction like an allergic reaction. For example, histamine can reach high levels in cheese, some wines, and certain kinds of fish such as tuna and mackerel.

In fish, histamine is believed to come from contamination by bacteria, particularly in fish that are not refrigerated properly. If you eat one of these foods with a high level of histamine, you could have a reaction that strongly resembles an allergic reaction to food. This reaction is called histamine toxicity.

Lactose intolerance. Another cause of food intolerance confused with a food allergy is lactose intolerance or lactase deficiency. This common food intolerance affects at least one out of ten people.

- Lactase is an enzyme that is in the lining of the gut.
- Lactase breaks down lactose, a sugar found in milk and most milk products.
- There is not enough lactase in the gut to digest lactose.
- Lactose, instead, is used by bacteria to form gas which causes bloating, abdominal pain, and sometimes diarrhea.

There are tests your health care provider can use to find out whether your body can digest lactose.

Food additives. Another type of food intolerance is a reaction to certain products that are added to food to enhance taste, provide color, or protect against the growth of microbes. Several compounds, such as MSG (monosodium glutamate) and sulfites, are tied to reactions that can be confused with food allergy.

MSG is a flavor enhancer, and when taken in large amounts, can cause some of the following signs.

- Flushing
- Sensations of warmth
- Headache
- Chest discomfort
- Feelings of detachment

These passing reactions occur rapidly after eating large amounts of food to which MSG has been added.

Sulfites occur naturally in foods or may be added to increase crispness or prevent mold growth. Sulfites in high concentrations sometimes pose problems for people with severe asthma. Sulfites can give off a gas called sulfur dioxide that the asthmatic inhales while eating the sulfite treated food. This irritates the lungs and can send an asthmatic into severe bronchospasm, a tightening of the lungs.

The Food and Drug Administration (FDA) has banned sulfites as spray-on preservatives in fresh fruits and vegetables. However, sulfites are still used in some foods and occur naturally during the fermentation of wine.

Gluten intolerance is associated with the disease called gluten-sensitive enteropathy or celiac disease. It happens if your immune system responds abnormally to gluten, which is a part of wheat and some other grains.

Psychological causes. Some people may have a food intolerance that has a psychological trigger. If your food intolerance is caused by this type of trigger, a careful psychiatric evaluation may identify an unpleasant event in your life, often during childhood, tied to eating a particular food. Eating that food years later, even as an adult, is associated with a rush of unpleasant sensations.

Other causes. There are several other conditions, including ulcers and cancers of the GI tract, which cause some of the same symptoms as food allergy. These problems include vomiting, diarrhea, and cramping abdominal pain made worse by eating.

Treatment

Food allergy is treated by avoiding the foods that trigger the reaction. Once you and your health care provider have identified the food(s) to which you are sensitive, you must remove them from your diet. To do this, you must read the detailed ingredient lists on each food you are considering eating.

Many allergy-producing foods such as peanuts, eggs, and milk, appear in foods one normally would not associate them with. Peanuts, for example, are often used as a protein source, and eggs are used in some salad dressings.

FDA requires ingredients in a packaged food to appear on its label. You can avoid most of the things to which you are sensitive if you read food labels carefully, and avoid restaurant-prepared foods that might have ingredients to which you are allergic.

If you are highly allergic, even the tiniest amounts of a food allergen (for example, a small portion of a peanut kernel), can prompt an allergic reaction.

If you have severe food allergies, you must be prepared to treat unintentional exposure. Even people who know a lot about what they are sensitive to occasionally make a mistake. To protect yourself, if you have had allergic reactions to a food, you should take these precautions:

- Wear a medical alert bracelet or necklace stating that you have a food allergy and are subject to severe reactions.

- Carry a syringe of adrenaline (epinephrine), obtained by prescription from your health care provider, and be prepared to give it to yourself if you think you are getting a food allergic reaction.

- Seek medical help immediately by either calling the rescue squad or by getting transported to an emergency room.

Anaphylactic allergic reactions can be fatal even when they start off with mild symptoms such as a tingling in the mouth and throat or GI discomfort.

Schools and day care centers must have plans in place to address any food allergy emergency. Parents and caregivers should take special care with children and learn how to follow these procedures:

- Protect children from foods to which they are allergic.
- Manage children if they eat a food to which they are allergic.
- Give children epinephrine.

Exercise-Induced Food Allergy

At least one situation may require more than simply eating food with allergens to start a reaction—exercise-induced food allergy. People who have this reaction only experience it after eating a specific food before exercising. As exercise increases and body temperature rises, itching and lightheadedness start, allergic reactions such as hives may appear, and even anaphylaxis may develop. The cure for exercised-induced food allergy is simple—avoid eating for a couple of hours before exercising.

There are several medicines that you can take to relieve food allergy symptoms that are not part of an anaphylactic reaction. These include the following:

- Antihistamines to relieve GI symptoms, hives, or sneezing and a runny nose
- Bronchodilators to relieve asthma symptoms

You should take these medicines if you have accidentally eaten a food to which you are allergic. They do not prevent an allergic reaction when taken before eating the food. No medicine in any form will reliably prevent an allergic reaction to that food before eating it.

Food Allergy in Infants and Children

Allergy to cow's milk is particularly common in infants and young children. In addition to causing hives and asthma, it can lead to colic and sleeplessness, and perhaps blood in the stool or poor growth. Infants are thought to be particularly susceptible to this allergic syndrome because their immune and digestive systems are immature. Milk allergy can develop within days to months of birth.

If your baby is on cow's milk formula, your provider may suggest a change to soy formula or an elemental formula if possible. Elemental formulas are produced from processed proteins with supplements added (basically sugars and amino acids). There are few if any allergens within these materials.

Health care providers sometimes prescribe glucocorticosteroid drugs to treat infants with very severe GI reactions to milk formulas. Fortunately, this food allergy tends to go away within the first few years of life.

Breast-feeding often helps babies avoid feeding problems related to allergic reactions. Therefore, health experts often suggest that mothers feed their baby only breast milk for the first 6 to 12 months of life to avoid milk allergy from developing within that time frame.

Some babies are very sensitive to a certain food. If you are nursing and eat that food, sufficient amounts can enter your breast milk to cause a food reaction in your baby. To keep possible food allergens out of your breast milk, you might try not eating those foods that could cause an allergic reaction in your baby, such as peanuts.

There is no conclusive evidence that breast-feeding prevents allergies from developing later in your child's life. It does, however, delay the start of food allergies by delaying your infant's exposure to those foods that can prompt allergies. Plus, it may avoid altogether food allergy problems sometimes seen in infants.

By delaying the introduction of solid foods until your baby is 6 months old or older, you can also prolong your baby's allergy-free period. In addition, the American Academy of Pediatrics recommends you delay adding eggs to your child's diet until he or she is 2 years old; and peanuts, tree nuts, and fish until he or she is 3 years old.

Some Controversial and Unproven Theories

There are several disorders that are popularly thought by some to be caused by food allergies. There is not enough scientific evidence to support the claims, or the evidence that does exist goes against such claims.

- **Migraine headaches.** There is controversy about whether migraine headaches can be caused by food allergy. Studies show people who are prone to migraines can have their headaches brought on by histamines and other substances in foods. The more difficult issue is whether food allergies actually cause migraines in such people.

- **Arthritis.** There is virtually no evidence that most rheumatoid arthritis or osteoarthritis can be made worse by foods, despite claims to the contrary.

- **Allergic tension fatigue syndrome.** There is no evidence that food allergies can cause a disorder called the allergic tension fatigue syndrome, in which people are tired, nervous, and may have problems concentrating, or have headaches.

- **Cerebral allergy.** Cerebral allergy is a term that has been given to people who have trouble concentrating and have headaches as well as other complaints. These symptoms are sometimes blamed on mast cells activated in the brain, but no other place in the body. Researchers have found no evidence that such a scenario can happen. Most health experts do not recognize cerebral allergy as a disorder.

- **Environmental illness.** In a seemingly pristine environment, some people have many non-specific complaints such as problems concentrating or depression. Sometimes this is blamed on small amounts of allergens or toxins in the environment. There is no evidence that such problems are due to food allergies.

- **Childhood hyperactivity.** Some people believe hyperactivity in children is caused by food allergies, but researchers have found that this behavioral disorder in children is only occasionally associated with food additives, and then only when such additives are consumed in large amounts. There is no evidence that a true food allergy can affect a child's activity except for the possibility that if a child itches, sneezes, and wheezes a lot, the child may be uncomfortable, and therefore, more difficult to guide. Also, children who are on antiallergy medicines that cause drowsiness may get sleepy in school or at home.

- **Controversial and unproven treatments.**
  - **Neutralization.** Putting a diluted solution of a particular food under your tongue about a half hour before you eat the food suspected of causing an allergic reaction. This is an attempt to neutralize the subsequent exposure to the food that you believe is harmful. The results of a carefully conducted clinical study show this procedure does not prevent an allergic reaction.
  - **Allergy shots.** Another unproven treatment for food allergy involves getting shots (immunotherapy) containing small quantities of the food extracts to which you are allergic. These shots are given regularly for a long period of time with the aim of desensitizing you to the food allergen. Researchers have not yet proven that allergy shots reliably relieve food allergies.

Research

The National Institute of Allergy and Infectious Diseases does research on food allergy and other allergic diseases. This research is focused on understanding what happens to the body during the allergic process—the sequence of events leading to the allergic response, and the factors responsible for allergic diseases.

One study by the Johns Hopkins Children's Center showed that simply washing your hands with soap and water will remove peanut allergens. Also, most household cleaners will remove them from surfaces such as food preparation areas at home as well as day care facilities and schools. These easy-to-do measures will help prevent peanut allergy reactions in children and adults.

Educating people, including patients, health care providers, school teachers, and day care workers, about the importance of food allergy is also an important research focus. The more people know about the disorder, the better equipped they will be to control food allergies.

Additional Information

American Academy of Allergy, Asthma, and Immunology
555 E. Wells St., Suite 1100
Milwaukee, WI 53202-3823
Toll-Free: 800-822-2762
Phone: 414-272-6071
Website: http://www.aaaai.org
E-mail: info@aaaai.org

American College of Allergy, Asthma, and Immunology
85 W. Algonquin Rd., Suite 550
Arlington Heights, IL 60005
Toll-Free: 800-842-7777
Phone: 847-427-1200
Fax: 847-427-1294
Website: http://allergy.mcg.edu
E-mail: mail@acaai.org

Asthma and Allergy Foundation of America
1233 20th Street, N.W., Suite 402
Washington, DC 20036
Toll-Free: 800-7-ASTHMA (800-727-8462)
Phone: 202-466-7643
Fax: 202-466-8940
Website: http://www.aafa.org
E-mail: info@aafa.org

The Food Allergy and Anaphylaxis Network
11781 Lee Jackson Highway, Suite 160
Fairfax, VA 22033
Toll-Free: 800-929-4040
Fax: 703-691-2713
Website: http://www.foodallergy.org
E-mail: faan@foodallergy.org

Chapter 57

Heart Health Nutrition: The DASH Eating Plan

Research has found that diet affects the development of high blood pressure, or hypertension (the medical term). Two studies, *DASH* and *DASH Sodium*, showed that blood pressure can be lowered by following a particular eating plan—called the Dietary Approaches to Stop Hypertension (DASH) eating plan—and reducing the amount of sodium consumed.

Results showed that reducing dietary sodium lowered blood pressure for both eating plans. At each sodium level, blood pressure was lower on the DASH eating plan than on the other eating plan. The biggest blood pressure reductions were for the DASH eating plan at the sodium intake of 1,500 milligrams per day. Those with hypertension saw the biggest reductions, but those without it also had large decreases. *DASH Sodium* shows the importance of lowering sodium intake—whatever your eating plan. But for a true winning combination, follow the DASH eating plan and lower your intake of salt and sodium.

DASH Eating Plan

The DASH eating plan in Table 57.1 is based on 2,000 calories a day. The number of daily servings in a food group may vary from those listed, depending on your caloric needs.

Excerpts from "Facts about the DASH Eating Plan," National Heart, Lung, and Blood Institute (NHLBI), NIH Publication No. 03–4082, Revised May 2003.

Table 57.1. Following the DASH Eating Plan

Food Group	Daily Serving (except as noted)	Serving Sizes	Examples and Notes	Significance of Each Food Group to the DASH Eating Plan
Grains and grain products	7–8	1 slice bread 1 oz dry cereal* ½ cup cooked rice, pasta, or cereal	Whole wheat bread, English muffin, pita bread, bagel, cereals, grits, oatmeal, crackers, unsalted pretzels, and popcorn	Major sources of energy and fiber
Vegetables	4–5	1 cup raw leafy vegetable ½ cooked vegetable 6 oz vegetable juice	Tomatoes, potatoes, carrots, green peas, squash, broccoli, turnip greens, collards, kale, spinach, artichokes, green beans, lima beans, sweet potatoes	Rich sources of potassium, magnesium, and fiber
Fruits	4–5	6 oz fruit juice 1 medium fruit ¼ cup dried fruit ½ cup fresh, frozen, or canned fruit	Apricots, bananas, dates, grapes, oranges, orange juice, grapefruit, grapefruit juice, mangoes, melons, peaches, pineapples, prunes, raisins, strawberries, tangerines	Important sources of potassium, magnesium, and fiber
Low-fat or fat free dairy foods	2–3	8 oz milk 1 cup yogurt 1½ oz cheese	Fat free (skim) or low-fat (1%) milk fat free or low-fat buttermilk, fat free or low-fat regular or frozen yogurt, low-fat and fat free cheese	Major sources of calcium and protein

Meats, poultry, and fish	2 or less	3 oz cooked meats, poultry, or fish	Select only lean; trim away visible fats; broil, roast, or boil, instead of frying; remove skin from poultry	Rich sources of protein and magnesium
Nuts, seeds, and dry beans	4–5 per week	1/3 cup or 1½ oz nuts, 2 Tbsp or ½ oz seeds, ½ cup cooked dry beans, peas	Almonds, filberts, mixed nuts, peanuts, walnuts, sunflower seeds, kidney beans, lentils	Rich sources of energy, magnesium, potassium, protein, and fiber
Fats and oils**	2–3	1 tsp soft margarine, 1 Tbsp low-fat mayonnaise, 2 Tbsp light salad dressing, 1 tsp vegetable oil	Soft margarine, low-fat mayonnaise, light salad dressing, vegetable oil (such as olive, corn, canola, or safflower)	DASH has 27 percent of calories as fat, including fat in or added to foods
Sweets	5 per week	1 Tbsp sugar, 1 Tbsp jelly or jam, ½ oz jelly beans, 8 oz lemonade	Maple syrup, sugar, jelly, jam, fruit-flavored gelatin, jelly beans, hard candy, fruit punch, sorbet, ices	Sweets should be low in fat

* Equals ½–1¼ cups, depending on cereal type. Check the product's Nutrition Facts label.

** Fat content changes serving counts for fats and oils: For example, 2 Tbsp of regular salad dressing equals 1 serving; 1 Tbsp of a low-fat dressing equals ½ serving; 1 Tbsp of a fat free dressing equals 0 servings.

How do I make the DASH?

The DASH eating plan used in the studies calls for a certain number of servings daily from various food groups. These are given in Table 57.1 for 2,000 calories per day. The number of servings you require may vary, depending on your caloric need.

The DASH eating plan was not designed to promote weight loss. But it is rich in lower calorie foods, such as fruits and vegetables. You can make it lower in calories by replacing higher calorie foods with more fruits and vegetables—and that also will make it easier for you to reach your DASH goals.

How to Lower Calories on the DASH Eating Plan

Increase Fruits

- Eat a medium apple instead of four shortbread cookies. You will save 80 calories.

- Eat 1/4 cup of dried apricots instead of a 2-ounce bag of pork rinds. You will save 230 calories.

Increase Vegetables

- Have a hamburger that is 3 ounces of meat instead of 6 ounces. Add 1/2 cup serving of carrots and 1/2 cup serving of spinach. You will save more than 200 calories.

- Instead of 5 ounces of chicken, have a stir-fry with 2 ounces of chicken and 1½ cups of raw vegetables. Use a small amount of vegetable oil. You will save 50 calories.

Increase Low-Fat or Fat Free Diary Products

- Have a 1/2 cup serving of low-fat frozen yogurt instead of a 1½ ounce milk chocolate bar. You will save about 110 calories.

Calorie-Saving Tips

- Use low-fat or fat free condiments.

- Use half as much vegetable oil, soft or liquid margarine, or salad dressing, or choose fat free versions.

- Eat smaller portions—cut back gradually.

- Choose low-fat or fat free dairy products to reduce total fat intake.

- Check the food labels to compare fat content in packaged foods—items marked low-fat or fat free are not always lower in calories than their regular versions.

- Limit foods with lots of added sugar, such as pies, flavored yogurts, candy bars, ice cream, sherbet, regular soft drinks, and fruit drinks.

- Eat fruits canned in their own juice.

- Add fruit to plain yogurt.

- Snack on fruit, vegetable sticks, unbuttered and unsalted popcorn, or bread sticks.

- Drink water or club soda.

Where is the sodium?

Only a small amount of sodium occurs naturally in foods. Most sodium is added during processing.

You should be aware that the DASH eating plan has more daily servings of fruits, vegetables, and whole grain foods than you may be used to eating. Because the plan is high in fiber, it can cause bloating and diarrhea in some persons. To avoid these problems, gradually increase your intake of fruit, vegetables, and whole grain foods.

Twenty-four hundred milligrams of sodium equals about 6 grams, or 1 teaspoon, of table salt (sodium chloride); 1,500 milligrams of sodium equals about 4 grams, or 2/3 teaspoon, of table salt. These amounts include all salt consumed—that in food products, used in cooking, and added at the table. Only small amounts of sodium occur naturally in food. Processed foods account for most of the salt and sodium Americans consume. So, be sure to read food labels to choose products lower in sodium. You may be surprised at many of the foods that have sodium. They include soy sauce, seasoned salts, monosodium glutamate (MSG), baking soda, and some antacids—the range is wide. Because it is rich in fruits and vegetables, which are naturally lower in sodium than many other foods, the DASH eating plan makes it easier to consume less salt and sodium. Still, you may want to begin by adopting the DASH eating plan at the level of 2,400 milligrams of sodium per day and then further lower your sodium intake to 1,500 milligrams per day.

Tips to Reduce Salt and Sodium

- Use reduced sodium or no-salt-added products. For example, choose low- or reduced-sodium, or no-salt-added versions of foods and condiments when available.

- Buy fresh, plain frozen, or canned with no-salt-added vegetables.

Table 57.2. Varying Amounts of Sodium in Foods

Food Groups	Sodium (mg)
Grains and grain products	
Cooked cereal, rice, pasta, unsalted, 1/2 cup	0–5
Ready-to-eat cereal, 1 cup	100–360
Bread, 1 slice	110–175
Vegetables	
Fresh or frozen, cooked without salt, 1/2 cup	1–70
Canned or frozen with sauce, 1/2 cup	140–460
Tomato juice, canned 3/4 cup	820
Fruit	
Fresh, frozen, canned, 1/2 cup	0–5
Low-fat or fat free dairy foods	
Milk, 1 cup	120
Yogurt, 8 oz	160
Natural cheeses, 1½ oz	110–450
Processed cheeses, 1½ oz	600
Nuts, seeds, and dry beans	
Peanuts, salted, 1/3 cup	120
Peanuts, unsalted, 1/3 cup	0–5
Beans, cooked from dried, or frozen, without salt, 1/2 cup	0–5
Beans, canned, 1/2 cup	400
Meats, fish, and poultry	
Fresh meat, fish, poultry, 3 oz	30–90
Tuna canned, water pack, no salt added, 3 oz	35–45
Tuna canned, water pack, 3 oz	250–350
Ham, lean, roasted, 3 oz	1,020

- Use fresh poultry, fish, and lean meat, rather than canned, smoked, or processed types.

- Choose ready-to-eat breakfast cereals that are lower in sodium.

- Limit cured foods (such as bacon and ham), foods packed in brine (such as pickles, pickled vegetables, olives, and sauerkraut), and condiments (such as MSG, mustard, horseradish, catsup, and barbecue sauce). Limit even lower sodium versions of soy sauce and teriyaki sauce—treat these condiments as you do table salt.

- Use spices instead of salt. In cooking, and at the table, flavor foods with herbs, spices, lemon, lime, vinegar, or salt-free seasoning blends. Start by cutting salt in half.

- Cook rice, pasta, and hot cereals without salt. Cut back on instant or flavored rice, pasta, and cereal mixes, which usually have added salt.

- Choose convenience foods that are lower in sodium. Cut back on frozen dinners, mixed dishes such as pizza, packaged mixes, canned soups or broths, and salad dressings—these often have a lot of sodium.

- Rinse canned foods, such as tuna, to remove some sodium.

The DASH eating plan requires no special foods and has no hard-to-follow recipes. One way to begin is by comparing food labels. Read the Nutrition Facts on food labels to compare the amount of sodium in products. Look for the sodium content in milligrams and the Percent Daily Value. Aim for foods that are less than 5 percent of the Daily Value of sodium. Compare the food labels of two versions of canned tomatoes. Regular canned tomatoes have ten times as much sodium as the unsalted canned tomatoes.

Reducing Sodium when Eating Out

- Ask how foods are prepared. Ask that they be prepared without added salt, MSG, or salt-containing ingredients. Most restaurants are willing to accommodate requests.

- Know the terms that indicate high sodium content: pickled, cured, soy sauce, broth.

- Move the salt shaker away.

- Limit condiments, such as mustard, catsup, pickles, and sauces with salt-containing ingredients.

- Choose fruits or vegetables instead of salty snack foods.

Remember that some days the foods you eat may add up to more than the recommended servings from one food group and less from another. Similarly, you may have too much sodium on a particular day. Do not worry. Just be sure that the average of several days or a week comes close to what is recommended for the food groups and for your chosen daily sodium level.

One important note: If you take medication to control high blood pressure, you should not stop using it. Follow the DASH eating plan, and talk with your doctor about your drug treatment.

Label Language

Food labels can help you choose items lower in sodium and saturated and total fat. Table 57.3 lists sodium and fat terms and meanings which

Table 57.3. Labels: Sodium, and Fat

Phrase	What It Means
Sodium	
Sodium free or salt free	Less than 5 mg per serving
Very low sodium	35 mg or less of sodium per serving
Low sodium	140 mg or less of sodium per serving
Low sodium meal	140 mg or less of sodium per 3½ oz (100 g)
Reduced or less sodium	At least 25 percent less sodium than the regular version
Light in sodium	50 percent less sodium than the regular version
Unsalted or no salt added	No salt added to the product during processing
Fat	
Fat free	Less than 0.5 g per serving
Low saturated fat	1 g or less per serving
Low-fat	3 g or less per serving
Reduced fat	At least 25 percent less fat than the regular version
Light in fat	Half the fat compared to the regular version

can be found on Nutrition Facts labels on cans, boxes, bottles, bags, and other packaging:

Getting Started

Make changes gradually.

- If you now eat one or two vegetables a day, add a serving at lunch and another at dinner.

- If you do not eat fruit now or have only juice at breakfast, add a serving to your meals or have it as a snack.

- Gradually increase your use of fat free and low-fat dairy products to three servings a day. For example, drink milk with lunch or dinner, instead of soda, sugar-sweetened tea, or alcohol. Choose low-fat (1 percent) or fat free (skim) dairy products to reduce your intake of saturated fat, total fat, cholesterol, and calories.

- Read food labels on margarines and salad dressings to choose those lowest in saturated fat and trans fat. Some margarine is now *trans* fat free.

Treat meat as one part of the whole meal, instead of the focus.

- Limit meat to 6 ounces a day (2 servings)—all that is needed. Three to four ounces is about the size of a deck of cards.

- If you now eat large portions of meat, cut them back gradually—by a half or a third at each meal.

- Include two or more vegetarian-style (meatless) meals each week.

- Increase servings of vegetables, rice, pasta, and dry beans in meals. Try casseroles, pasta, and stir-fry dishes, which have less meat and more vegetables, grains, and dry beans. Use fruits or other foods low in saturated fat, cholesterol, and calories as desserts and snacks.

- Fruits and other low-fat foods offer great taste and variety. Use fruits canned in their own juice. Fresh fruits require little or no preparation. Dried fruits are a good choice to carry with you or to have ready in the car.

- Try these snack ideas: unsalted pretzels or nuts mixed with raisins; graham crackers; low-fat and fat free yogurt and frozen yogurt; popcorn with no salt or butter added; and raw vegetables.

Here are some other tips.

- Choose whole grain foods to get added nutrients, such as minerals and fiber. For example, choose whole wheat bread or whole grain cereals.

- If you have trouble digesting dairy products, try taking lactase enzyme pills or drops (available at drugstores and groceries) with the dairy foods. Or, buy lactose-free milk or milk with lactase enzyme added to it.

- Use fresh, frozen, or no-salt-added canned vegetables.

Making the DASH to Good Health

The DASH plan is a new way of eating—for a lifetime. If you slip from the eating plan for a few days, do not let it keep you from reaching your health goals. Get back on track. Here is how:

- Ask yourself why you got off the track. Was it at a party? Were you feeling stress at home or work? Find out what triggered your sidetrack—and start again with the DASH plan.

- Do not worry about a slip. Everyone slips—especially when learning something new. Remember that changing your lifestyle is a long-term process.

- See if you tried to do too much at once. Often, those starting a new lifestyle try to change too much at once. Instead, change one or two things at a time. Slowly, but surely, is the best way to succeed.

- Break the process down into small steps. This not only keeps you from trying to do too much at once, but also keeps the changes simpler. Break complex goals into smaller, simpler steps, each of which is attainable.

- Write it down. Keep track of what you eat. This can help you find the problem. Besides noting what you eat, also record: where you are, what you are doing, and how you feel. Keep track for several days. You may find, for instance, that you eat high-fat foods while watching television. If so, you could start keeping a substitute snack on hand to eat instead of the high-fat foods. This record also helps you be sure you're getting enough of each food group.

- Celebrate success. Treat yourself to a nonfood treat for your accomplishments.

Additional Information

National Heart, Lung, and Blood Institute
P.O. Box 30105
Bethesda, MD 20824-0105
Toll-Free: 800-575-9355
Phone: 301-592-8573
TTY: 240-629-3255
Fax: 301-592-8563
Website: http://www.nhlbi.nih.gov
E-mail: nhlbiinfo@nhlbi.nih.gov

Chapter 58

Hemodialysis: Eat Right to Feel Right

When you start hemodialysis, you must make many changes in your life. Watching the foods you eat will make you healthier.

How does food affect my hemodialysis?

Food gives you energy and helps your body repair itself. Food is broken down in your stomach and intestines. Your blood picks up nutrients from the digested food and carries them to all your body cells. These cells take nutrients from your blood and put waste products back into the bloodstream. When your kidneys were healthy, they worked around the clock to remove wastes from your blood. The wastes left your body when you urinated. Other wastes are removed in bowel movements.

Now your kidneys have stopped working. Hemodialysis removes wastes from your blood. But between sessions, wastes can build up in your blood and make you sick. You can reduce the amount of wastes by watching what you eat and drink. A good meal plan can improve your dialysis and your health.

What do I need to know about fluids?

You already know you need to watch how much you drink. Any food that is liquid at room temperature also contains water. These foods

Excerpted from "Eat Right to Feel Right on Hemodialysis," National Institute of Diabetes and Digestive and Kidney Diseases (NIDDK), NIH Publication No. 03–4274, April 2003.

include soup, gelatin, and ice cream. Many fruits and vegetables contain lots of water, too. They include melons, grapes, apples, oranges, tomatoes, lettuce, and celery. All these foods add to your fluid intake.

Fluid can build up between dialysis sessions, causing swelling and weight gain. The extra fluid affects your blood pressure and can make your heart work harder. You could get serious heart trouble from overloading your system with fluid.

Your dry weight is your weight after a dialysis session when all of the extra fluid in your body has been removed. If you let too much fluid build up between sessions, it is harder to get down to your proper dry weight. Your dry weight may change over a period of 3 to 6 weeks. Talk to your doctor regularly about what your dry weight should be.

Control Your Thirst: You can keep your fluids down by drinking from smaller cups or glasses. Freeze juice in an ice cube tray and eat it like a popsicle. (Remember to count the popsicle in your fluid allowance.) A dietitian will be able to give you other tips for managing your thirst.

What do I need to know about potassium?

Potassium is a mineral found in many foods, especially milk, fruits, and vegetables. It affects how steadily your heart beats. Healthy kidneys keep the right amount of potassium in the blood to keep the heart beating at a steady pace. Potassium levels can rise between dialysis sessions and affect your heartbeat. Eating too much potassium can be very dangerous to your heart. It may even cause death.

To control potassium levels in your blood, avoid foods like avocados, bananas, kiwis, and dried fruit, which are very high in potassium. Also, eat smaller portions of other high-potassium foods. For example, eat half a pear instead of a whole pear. Eat only very small portions of oranges and melons.

You can remove some of the potassium from potatoes and other vegetables by peeling them, then soaking them in a large amount of water for several hours. Drain and rinse before cooking. Your dietitian can give you more specific information about the potassium content of foods.

Make a food plan that reduces the potassium in your diet. Start by noting the high-potassium foods that you now eat. A dietitian can help you add other foods to the list.

High-potassium foods include the following:

- apricots
- avocados
- bananas
- beets
- brussel sprouts
- cantaloupe
- clams
- dates
- figs
- kiwi fruit
- lima beans
- melons
- milk
- nectarines
- orange juice
- oranges
- peanuts
- pears (fresh)
- potatoes
- prune juice
- prunes
- raisins
- sardines
- spinach
- tomatoes
- winter squash
- yogurt

What do I need to know about phosphorus?

Phosphorus is a mineral found in many foods. If you have too much phosphorus in your blood, it pulls calcium from your bones. Losing calcium will make your bones weak and likely to break. Also, too much phosphorus may make your skin itch. Foods like milk and cheese, dried beans, peas, colas, nuts, and peanut butter are high in phosphorus. Usually, people on dialysis are limited to 1½ cup of milk per day. The renal dietitian will give you more specific information regarding phosphorus.

You probably will need to take a phosphate binder like Renagel, PhosLo, Tums, or calcium carbonate to control the phosphorus in your blood between dialysis sessions. These medications act like sponges to soak up, or bind, phosphorus while it is in the stomach. Because it is bound, the phosphorus does not get into the blood. Instead, it is passed out of the body in the stool.

What do I need to know about protein?

Before you were on dialysis, your doctor may have told you to follow a low-protein diet. Being on dialysis changes this. Most people on dialysis are encouraged to eat as much high-quality protein as they can. The better nourished you are, the healthier you will be. You will also have greater resistance to infection and recover from surgery more quickly.

Protein helps you keep muscle and repair tissue. In your body, protein breaks down into a waste product called urea. If urea builds up in your blood, you can become very sick. Some sources of protein produce less waste than others. These are called high-quality proteins. High-quality proteins come from meat, fish, poultry, and eggs (especially egg whites). Getting most of your protein from these sources can reduce the amount of urea in your blood.

What do I need to know about sodium?

Sodium is found in salt and other foods. Most canned foods and frozen dinners contain large amounts of sodium. Too much sodium makes you thirsty. But if you drink more fluid, your heart has to work harder to pump the fluid through your body. Over time, this can cause high blood pressure and congestive heart failure.

Try to eat fresh foods that are naturally low in sodium. Look for products labeled low sodium. Do not use salt substitutes because they contain potassium. Talk to a dietitian about spices you can use to flavor your food. The dietitian can help you find spice blends without sodium or potassium.

What do I need to know about calories?

Calories provide energy for your body. If your doctor recommends it, you may need to cut down on the calories you eat. A dietitian can help you plan ways to cut calories in the best possible way.

But some people on dialysis need to gain weight. You may need to find ways to add calories to your diet. Vegetable oils—like olive oil, canola oil, and safflower oil—are good sources of calories. Use them generously on breads, rice, and noodles.

Butter and margarines are rich in calories. But these fatty foods can also clog your arteries. Use them less often. Soft margarine that comes in tubs is better than stick margarine. Vegetable oils are the healthiest way to add fat to your diet if you need to gain weight.

Hard candy, sugar, honey, jam, and jelly provide calories and energy without clogging arteries or adding other things that your body does not need.

Note: If you have diabetes, be very careful about eating sweets. A dietitian's guidance is very important for people with diabetes.

Should I take vitamins and minerals?

Vitamins and minerals may be missing from your diet because you have to avoid so many foods. Your doctor may prescribe a vitamin and mineral supplement like Nephrocaps.

Warning: Do not take vitamins that you can buy off the store shelf. They may contain vitamins or minerals that are harmful to you.

Cookbooks with Recipes for People on Dialysis

The Renal Gourmet.
Author: Mardy Peters
ISBN: 0-9641730-0-X
Publisher: Emenar Inc.
13n625 Coombs Road
Elgin, IL 60123
Toll-Free: 800-445-5653

Southwest Cookbook for People on Dialysis
National Kidney Foundation of Texas
13500 Midway Road
Suite 101
Dallas, TX 75244
Phone: 972-934-8057

Creative Cooking for Renal Diets
Cleveland Clinic Foundation
ISBN: 0-941511-00-6
Senay Publishing
P.O. Box 397
Chesterland, OH 44026
Phone: 440-256-4435

Creative Cooking for Renal Diabetic Diets
Cleveland Clinic Foundation
ISBN: 0-941511-01-4
Senay Publishing
P.O. Box 397
Chesterland, OH 44026
Phone: 440-256-4435

Additional Information

American Association of Kidney Patients
3503 E. Frontage Rd., Ste. 315
Tampa, FL 33607
Toll-Free: 800-749-2257
Fax: 813-636-8122
Website: http://www.aakp.org
E-mail: info@aakp.org

National Kidney Foundation
30 East 33rd St.
New York, NY 10016
Toll-Free: 800-622-9010
Phone: 212-889-2210
Fax: 212-689-9261
Website: http://www.kidney.org.
E-mail: info@kidney.org

National Kidney and Urologic Diseases Information Clearinghouse
3 Information Way
Bethesda, MD 20892-3580
Toll-Free: 800-891-5390
Fax: 703-738-4929
Website: http://kidney.niddk.nih.gov
E-mail: nkudic@info.niddk.nih.gov

Chapter 59

Inborn Errors of Metabolism

Definition

Inborn errors of metabolism are rare genetic disorders in which the body cannot turn food into energy (metabolize food) normally. The disorders are usually caused by defects in the enzymes involved in the biochemical pathways that break down food components.

Side Effects

The food product that is unable to be metabolized (broken down into energy) can build up in your body and cause a wide array of symptoms. Several inborn errors of metabolism cause mental retardation if not controlled.

Recommendations

Inborn errors of metabolism often demand diet changes. The type and extent of the changes depends on the specific metabolic error. Registered dietitians and physicians can help with the diet modifications needed for each disease.

The following are some examples of inborn errors of metabolism.

Fructose Intolerance

- A genetic disorder in the breakdown of the carbohydrate fructose. It is potentially life-threatening, but may be treated by diet changes.

- Food sources of fructose include fruits, fruit juices, sucrose (all sugars—cane, beet, white, brown, etc.), corn syrups, honey, sorbitol, levulose, invert sugar, some vegetable and starches.

- All fructose should be avoided in the diet. The severity of the restriction depends on individual tolerance. Sugar and fructose are found in many foods, making the diet difficult to follow.

Galactosemia

- A genetic disorder in the breakdown of the carbohydrate galactose to glucose. It can result in cataracts, enlarged liver, enlarged spleen, and mental retardation. Typically, the disease is found in milk-fed infants shortly after birth. This is because milk contains large amounts of galactose.

- Food sources of galactose include mammalian milks, dairy products, and foods containing them.

- It is recommended that milk and milk products should be avoided, including yogurt, cheese, ice cream. Galactose and lactose-free milk substitutes and foods should be used. Other sources of galactose may include sugar beets, gums, seaweed, flaxseed, mucilage, whey, some vegetables, etc. Women who carry the genetic trait should also follow the diet since galactose may cause mental retardation to the fetus. Contact a registered dietitian for complete information on a galactose-free diet.

Maple Sugar Urine Disease (MSUD)

- A rare genetic disorder in the breakdown of the branch chain amino acids valine, leucine, and isoleucine. Typically the disease is found shortly after birth and is characterized by maple syrup odor of the urine, vomiting, refusal to eat, and increased reflex actions. If left untreated, life-threatening neurological damage may result.

- Treatment includes a special diet. Strict compliance is necessary to prevent neurological damage. This requires close supervision by a registered dietitian or physician, and cooperation by parent(s).

Phenylketonuria (PKU)

- A rare genetic disorder that can result in severe progressive mental retardation if untreated by diet. Most states require blood or urine testing for PKU is all newborns.

- A low phenylalanine diet is required. Strict compliance to the diet is necessary to reduce or prevent mental retardation. This requires close supervision by a registered dietitian or physician, and cooperation of the parent(s) and child.

Chapter 60

Ketogenic Diet for Seizures

Common Questions about the Ketogenic Diet

What is the ketogenic diet?

The ketogenic diet is a special diet used to treat seizures. It was initially studied in the 1920s as a treatment option for those with intractable epilepsy. Since then, medications have replaced the diet, but there is now a resurgence of interest in the Ketogenic diet. The diet is high in fat and low in carbohydrate and protein, which results in ketosis. In addition, fluids are limited which helps contribute to the diet's success. This ketotic state exerts an anti-epileptic effect, though its precise mechanism of action is not completely understood.

How does the ketogenic diet work?

The diet is high in fat and low in carbohydrate and protein which results in ketosis. In addition, fluids are limited which helps contribute to the diet's success. This ketotic state exerts an anti-epileptic effect, though its precise mechanism of action is not completely understood.

"Frequently Asked Questions about the Ketogenic Diet," reprinted with permission from the Ketogenic Diet Program at Lucile Packard Children's Hospital–Stanford University, © 2000. Updated in August 2005 by Dr. David A. Cooke, M.D., Diplomate, American Board of Internal Medicine.

What type of seizures is the ketogenic diet effective for?

It appears to be effective for multiple types of seizures. However, we have found it to be most effective for myoclonic seizures and "minor motor" seizures. The diet also seems to be helpful for other types of seizures, such as tonic-clonic seizures and complex partial seizures.

Is my child a good candidate for the ketogenic diet?

We recommend that you consult your physician or neurologist about the appropriateness of the ketogenic diet for your child's seizure disorder. You should also contact other keto providers and families who have been on the diet. Usually the ketogenic diet is used as a secondary method of treatment, that is, when conventional anti-seizure medications do not seem to adequately control seizures. Also, if the adverse effects of the anti-seizure medications are too great, the diet can also be considered (so that medications can be reduced).

How do I locate an institution that is currently treating children successfully with the ketogenic diet?

Ask your child's neurologist for a referral to a site, preferably close to home, that will evaluate your child for appropriateness to start the ketogenic diet. Please note that as there are a limited number of institutions that have an active keto team, your child may have to wait a month or more to be admitted.

How long will my child have to be in the hospital?

Uncomplicated hospital admissions scheduled to initiate the ketogenic diet are typically 4–5 days in duration (Monday–Friday).

How long does my child stay on the diet?

If the diet proves to be a worthwhile form of therapy, the diet usually is followed for two years and weaned in the third year.

How soon will we know if the diet is working?

The diet's effectiveness is seen in varying amounts of time among individuals. It can be immediate, while the diet is being initiated in the hospital, or it may take several months. Remember, seizures are different for each child; some children have several daily and others only once every 6 months.

How can my child go on diet if he is allergic or intolerant to dairy products?

The ketogenic diet can be planned for children who cannot tolerate milk or milk products; this is true for either oral or gastrostomy fed keto kids. Heavy whip cream does not need to be a component of the diet; it can be replaced with other food sources of carbohydrate, fat, and protein and produce the same degree of ketosis. For children fed by a gastrostomy, nasogastric or jejunal feeding tube, RCF® (Ross Carbohydrate Free) is recommended. The protein in dairy products, which is the allergen, is replaced by a soy protein in RCF.

How will we be able to manage birthdays and holidays?

Most of us are used to celebrating special occasions with friends, family, fun, and food. These days can still be special, but they do not need to be food centered for the ketogenic kids. For instance, at Halloween, trick or treat candy can be traded in for nickels to buy a new toy or rent a video. Birthday candles can be stuck into clay and placed on a gift or the table. The rest of the family need not suffer through holidays; however, being sensitive to a keto kid's unique diet therapy is warranted.

How will my child feel on this diet?

Children do seem to respond differently to the different stages of the ketogenic diet. A lot of this depends on what the child's baseline awake state is. Most often, during the fasting your child may feel sleepy, lethargic, and cranky. Then as the diet begins, lethargy may continue as well as nausea and vomiting, this may be due to excessive ketosis, or the side effects of the change in metabolism from using glucose as a primary energy source to using fats instead. It may be also related to a change in drug levels. In time, children should return to their normal, or close to normal activity level. One common side effect of a high fat diet for everyone is a slower gastric emptying time, thus even though the portions may look smaller, the food will stay in the stomach longer and give a longer feeling of satiety.

Are there any risks to the ketogenic diet?

Overall, the ketogenic diet appears to be relatively safe. However, a number of complications have been reported in children on the diet. Most are manageable, but they should be taken into consideration when discussing a trial of this diet.

513

Dehydration during the early phase of the diet is the most common complication. This can usually be prevented by ensuring fluid intake is adequate. Multiple metabolic abnormalities including altered levels of uric acid, protein, magnesium, and sodium in the blood have been reported. These are detectable with routine blood tests, and are correctable with supplementation or discontinuation of the ketogenic diet.

The risk for kidney stones appears to be increased, but this can also be minimized by giving plenty of fluids. Osteopenia (thinning of bones) has been reported with longer-term use, and there have been rare occurrences of heart and pancreas problems in children on the ketogenic diet.

What if my child cheats on the diet?

Cheating, or mistakes happen for various reasons, it can be purposeful by the child, or an incorrect amount of food weighed out and realized retrospectively. Trying to minimize this is important, but being prepared for what might likely occur at least once is equally important. Depending on how big the extra amount of food is/was depends on the treatment. Often times, it is safe just to recognize the mistake and pick up with the regular ketogenic meal plan at the next meal.

Will anti-seizure medications be discontinued after my child goes on the diet?

That depends on the individual circumstances. In most patients, anti-seizure medications are reduced.

If the diet seems to be working, how long will my child be on the diet?

If your child remains seizure-free for two years, most neurologists would recommend switching back to a normal diet. This weaning off the ketogenic diet is analogous to weaning anti-seizure medication after a seizure-free interval. The success rates of the ability of children to remain seizure-free off the diet after a successful treatment (with the diet) have not been well studied.

Can the ketogenic diet be used in adults?

In general, the diet does not seem to be as effective in adults. Most studies have been restricted to children and a few adolescents. In these studies, people have pointed out that the diet does not seem to work as well in older children, and seems to work best in children aged 1–10 years. The reason is not clear, but some have felt that older adolescents and adults may not make or use ketones quite as well. There are currently no published adult studies.

Is the ketogenic diet used for conditions other than epilepsy?

So far, the only condition for which the diet seems to be effective is epilepsy, with one exception of treating seizures in a rare metabolic condition that begins in infancy (such as glucose transport protein defects). In this condition inadequate amounts of glucose (sugar) gets transported to the brain. There is very little information on the use of the diet in other conditions, such as multiple sclerosis, diabetes, or obesity.

Can the ketogenic diet be used for epilepsy in animals?

The use of the ketogenic diet in animals is as yet undefined. Experimental models using rats have been developed, but the efficacy and side effects of the diet in other animals is not known. We would recommend that people consult with their veterinarian about the ketogenic diet for their pets.

Chapter 61

Lactose Intolerance

Lactose intolerance is the inability to digest significant amounts of lactose, the predominant sugar of milk. This inability results from a shortage of the enzyme lactase, which is normally produced by the cells that line the small intestine. Lactase breaks down milk sugar into simpler forms that can then be absorbed into the bloodstream. When there is not enough lactase to digest the amount of lactose consumed, the results, although not usually dangerous, may be very distressing. While not all persons deficient in lactase have symptoms, those who do are considered to be lactose intolerant.

Common symptoms include nausea, cramps, bloating, gas, and diarrhea, which begin about 30 minutes to 2 hours after eating or drinking foods containing lactose. The severity of symptoms varies depending on the amount of lactose each individual can tolerate.

Some causes of lactose intolerance are well-known. For instance, certain digestive diseases and injuries to the small intestine can reduce the amount of enzymes produced. In rare cases, children are born without the ability to produce lactase. For most people, though, lactase deficiency is a condition that develops naturally over time. After about the age of 2 years, the body begins to produce less lactase. However, many people may not experience symptoms until they are much older.

Excerpted from "Lactose Intolerance," National Institute of Diabetes and Digestive and Kidney Diseases (NIDDK), NIH Publication No. 03–2751, March 2003.

Between 30 and 50 million Americans are lactose intolerant. Certain ethnic and racial populations are more widely affected than others. As many as 75 percent of all African-Americans and American Indians and 90 percent of Asian-Americans are lactose intolerant. The condition is least common among persons of northern European descent.

Researchers have identified a genetic variation associated with lactose intolerance; this discovery may be useful in developing a diagnostic test to identify people with this condition.

How is lactose intolerance treated?

Fortunately, lactose intolerance is relatively easy to treat. No treatment can improve the body's ability to produce lactase, but symptoms can be controlled through diet.

Young children with lactase deficiency should not eat any foods containing lactose. Most older children and adults need not avoid lactose completely, but people differ in the amounts and types of foods they can handle. For example, one person may have symptoms after drinking a small glass of milk, while another can drink one glass, but not two. Others may be able to manage ice cream and aged cheeses, such as cheddar and swiss, but not other dairy products. Dietary control of lactose intolerance depends on people learning through trial and error how much lactose they can handle.

For those who react to very small amounts of lactose or have trouble limiting their intake of foods that contain it, lactase enzymes are available without a prescription to help people digest foods that contain lactose. The tablets are taken with the first bite of dairy food. Lactase enzyme is also available as a liquid. Adding a few drops of the enzyme will convert the lactose in milk or cream, making it more digestible for people with lactose intolerance.

Lactose-reduced milk and other products are available at most supermarkets. The milk contains all of the nutrients found in regular milk and remains fresh for about the same length of time, or longer if it is super-pasteurized.

How is nutrition balanced?

Milk and other dairy products are a major source of nutrients in the American diet. The most important of these nutrients is calcium. Calcium is essential for the growth and repair of bones throughout life. In the middle and later years, a shortage of calcium may lead to thin, fragile bones that break easily, a condition called osteoporosis.

A concern, then, for both children and adults with lactose intolerance, is getting enough calcium in a diet that includes little or no milk.

In 1997, the Institute of Medicine released a report recommending new requirements for daily calcium intake. How much calcium a person needs to maintain good health varies by age group. Recommendations from the report are shown in Table 61.1.

In planning meals, making sure that each day's diet includes enough calcium is important, even if the diet does not contain dairy products. Many nondairy foods are high in calcium. Excellent sources of calcium include green vegetables such as broccoli and kale, and fish with soft, edible bones such as salmon and sardines.

Recent research shows that yogurt with active cultures may be a good source of calcium for many people with lactose intolerance, even though it is fairly high in lactose. Evidence shows that the bacterial cultures used to make yogurt produce some of the lactase enzyme required for proper digestion.

Clearly, many foods can provide the calcium and other nutrients the body needs, even when intake of milk and dairy products is limited. However, factors other than calcium and lactose content should be kept in mind when planning a diet. Some vegetables that are high in calcium (Swiss chard, spinach, and rhubarb, for instance) are not good choices because the body cannot use the calcium they contain. They also contain substances called oxalates, which stop calcium absorption. Calcium is absorbed and used only when there is enough vitamin D in the body. A balanced diet should provide an adequate supply of vitamin

Table 61.1. Recommended Calcium Consumption by Age Group

Age group	Amount of calcium to consume daily, in milligrams (mg)
0–6 months	210 mg
7–12 months	270 mg
1–3 years	500 mg
4–8 years	800 mg
9–18 years	1,300 mg
19–50 years	1,000 mg
51–70+ years	1,200 mg
Pregnant and nursing women under 19	1,300 mg
Pregnant and nursing women over 19	1,000 mg

D. Sources of vitamin D include eggs and liver. However, sunlight helps the body naturally absorb or synthesize vitamin D, and with enough exposure to the sun, food sources may not be necessary.

Some people with lactose intolerance may think they are not getting enough calcium and vitamin D in their diet. Consultation with a doctor or dietitian may be helpful in deciding whether any dietary supplements are needed. Taking vitamins or minerals of the wrong kind or in the wrong amounts can be harmful. A dietitian can help in planning meals that will provide the most nutrients with the least chance of causing discomfort.

What is hidden lactose?

Although milk and foods made from milk are the only natural sources, lactose is often added to prepared foods. People with very low tolerance for lactose should know about the many food products that may contain even small amounts of lactose such as the following:

- bread and other baked goods
- processed breakfast cereals
- instant potatoes, soups, and breakfast drinks
- margarine
- lunch meats (other than kosher)
- salad dressings
- candies and other snacks
- mixes for pancakes, biscuits, and cookies
- powdered meal-replacement supplements

Some products labeled nondairy, such as powdered coffee creamer and whipped toppings, may also include ingredients that are derived from milk, and therefore, contain lactose.

Smart shoppers learn to read food labels with care, looking not only for milk and lactose among the contents, but also for such words as whey, curds, milk by-products, dry milk solids, and nonfat dry milk powder. If any of these are listed on a label, the product contains lactose.

In addition, lactose is used as the base for more than 20 percent of prescription drugs and about 6 percent of over-the-counter medicines. Many types of birth control pills, for example, contain lactose, as do some tablets for stomach acid and gas. However, these products typically affect only people with severe lactose intolerance.

Summary

Even though lactose intolerance is widespread, it need not pose a serious threat to good health. People who have trouble digesting lactose can learn which dairy products and other foods they can eat without discomfort, and which ones they should avoid. Many will be able to enjoy milk, ice cream, and other such products if they take them in small amounts or eat other food at the same time. Others can use lactase liquid or tablets to help digest the lactose. Even older women at risk for osteoporosis, and growing children who must avoid milk and foods made with milk, can meet most of their special dietary needs by eating greens, fish, and other calcium-rich foods that are free of lactose. A carefully chosen diet, with calcium supplements—if the doctor or dietitian recommends them—is the key to reducing symptoms and protecting future health.

Additional Information

American Dietetic Association (ADA)
120 South Riverside Plaza, Suite 2000
Chicago, IL 60606-6995
Toll-Free: 800-877-1600
Fax: 312-899-4899
Website: http://www.eatright.org
E-mail: hotline@eatright.org

International Foundation for Functional Gastrointestinal Disorders (IFFGD)
P.O. Box 170864
Milwaukee, WI 53217
Toll-Free: 888-964-2001
Phone: 414-964-1799
Fax: 414-964-7176
Website: http://www.iffgd.org
E-mail: iffgd@iffgd.org

National Digestive Diseases Information Clearinghouse
2 Information Way
Bethesda, MD 20892-3570
Toll-Free: 800-891-5389
Fax: 703-738-4929
Website: http://digestive.niddk.nih.gov
E-mail: nddic@info.niddk.nih.gov

Chapter 62

Malnutrition

Malnutrition is a disparity between the amount of food and other nutrients that the body needs, and the amount that it is receiving. This imbalance is most frequently associated with undernutrition, the primary focus of this chapter, but it may also be due to overnutrition.

Chronic overnutrition can lead to obesity and to metabolic syndrome, a set of risk factors characterized by abdominal obesity, a decreased ability to process glucose (insulin resistance), dyslipidemia (unhealthy lipid levels), and hypertension. Those with metabolic syndrome have been shown to be at a greater risk of developing type 2 diabetes and cardiovascular disease. Another relatively uncommon form of overnutrition is vitamin or mineral toxicity. This is usually due to excessive supplementation, for instance, high doses of fat-soluble vitamins such as Vitamin A, rather than the ingestion of food. Toxicity symptoms depend on the substance(s) ingested, the severity of the overdose, and whether it is acute or chronic.

Undernutrition occurs when one or more vital nutrients are not present in the quantity that is needed for the body to develop and function normally. This may be due to insufficient intake, increased loss, increased demand, or a condition or disease that decreases the body's ability to digest and absorb nutrients from available food. While the need for adequate nutrition is a constant, the demands of the body will vary, both on a daily and yearly basis.

- **During infancy, adolescence, and pregnancy** additional nutritional support is crucial for normal growth and development. A severe shortage of food will lead to a condition in children called marasmus that is characterized by a thin body and stunted growth. If enough calories are given, but the food is lacking in protein, a child may develop kwashiorkor—a condition characterized by edema (fluid retention), an enlarged liver, apathy, and delayed development. Deficiencies of specific vitamins can affect bone and tissue formation. A lack of Vitamin D, for instance, can affect bone formation—causing rickets in children and osteomalacia in adults, while a deficiency in folic acid during pregnancy can cause birth defects.

- **Acute conditions** such as surgery, severe burns, infections, and trauma can drastically increase short-term nutritional requirements. Those patients who have been malnourished for some time may have compromised immune systems and a poorer prognosis. They frequently take longer to heal from surgical procedures and must spend more days in the hospital. For this reason, many doctors screen and then monitor the nutritional status of their hospitalized patients. Patients having surgery are frequently evaluated both prior to surgery and during their recovery process.

- **Chronic diseases** may be associated with nutrient loss, nutrient demand, and with malabsorption (the inability of the body to use one or more available nutrients). Malabsorption may occur with chronic diseases such as celiac disease, cystic fibrosis, pancreatic insufficiency, and pernicious anemia. An increased loss of nutrients may be seen with chronic kidney disease, diarrhea, and hemorrhaging. Sometimes conditions and their treatments can both cause malnutrition through decreased intake. Examples of this are the decreased appetite, difficulty swallowing, and nausea associated both with cancer (and chemotherapy), and with human immunodeficiency virus/acquired immunodeficiency syndrome (HIV/AIDS) and its drug therapies. Increased loss, malabsorption, and decreased intake may also be seen in patients who chronically abuse drugs and/or alcohol.

- **Elderly patients** require fewer calories, but continue to require adequate nutritional support. They are often less able to absorb nutrients due in part to decreased stomach acid production, and are more likely to have one or more chronic ailments that may affect their nutritional status. At the same time, they may have more difficulty preparing meals, and may have less access to a variety of nutritious foods. Older patients also frequently eat less due to a decreased appetite, decreased sense of smell, and/or mechanical difficulties with chewing or swallowing.

Treatments

Treatment of undernutrition includes the following:

- Restoring the nutrients that are missing, making nutrient-rich foods available, and providing supplements for specific deficiencies. In someone who is severely malnourished, this must be done slowly until the body has had time to adjust to the increased intake, and then maintained at a higher than normal level until a normal or near normal weight has been achieved.

- Regular monitoring of those patients who have chronic malabsorption disorders or protein- or nutrient-losing conditions. Once the deficiencies have been addressed, putting a treatment plan into place is needed to prevent the malnutrition from recurring.

- Addressing any social, psychological, educational, and financial issues that may be causing or exacerbating the malnutrition, such as access to nutritious food.

Part Eight

National Government Nutrition Support Programs

Chapter 63

Food Stamp Program

What is the Food Stamp Program for?

The Food Stamp Program helped put food on the table for some 10.3 million households and 23.9 million individuals each day in Fiscal Year 2004. It provides low-income households with coupons or electronic benefits they can use like cash at most grocery stores to ensure that they have access to a healthy diet. The Food Stamp Program is the cornerstone of the Federal food assistance programs, and provides crucial support to needy households, and to those making the transition from welfare to work. It provided an average of $2.1 billion a month in benefits in Fiscal Year 2004.

The U.S. Department of Agriculture administers the Food Stamp Program at the Federal level through its Food and Nutrition Service (FNS). State agencies administer the program at State and local levels, including determination of eligibility, allotments, and distribution of benefits.

Who is the Food Stamp Program for?

Households must meet eligibility requirements and provide information—and verification—about their household circumstances. U.S. citizens and some aliens who are admitted for permanent residency

Excerpts from "Food Stamp Program, Frequently Asked Questions," U.S. Department of Agriculture (USDA), June 21, 2005.

may qualify. The welfare reform act of 1996 ended eligibility for many legal immigrants, though Congress later restored benefits to many children and elderly immigrants, as well as some specific groups. The welfare reform act also placed time limits on benefits for unemployed, able-bodied, childless adults.

Local food stamp offices can provide information about eligibility, and USDA operates a toll-free number (800-221-5689) for people to receive information about the Food Stamp Program. Most states also have a toll-free information/hotline number.

To Participate in the Food Stamp Program

• Households may have no more than $2,000 in countable re-sources, such as a bank account ($3,000 if at least one person in the household is age 60 or older, or is disabled). Certain re-sources are not counted, such as a home and lot. Special rules are used to determine the resource value of vehicles owned by household members.

• The gross monthly income of most households must be 130 percent or less of the Federal poverty guidelines ($1,698 per month for a family of three in most places, effective Oct. 1, 2004 through Sept. 30, 2005). Gross income includes all cash payments to the household, with a few exceptions specified in the law or the program regulations.

• Net monthly income must be 100 percent or less of Federal poverty guidelines ($1,306 per month for a household of three in most places, effective Oct. 1, 2004 through Sept. 30, 2005). Net income is figured by adding all of a household's gross in-come, and then taking a number of approved deductions for child care, some shelter costs, and other expenses. Households with an elderly or disabled member are subject only to the net income test.

• Most able-bodied adult applicants must meet certain work re-quirements.

• All household members must provide a Social Security number or apply for one.

Federal poverty guidelines are established by the Office of Man-agement and Budget, and are updated annually by the Department of Health and Human Services.

How do I obtain food stamps?

Go to the local food stamp office and fill out an application. You have the right to submit the application the same day. You can also call the office and ask them to send you an application, fill it in, and send it in by mail, or in some cases, by fax. The local office will give you an appointment for an interview. One thing to keep in mind is that the Food Stamp Program prorates the first month's benefits from the day the local office gets your application, so it is to your advantage to get the application to the office quickly, even if you have not had time to fill it out completely. Just give the local office your name, address, and signature if you cannot complete the form immediately.

How is each household's food stamp allotment determined?

Eligible households are issued a monthly allotment of food stamps based on the Thrifty Food Plan (TFP), a low-cost model diet plan. The TFP is based on National Academy of Sciences' Recommended Dietary Allowances (RDA), and on food choices of low-income households.

An individual household's food stamp allotment is equal to the maximum allotment for that household's size, less 30 percent of the household's net income. Households with no countable income receive the maximum allotment ($393 per month in Fiscal Year 2005 for a household of three people). Allotment levels are higher for Alaska, Hawaii, Guam, and the Virgin Islands, reflecting higher food prices in those areas.

What is the average benefit from the Food Stamp Program?

The average monthly benefit was about $86 per person and about $200 per household in FY 2004.

What foods are eligible for purchase with food stamps?

Households can use food stamp benefits to buy the following items:

- Foods for the household to eat, such as:
  - breads and cereals;
  - fruits and vegetables;
  - meats, fish, and poultry; and

- dairy products.

- Seeds and plants which produce food for the household to eat.

Households cannot use food stamp benefits to buy the following items:

- Beer, wine, liquor, cigarettes, or tobacco

- Any nonfood items, such as: pet foods, soaps, paper products, or household supplies

- Vitamins and medicines

- Food that will be eaten in the store

- Hot foods

In some areas, restaurants can be authorized to accept food stamp benefits from qualified homeless, elderly, or disabled people in exchange for low-cost meals. Food stamp benefits cannot be exchanged for cash.

What keeps unqualified people from getting food stamps?

As part of the commitment to program integrity, USDA works closely with the States to ensure that they issue their benefits correctly. State workers carefully evaluate each application to determine eligibility and the appropriate level of benefits. USDA monitors the accuracy of eligibility and benefit determinations. States that fail to meet standards for issuing their food stamp benefits correctly can be sanctioned by USDA, and those that exceed the standard for payment accuracy can be eligible for additional funding support. People who receive food stamp benefits in error must repay any benefits for which they did not qualify.

What are some characteristics of food stamp households?

The following statistics are based on a study of data gathered in Fiscal Year 2003:

- 51 percent of all participants are children (18 or younger), and 65 percent of them live in single-parent households.

- 55 percent of food stamp households include children.

- 9 percent of all participants are elderly (age 60 or over).

- 79 percent of all benefits go to households with children, 16 percent go to households with disabled persons, and 7 percent go to households with elderly persons.

- 36 percent of households with children were headed by a single parent, the overwhelming majority of whom were women.

- The average household size is 2.3 persons.

- The average gross monthly income per food stamp household is $640.

- 41 percent of participants are white; 36 percent are African-American, non-Hispanic; 18 percent are Hispanic; 3 percent are Asian; 2 percent are Native American; and 1 percent are of unknown race or ethnicity.

How many people get food stamps, and at what cost?

The Food Stamp Program served an average of 23.9 million people each month during Fiscal Year 2004 and cost $27.2 billion for the year. By comparison:

- in 2000, it served 17.2 million people a month and cost $17.1 billion.

Table 63.1. Gross and Net Income Eligibility Standards for the Continental U.S.,* Guam, and the Virgin Islands, Oct. 1, 2004 to Sept. 30, 2005

Household size	Gross monthly income (130 percent of poverty)	Net monthly income (100 percent of poverty)
1	1,009	776
2	1,354	1,041
3	1,698	1,306
4	2,043	1,571
5	2,387	1,836
6	2,732	2,101
7	3,076	2,366
8	3,421	2,631
Each additional member	+345	+265

* Eligibility levels are slightly higher for Alaska and Hawaii.

- in 1995, it served 26.6 million people a month and cost $24.6 billion.

- in 1990, it served 20.1 million people and cost $15.5 billion.

- in 1985, it served 19.9 million people and cost $11.7 billion.

- in 1980, it served 21.1 million people and cost $9.2 billion.

- in 1975, it served 17.1 million people and cost $4.6 billion.

- in 1970, it served 4.3 million people and cost $577 million.

The program's all-time high participation was 27.97 million people in March of 1994.

Table 63.2. Maximum Allotment Levels for the Continental United States, from October 1, 2004 to September 30, 2005

Household size	Maximum allotment level
1	$149
2	274
3	393
4	499
5	592
6	711
7	786
8	898
Each additional member	+112

Additional Information

Food, Nutrition, and Consumer Service
3101 Park Center Drive
Alexandria, VA 22302
Toll-Free: 800-221-5689
Phone: 703-305-2286
Website: http://www.fns.usda.gov
E-mail: FSPHQ-WEB@fns.usda.gov

Chapter 64

Women, Infants, and Children (WIC) Supplemental Nutrition Program

WIC provides nutritious foods, nutrition counseling, and referrals to health and other social services to participants at no charge. WIC serves low-income pregnant, postpartum, and breast-feeding women; and infants and children up to age 5 who are at nutrition risk. WIC is not an entitlement program; that is, Congress does not set aside funds to allow every eligible individual to participate in the program. Instead, WIC is a Federal grant program for which Congress authorizes a specific amount of funding each year for program operations. The Food and Nutrition Service, which administers the program at the Federal level, provides these funds to WIC State agencies (State health departments or comparable agencies) to pay for WIC foods, nutrition counseling and education, and administrative costs.

Where is WIC available?

The program is available in all 50 States, 33 Indian Tribal Organizations, America Samoa, District of Columbia, Guam, Puerto Rico, and the Virgin Islands. These 88 WIC State agencies administer the program through 2,200 local agencies and 9,000 clinic sites.

Who is eligible?

Pregnant or postpartum women, infants, and children up to age 5 are eligible. They must meet income guidelines, a State residency

"WIC: The Special Supplemental Nutrition Program for Women, Infants and Children," U.S. Department of Agriculture (USDA), December 2004.

requirement, and be individually determined to be at nutrition risk by a health professional. To be eligible on the basis of income, applicants' income must fall at or below 185 percent of the U.S. Poverty Income Guidelines (currently $34,873 for a family of four). A person who participates or has family members who participate in certain other benefit programs, such as the Food Stamp Program, Medicaid, or Temporary Assistance for Needy Families, automatically meets the income eligibility requirement.

What is nutrition risk?

Two major types of nutrition risk are recognized for WIC eligibility:

- Medically-based risks such as anemia, underweight, overweight, history of pregnancy complications, or poor pregnancy outcomes.

- Dietary risks, such as failure to meet the dietary guidelines, or inappropriate nutrition practices.

Nutrition risk is determined by a health professional such as a physician, nutritionist, or nurse, and is based on Federal guidelines. This health screening is free to program applicants.

How many people does WIC serve?

More than 7.5 million people get WIC benefits each month. In 1974, the first year WIC was permanently authorized, 88,000 people participated. By 1980, participation was at 1.9 million; by 1985 it was 3.1 million; and by 1990 it was 4.5 million. Average monthly participation for Fiscal Year (FY) 2003 was approximately 7.63 million. Children have always been the largest category of WIC participants. Of the 7.63 million people who received WIC benefits each month in FY 2003, approximately 3.82 million were children, 1.95 million were infants, and 1.86 million were women.

What food benefits do WIC participants receive?

In most WIC State agencies, WIC participants receive checks or vouchers to purchase specific foods each month that are designed to supplement their diets. A few WIC State agencies distribute the WIC foods through warehouses or deliver the foods to participants' homes. The foods provided are high in one or more of the following nutrients: protein, calcium, iron, and vitamins A and C. These are the nutrients frequently lacking in the diets of the program's target population. Different food packages are provided for different categories of participants. WIC foods include iron-fortified infant formula and infant cereal, iron-fortified adult cereal, vitamin C-rich fruit or vegetable juice, eggs, milk, cheese, peanut butter, dried beans/peas, tuna fish, and carrots. Special therapeutic infant formulas and medical foods are provided when prescribed by a physician for a specified medical condition.

Who gets first priority for participation?

WIC cannot serve all eligible people, so a system of priorities has been established for filling program openings. Once a local WIC agency has reached its maximum caseload, vacancies are filled in the order of the following priority levels:

- Pregnant women, breast-feeding women, and infants determined to be at nutrition risk because of a nutrition-related medical condition.

- Infants up to 6 months of age whose mothers participated in WIC or could have participated, and had a serious medical problem.

- Children at nutrition risk because of a nutrition-related medical problem.

- Pregnant or breast-feeding women and infants at nutrition risk because of an inadequate dietary pattern.

- Children at nutrition risk because of an inadequate dietary pattern.

- Postpartum women who are not breast-feeding with any nutrition risk.

- Individuals at nutrition risk only because they are homeless or migrants, and

- Current participants who, without WIC foods, could continue to have medical and/or dietary problems.

What is the WIC infant formula rebate system?

Mothers participating in WIC are encouraged to breast-feed their infants if possible, but WIC State agencies provide infant formula for mothers who choose to use bottle-feeding. WIC State agencies are required by law to have competitively bid infant formula rebate contracts with infant formula manufacturers. This means WIC State agencies agree to provide one brand of infant formula and in return the manufacturer gives the State agency a rebate for each can of infant formula purchased by WIC participants. The brand of infant formula provided by WIC varies from State agency to State agency depending on which company has the rebate contract in a particular State. By negotiating rebates with formula manufacturers, States are able to serve more people. For FY 2003, rebate savings were $1.52 billion, supporting an average of 1.9 million participants each month, or 25 percent of the estimated average monthly caseload.

What is WIC's current funding level?

Congress appropriated $5.235 billion for WIC in FY 2005. By comparison, the WIC Program appropriation was $20.6 million in 1974; $750 million in 1980; $1.5 billion in 1985; and $2.1 billion in 1990.

Additional Information

Food, Nutrition, and Consumer Service
3101 Park Center Drive
Alexandria, VA 22302
Toll-Free: 800-221-5689
Phone: 703-305-2286
Website: http://www.fns.usda.gov
E-mail: FSPHQ-WEB@fns.usda.gov

Chapter 65

School Nutrition Programs

National School Lunch Program

The National School Lunch Program is a federally assisted meal program operating in more than 99,800 public and non-profit private schools and residential child care institutions. It provides nutritionally balanced, low-cost or free lunches to more than 26 million children each school day. In 1998, Congress expanded the National School Lunch Program to include reimbursement for snacks served to children in after-school educational and enrichment programs to include children through 18 years of age.

The Food and Nutrition Service administers the program at the Federal level. At the State level, the National School Lunch Program is usually administered by State education agencies, which operate the program through agreements with school food authorities.

How does the National School Lunch Program work?

Generally, public or nonprofit private schools of high school grade or under, and public or nonprofit private residential child care institutions may participate in the school lunch program. School districts and independent schools that choose to take part in the lunch program, get cash subsidies and donated commodities from the U.S. Department

This chapter includes, "National School Lunch Program," "The School Breakfast Program," and "Special Milk Program," from the U.S. Department of Agriculture (USDA), December 2004.

of Agriculture (USDA) for each meal they serve. In return, they must serve lunches that meet Federal requirements, and they must offer free or reduced price lunches to eligible children. School food authorities can also be reimbursed for snacks served to children through age 18 in after-school educational or enrichment programs.

What are the nutritional requirements for school lunches?

School lunches must meet the applicable recommendations of the *Dietary Guidelines for Americans*, which recommend that no more than 30 percent of an individual's calories come from fat, and less than 10 percent from saturated fat. Regulations also establish a standard for school lunches to provide one-third of the Recommended Dietary Allowances (RDA) of protein, vitamin A, vitamin C, iron, calcium, and calories. School lunches must meet Federal nutrition requirements, but decisions about what specific foods to serve and how they are prepared are made by local school food authorities.

How do children qualify for free and reduced-price meals?

Any child at a participating school may purchase a meal through the National School Lunch Program. Children from families with incomes at or below 130 percent of the poverty level are eligible for free meals. Those with incomes between 130 percent and 185 percent of the poverty level are eligible for reduced-price meals, for which students can be charged no more than 40 cents. (For the period July 1, 2004 through June 30, 2005, 130 percent of the poverty level is $24,505 for a family of four; 185 percent is $34,873.)

Children from families with incomes over 185 percent of poverty pay a full price, though their meals are still subsidized to some extent. Local school food authorities set their own prices for full-price (paid) meals, but must operate their meal services as non-profit programs.

After-school snacks are provided to children on the same income eligibility basis as school meals. However, programs that operate in areas where at least 50 percent of students are eligible for free or reduced-price meals may serve all their snacks for free.

How much reimbursement do schools get?

Most of the support USDA provides to schools in the National School Lunch Program comes in the form of a cash reimbursement for each meal served. The current (July 1, 2004 through June 30, 2005) basic cash reimbursement rates are as follows:

- Free lunches: $2.24
- Reduced-price lunches: $1.84
- Paid lunches: $0.21
- Free snacks: $0.61
- Reduced-price snacks: $0.30
- Paid snacks: $0.05

Higher reimbursement rates are in effect for Alaska and Hawaii, and for some schools with high percentages of low-income children.

What other support do schools get from USDA?

In addition to cash reimbursements, schools are entitled by law to receive commodity foods, called entitlement foods, at a value of 17.25 cents for each meal served. Schools can also get bonus commodities as they are available from surplus agricultural stocks.

Through Team Nutrition, USDA provides schools with technical training and assistance to help school food service staffs prepare healthful meals, and with nutrition education to help children understand the link between diet and health.

What types of foods do schools get from USDA?

States select entitlement foods for their schools from a list of various foods purchased by USDA and offered through the school lunch program. Bonus foods are offered only as they become available through agricultural surplus. The variety of both entitlement and bonus commodities schools can get from USDA depends on quantities available and market prices.

A very successful project between USDA and the Department of Defense has helped provide schools with fresh produce purchased through Department of Defense. USDA has also worked with schools to help promote connections with local small farmers who may be able to provide fresh produce.

How many children have been served over the years?

The National School Lunch Act in 1946 created the modern school lunch program, though USDA had provided funds and food to schools for many years prior to that. About 7.1 million children were participating in the National School Lunch Program by the end of its first year, 1946–47. By 1970, 22 million children were participating, and by 1980 the figure was nearly 27 million. In 1990, an average of 24 million children ate school lunch every day. In Fiscal Year 2003, more than 28.4 million children each day got their lunch through the National School Lunch Program. Since the modern program began, more than 187 billion lunches have been served.

How much does the program cost?

The National School Lunch Program cost $7.1 billion in FY 2003. By comparison, the lunch program's total cost in 1947 was $70 million; in 1950, $119.7 million; 1960, $225.8 million; 1970, $565.5 million; 1975, $1.7 billion; 1980, $3.2 billion; 1985, $3.4 billion; and 1990, $3.7 billion.

The School Breakfast Program

The School Breakfast Program is a federally assisted meal program operating in public and nonprofit private schools and residential child care institutions. It began as a pilot project in 1966, and was made permanent in 1975.

The School Breakfast Program is administered at the Federal level by the Food and Nutrition Service. At the State level, the program is usually administered by State education agencies, which operate the program through agreements with local school food authorities in more than 78,000 schools and institutions.

How does the School Breakfast Program work?

The School Breakfast Program operates in the same manner as the National School Lunch Program. Generally, public or nonprofit private schools of high school grade or under and public or nonprofit private residential child care institutions may participate in the School Breakfast Program. School districts and independent schools that choose to take part in the breakfast program receive cash subsidies from the U.S. Department of Agriculture (USDA) for each meal they serve. In return, they must serve breakfasts that meet Federal requirements, and they must offer free or reduced price breakfasts to eligible children.

What are the nutritional requirements for school breakfasts?

School breakfasts must meet the applicable recommendations of the *Dietary Guidelines for Americans* which recommend that no more than 30 percent of an individual's calories come from fat, and less than 10 percent from saturated fat. In addition, breakfasts must provide one-fourth of the Recommended Dietary Allowance (RDA) for protein, calcium, iron, vitamin A, vitamin C and calories. The decisions about what specific food to serve and how they are prepared are made by local school food authorities.

How do children qualify for free and reduced price breakfasts?

Any child at a participating school may purchase a meal through the School Breakfast Program. Children from families with incomes at or below 130 percent of the Federal poverty level are eligible for free meals. Those with incomes between 130 percent and 185 percent of the poverty level are eligible for reduced-price meals. (For the period July 1, 2004 through June 30, 2005, 130 percent of the poverty level is $24,505 for a family of four; 185 percent is $34,873.) Children from families over 185 percent of poverty pay full price, though their meals are still subsidized to some extent.

How much reimbursement do schools get?

Most of the support USDA provides to schools in the School Breakfast Program comes in the form of a cash reimbursement for each breakfast served. The current (July 1, 2004 through June 30, 2005) basic cash reimbursement rates are as follows:

- Free breakfasts: $1.23
- Reduced-price breakfasts: $0.93
- Paid breakfasts: $0.23

Schools may qualify for higher severe need reimbursements if a specified percentage of their lunches are served free or at a reduced price. Severe need payments are up to 23 cents higher than the normal reimbursements for free and reduced-price breakfasts. About 65 percent of the breakfasts served in the School Breakfast Program receive severe need payments. Higher reimbursement rates are in effect for Alaska and Hawaii.

Schools may charge no more than 30 cents for a reduced-price breakfast. Schools set their own prices for breakfasts served to students who pay the full meal price (paid), though they must operate their meal services as non-profit programs.

How many children have been served over the years?

In Fiscal Year 2002, an average of 8.1 million children participated every day. That number grew to 8.4 million in Fiscal Year 2003. Of those, 6.9 million received their meals free or at a reduced-price.

Participation has slowly, but steadily grown over the years: 1970, 0.5 million children; 1975, 1.8 million children; 1980, 3.6 million children; 1985, 3.4 million children; 1990, 4.1 million children; 1995, 6.3 million children; 2000, 7.6 million children.

Special Milk Program

What is the Special Milk Program?

The Special Milk Program provides milk to children in schools, child care institutions, and eligible camps that do not participate in other Federal child nutrition meal service programs. The program reimburses schools and institutions for the milk they serve. In 2003, nearly 6,159 schools and residential child care institutions participated, along with 1,157 summer camps, and 559 non-residential child care institutions.

Schools in the National School Lunch or School Breakfast Programs may also participate in the Special Milk Program to provide milk to children in half-day pre-kindergarten and kindergarten programs where children do not have access to the school meal programs.

The Food and Nutrition Service administers the program at the Federal level. At the State level, the Special Milk Program is usually administered by State education agencies which operate the program through agreements with school food authorities.

How does the Special Milk Program work?

Generally, public or nonprofit private schools of high school grade or under and public or nonprofit private residential child care institutions and eligible camps may participate in the Special Milk Program provided they do not participate in other Federal child nutrition meal service programs, except to serve milk to pre-kindergarten and kindergarten children. Participating schools and institutions receive reimbursement from the U.S. Department of Agriculture (USDA) for each half pint of milk served. They must operate their milk programs on a non-profit basis. They agree to use the Federal reimbursement to reduce the selling price of milk to all children.

Any child at a participating school or half-day pre-kindergarten program can get milk through the Special Milk Program. Children may buy milk or receive it free, depending on the school's choice of program options.

What types of milk can be offered and what are the nutritional requirements for the milk program?

Schools or institutions may choose pasteurized fluid types of unflavored or flavored whole milk, low-fat milk, skim milk, and cultured buttermilk that meet State and local standards. All milk should contain vitamins A and D at levels specified by the Food and Drug Administration.

How do children qualify for free milk?

When local school officials offer free milk under the program to low-income children, any child from a family that meets income guidelines for free meals is eligible. Each child's family must apply annually for free milk eligibility.

How much reimbursement do schools get?

The Federal reimbursement for each half-pint of milk sold to children in School Year 2004–2005 is 17.0 cents. For children who receive their milk free, the USDA reimburses schools the net purchase price of the milk.

How much milk is served annually in the Special Milk Program?

In 2003, over 107.8 million half pints of milk were served through the Special Milk Program. Expansion of the National School Lunch and School Breakfast Programs, which include milk, has led to a substantial reduction in the Special Milk Program since its peak in the late 1960s. The program served nearly 3 billion half pints of milk in 1969; 1.8 billion in 1980; and 179 million in 1990.

How much does the program cost?

Congress appropriated $14.4 million for the Special Milk Program in Fiscal Year 2003. By comparison, the program cost $101.2 million in 1970; $145.2 million in 1980; and $19.2 million in 1990.

Additional Information

Food, Nutrition, and Consumer Services
3101 Park Center Drive, Room 914
Alexandria, VA 22302
Toll-Free: 800-221-5689
Phone: 703-305-2286
Website: http://www.fns.usda.gov/cnd
E-mail: FSPHQ-WEB@fns.usda.gov

For information on the operation of all the Child Nutrition Programs, contact the State agency in your state that is responsible for the administration of the programs. A listing of all our State agencies may be found on the USDA Food and Nutrition Service website.

Chapter 66

Senior Adult Nutrition Programs

Elderly Nutrition Program

With the aging of the U.S. population, increased attention is being given to delivering health and related services to older persons in the community. Since adequate nutrition is critical to health, functioning, and the quality of life, it is an important component of home- and community-based services for older people.

The Administration on Aging's (AoA) Elderly Nutrition Program provides grants to support nutrition services to older people throughout the country. The Elderly Nutrition Program, authorized under Title III, Grants for State and Community Programs on Aging, and Title VI, Grants for Native Americans, under the Older Americans Act, is intended to improve the dietary intakes of participants, and to offer participants opportunities to form new friendships and to create informal support networks.

The Elderly Nutrition Program provides for congregate and home-delivered meals. These meals and other nutrition services are provided in a variety of settings, such as senior centers, schools, and in individual homes.

Meals served under the program must provide at least one-third of the daily Recommended Dietary Allowances (RDA) established by the Food and Nutrition Board of the National Academy of Science–

This chapter includes "The Elderly Nutrition Program," Administration on Aging (AOA), updated September 9, 2004; and "Senior Farmers' Market Nutrition Program," U. S. Department of Agriculture (USDA), December 2004.

National Research Council. In practice, the Elderly Nutrition Program's 3.1 million elderly participants are receiving an estimated 40 to 50 percent of most required nutrients.

The Elderly Nutrition Program also provides a range of related services, by some of the aging network's estimated 4,000 nutrition service providers, including nutrition screening, assessment, education, and counseling. These services help older participants to identify their general and special nutrition needs, as they may relate to health concerns such as hypertension and diabetes.

The services help older participants to learn to shop for, and/or to plan and prepare, meals that are economical, and which help to manage or ameliorate specific health problems, as well as enhancing their health and well-being. The congregate meal programs also provide older people with positive social contacts with other seniors at the group meal sites.

Volunteers who deliver meals to older persons who are homebound are encouraged to spend some time with the elderly. The volunteers also offer an important opportunity to check on the welfare of the homebound elderly, and are encouraged to report any health or other problems that they may note during their visits.

In addition to providing nutrition and nutrition-related services, the Elderly Nutrition Program provides an important link to other needed supportive in-home and community-based services such as homemaker and home health aide services, transportation, fitness programs, and even home repair and home modification programs.

Eligibility

While there is no means test for participation in the Elderly Nutrition Program, services are targeted to older people with the greatest economic or social need, with special attention given to low-income minorities. In addition to focusing on low-income and other older persons at risk of losing their independence, the individuals who may receive services include:

- a spouse of any age;
- disabled persons under age 60 who reside in housing facilities occupied primarily by the elderly where congregate meals are served;
- disabled persons who reside at home and accompany older persons to meals; and
- nutrition service volunteers.

Since American Indians, Alaskan Natives, and Native Hawaiians tend to have lower life expectancies and higher rates of illness at younger ages, Tribal Organizations are given the option of setting the age at which older people can participate in the program.

Program Outcomes

A congressionally-mandated evaluation of the Elderly Nutrition Program, released in fiscal year (FY) 1996, found that its participants have higher daily intakes of key nutrients than similar nonparticipants, and that they have more social contacts as a result of the program.

Among Elderly Nutrition Program participants, 80 to 90 percent have incomes below 200 percent of the Department of Health and Human Services' poverty level index, which is twice the rate for the overall elderly population. More than twice as many Title III participants live alone; and two-thirds of participants are either over or under their desired weight, placing them at risk for nutrition and health problems. Title III home-delivered meals participants have twice as many physical impairments compared with the overall elderly population.

For every $1 of federal congregate funds, $1.70 additional funding is leveraged; for every $1 of federal home-delivered funds, $3.35 additional funding is leveraged. The leveraged funds come from other sources including state, tribal, local, and other federal moneys and services, as well as through donations from participants. Nationally, total contributions amounted to $170 million.

The average cost of a meal, including the value of donated labor and supplies, was $5.17 for a group meal and $5.31 for a home-delivered meal under Title III. Comparable costs for a meal under Title VI were $6.19 and $7.18, respectively.

Senior Farmers' Market Nutrition Program

The Senior Farmers' Market Nutrition Program (SFMNP) is a program in which grants are awarded to States, United States territories, and federally-recognized Indian tribal governments to provide low-income seniors with coupons that can be exchanged for eligible foods at farmers' markets, roadside stands, and community supported agriculture programs. The grant funds may be used only to support the costs of the foods that are provided under the SFMNP; no administrative funding is available.

What is the purpose of the SFMNP?

The Senior Farmers' Market Nutrition Program has the following purposes:

1. Provide fresh, nutritious, unprepared, locally grown fruits, vegetables, and herbs from farmers' markets, roadside stands, and community supported agriculture programs to low-income seniors.

2. Increase the consumption of agricultural commodities by expanding, developing, or aiding in the development and expansion of domestic farmers' markets, roadside stands, and community supported agriculture programs.

Who is eligible for SFMNP benefits?

Low-income seniors, generally defined as individuals who are at least 60 years old, and who have household incomes of not more than 185% of the federal poverty income guidelines (published each year by the Department of Health and Human Services) are the targeted recipients of SFMNP benefits. Some State agencies accept proof of participation or enrollment in another means-tested program, such as the Commodity Supplemental Food Program or Food Stamps, for SFMNP eligibility.

When does the SFMNP operate?

SFMNP benefits are provided to eligible recipients for use during the harvest season. In some States, the SFMNP season is relatively short because the growing season in that area is not very long. In other States with longer growing seasons, recipients have a longer period of time in which to use their SFMNP benefits.

Where does the SFMNP operate?

For Fiscal Year (FY) 2004, grants were awarded to 47 State agencies and federally recognized Indian tribal governments to operate the SFMNP: Alabama, Alaska, Arkansas, California, the Chickasaw Nation in Oklahoma, Colorado, Connecticut, the District of Columbia, Five Sandoval Pueblos (New Mexico), Florida, the Grand Traverse Indians in Michigan, Hawaii, Illinois, Indiana, Iowa, Kansas, Kentucky, Louisiana, Maine, Maryland, Massachusetts, Michigan, Minnesota, Mississippi, the Mississippi Band of Choctaw Indians, Missouri, Montana,

Nebraska, Nevada, New Hampshire, New Jersey, New York, North Carolina, Ohio, Oregon, the Osage Tribal Council in Oklahoma, Pennsylvania, Puerto Rico, Rhode Island, San Felipe Pueblo (New Mexico), South Carolina, Tennessee, Vermont, Virginia, Washington, West Virginia, and Wisconsin.

How does the SFMNP operate?

Once the SFMNP benefits have been issued to eligible seniors, they can be used to purchase fresh, nutritious, unprepared, locally grown fruits, vegetables, and herbs at authorized farmers' markets, roadside stands, and community supported agriculture programs. In 2003, these products were available from almost 14,000 farmers at more than 2,000 farmers' markets as well as close to 1,800 roadside stands and 200 community supported agriculture programs.

What foods are available through the SFMNP?

Fresh, nutritious, unprepared fruits, vegetables, and fresh-cut herbs can be purchased with SFMNP benefits. State agencies may limit SFMNP sales to specific foods that are locally grown in order to encourage SFMNP recipients to support the farmers in their own States. Certain foods are not eligible for purchase with SFMNP benefits; these include dried fruits or vegetables, such as prunes (dried plums), raisins (dried grapes), sun-dried tomatoes, or dried chili peppers. Potted fruit or vegetable plants, potted or dried herbs, wild rice, nuts of any kind (even raw), honey, maple syrup, cider, and molasses are also not allowed.

Who has the administrative responsibility for the SFMNP?

USDA's Food and Nutrition Service administers the SFMNP grants.

What is the current funding level?

For FY 2002–2007, Congress provided a total of $15 million for the SFMNP.

How many recipients are served in the SFMNP?

In FY 2003, approximately 800,000 people received SFMNP coupons.

Additional Information

Administration on Aging
Washington, DC 20201
Toll-Free Eldercare Locator: 800-677-1116, Monday–Friday, 9 a.m. to 8 p.m. ET
Phone: 202-619-0724
Fax: 202-357-3560
Website: http://www.aoa.gov
E-mail: aoainfo@aoa.gov

Food, Nutrition, and Consumer Services
3101 Park Center Drive
Alexandria, VA 22302
Toll-Free: 800-221-5689
Phone: 703-305-2286
Website: http://www.fns.usda.gov
E-mail: FSPHQ-WEB@fns.usda.gov

Part Nine

Additional Help
and Information

Chapter 67

Glossary of Nutrition and Dietary Terms

Acceptable Macronutrient Distribution Ranges (AMDR): Range of intake for a particular energy source that is associated with reduced risk of chronic disease while providing intakes of essential nutrients. If an individual consumes in excess of the AMDR, there is a potential of increasing the risk of chronic diseases and/or insufficient intakes of essential nutrients.

Added Sugars: Sugars and syrups that are added to foods during processing or preparation. Added sugars do not include naturally occurring sugars such as those that occur in milk and fruits.

Adequate Intakes (AI): A recommended average daily nutrient intake level based on observed or experimentally determined approximations or estimates of mean nutrient intake by a group (or groups) of apparently healthy people. The AI is used when the Estimated Average Requirement (EAR) cannot be determined.

Basic Food Groups: In the USDA food intake patterns, the basic food groups are grains; fruits; vegetables; milk, yogurt, and cheese; and meat, poultry, fish, dried peas and beans, eggs, and nuts. In the DASH

Unmarked definitions in this chapter are from *Dietary Guidelines for Americans, 2005*, U.S. Department of Health and Human Services (HHS) and U.S. Department of Agriculture (USDA). Terms marked [1] are from *Report of the Dietary Guidelines Advisory Committee of the Dietary Guidelines for Americans, 2005*, HHS and USDA.

Eating Plan, nuts, seeds, and dry beans are a separate food group from meat, poultry, fish, and eggs.

Body Mass Index (BMI): BMI is a practical measure for approximating total body fat and is a measure of weight in relation to height. It is calculated as weight in kilograms divided by the square of the height in meters.

Calorie Compensation (or Energy Compensation): The ability to regulate energy intake with minimal conscious effort, such as reducing the amount of food consumed on some occasions to compensate for increased consumption at other times. [1]

Cardiovascular Disease: Refers to diseases of the heart and diseases of the blood vessel system (arteries, capillaries, veins) throughout a person's entire body such as the brain, legs, and lungs.

Cholesterol: A sterol present in all animal tissues. Free cholesterol is a component of cell membranes and serves as a precursor for steroid hormones, including estrogen, testosterone, aldosterone, and bile acids. Humans are able to synthesize sufficient cholesterol to meet biologic requirements, and there is no evidence for a dietary requirement for cholesterol.

- **Dietary cholesterol:** Consumed from foods of animal origin, including meat, fish, poultry, eggs, and dairy products. Plant foods, such as grains, fruits and vegetables, and oils from these sources contain no dietary cholesterol.

- **Serum cholesterol:** Travels in the blood in distinct particles containing both lipids and proteins. Three major classes of lipoproteins are found in the serum of a fasting individual: low-density lipoprotein (LDL), high density lipoprotein (HDL), and very-low-density lipoprotein (VLDL). Another lipoprotein class, intermediate-density lipoprotein (IDL), resides between VLDL and LDL; in clinical practice, IDL is included in the LDL measurement.

Chronic Diseases: Long-term duration diseases, such as heart disease, cancer, and diabetes, are the leading causes of death and disability in the U.S. Although chronic diseases are among the most common and costly health problems, they are also among the most preventable. Adopting healthy behaviors such as eating nutritious foods, being physically active, and avoiding tobacco use can prevent or control the devastating effects of these diseases.

Complex Carbohydrates: Large chains of sugar units arranged to form starches and fiber. Complex carbohydrates include vegetables, whole fruits, rice, pasta, potatoes, grains (brown rice, oats, wheat, barley, corn), and legumes (chick peas, black-eyed peas, lentils, as well as beans such as lima, kidney, pinto, soy, and black beans). [1]

Coronary Heart Disease: A narrowing of the small blood vessels that supply blood and oxygen to the heart (coronary arteries).

Daily Food Intake Pattern: Identifies the types and amounts of foods that are recommended to be eaten each day and that meet specific nutritional goals.

Danger Zone: The temperature that allows bacteria to multiply rapidly and produce toxins, between 40° F and 140° F. To keep food out of this danger zone, keep cold food cold and hot food hot.

Dietary Fiber: Non-starch polysaccharides and lignin that are not digested by enzymes in the small intestine. Dietary fiber typically refers to nondigestible carbohydrates from plant foods.

Dietary Reference Intakes (DRI): A set of nutrient-based reference values that expand upon and replace the former Recommended Dietary Allowances (RDA) in the United States and the Recommended Nutrient Intakes (RNI) in Canada. They are actually a set of four reference values: Estimated Average Requirements (EAR), RDA, AI, and Tolerable Upper Intake Levels (UL).

Discretionary Calorie Allowance: The balance of calories remaining in a person's energy allowance after accounting for the number of calories needed to meet recommended nutrient intakes through consumption of foods in low-fat or no added sugar forms. The discretionary calorie allowance may be used in selecting forms of foods that are not the most nutrient-dense (e.g., whole milk rather than fat-free milk) or may be additions to foods (e.g., salad dressing, sugar, butter).

Energy Allowance: A person's energy allowance is the calorie intake at which weight maintenance occurs.

Energy Density: The calories contained in 100 grams of a particular food defines that food's energy density. [1]

Estimated Average Requirements (EAR): The average daily nutrient intake level estimated to meet the requirement of half the healthy individuals in a particular life stage and gender group.

Estimated Energy Requirement (EER): Represents the average dietary energy intake that will maintain energy balance in a healthy person of a given gender, age, weight, height, and physical activity level.

Foodborne Disease: Caused by consuming contaminated foods or beverages. Many different disease-causing microbes, or pathogens, can contaminate foods, so there are many different foodborne infections. In addition, poisonous chemicals, or other harmful substances, can cause foodborne diseases if they are present in food. The most commonly recognized foodborne infections are those caused by the bacteria *Campylobacter*, *Salmonella*, and *E. coli* O157:H7, and by a group of viruses called calicivirus, also known as the Norwalk and Norwalk-like viruses.

Food Pattern Modeling: The process of developing and adjusting daily intake amounts from each food group and subgroup to meet specific criteria. The criteria may be meeting nutrient intake goals, limitations by food component (such as limiting saturated fats), or limiting or eliminating certain types of foods (such as no meats or no legumes). [1]

Functional Fiber: Isolated, nondigestible carbohydrates that have beneficial physiological effects in humans. [1]

Glycemic Index: A classification proposed to quantify the relative blood glucose response to carbohydrate-containing foods. Operationally, it is the area under the curve for the increase in blood glucose after the ingestion of a set amount of carbohydrate in a food (e.g., 50 grams) during the 2-hour postprandial period relative to the same amount of carbohydrate from a reference food (white bread or glucose) tested in the same individual under the same conditions using the initial blood glucose concentration as a baseline. [1]

Glycemic Load: An indicator of glucose response or insulin demand that is induced by total carbohydrate intake. It is calculated by multiplying the weighted mean of the dietary glycemic index by the percentage of total energy from carbohydrate. [1]

Glycemic Response: The effects that carbohydrate-containing foods have on blood glucose concentration during the digestion process. [1]

Glycerol: A three-carbon substance that forms the backbone of fatty acids in fats. [1]

Heme Iron: One of two forms of iron occurring in foods. Heme iron is bound within the iron-carrying proteins (hemoglobin and myoglobin) found in meat, poultry, and fish. While it contributes a smaller portion of iron to typical American diets than non-heme iron, a larger proportion of heme iron is absorbed.

High Fructose Corn Syrup (HFCS): A corn sweetener derived from the wet milling of corn. Cornstarch is converted to syrup that is nearly all dextrose. HFCS is found in numerous foods and beverages on the grocery store shelves.

Hydrogenation: A chemical reaction that adds hydrogen atoms to an unsaturated fat, thus saturating it and making it solid at room temperature.

Leisure-Time Physical Activity: Physical activity that is performed during exercise, recreation, or any additional time other than that associated with one's regular job duties, occupation, or transportation.

Listeriosis: A serious infection caused by eating food contaminated with the bacterium *Listeria monocytogenes*, which has recently been recognized as an important public health problem in the U.S. The disease affects primarily pregnant women, their fetuses, newborns, and adults with weakened immune systems. Listeria is killed by pasteurization and cooking; however, in certain ready-to-eat foods, such as hot dogs and deli meats, contamination may occur after cooking/manufacture, but before packaging. *Listeria monocytogenes* can survive at refrigerated temperatures.

Macronutrient: The dietary macronutrient groups are carbohydrates, proteins, and fats.

Metabolic Equivalent (MET): A way of measuring physical activity intensity. This unit is used to estimate the amount of oxygen used by the body during physical activity. 1 MET = the energy (oxygen) used by the body as you sit quietly, perhaps while talking on the phone or reading a book. The harder your body works during the activity, the higher the MET. [1]

Metabolic Syndrome: A collection of metabolic risk factors in one individual. The root causes of metabolic syndrome are excessive weight, obesity, physical activity, and genetic factors. Various risk factors have been included in metabolic syndrome. Factors generally accepted as being characteristic of this syndrome include abdominal obesity, atherogenic dyslipidemia, raised blood pressure, insulin resistance with or without glucose intolerance, prothrombotic state, and proinflammatory state. [1]

Micronutrient: Vitamins and minerals that are required in the human diet in very small amounts.

Moderate Physical Activity: Any activity that burns 3.5 to 7 kcal/min or the equivalent of 3 to 6 metabolic equivalents (MET), and results in achieving 60 to 73 percent of peak heart rate. An estimate of a person's peak heart rate can be obtained by subtracting the person's age from 220. Examples of moderate physical activity include walking briskly, mowing the lawn, dancing, swimming, or bicycling on level terrain. A person should feel some exertion, but should be able to carry on a conversation comfortably during the activity.

Monounsaturated Fatty Acids (MUFA): Monounsaturated fatty acids have one double bond. Plant sources that are rich in MUFA include vegetable oils (e.g., canola oil, olive oil, high oleic safflower oil, and sunflower oil) that are liquid at room temperature and nuts.

Nutrient Adequacy: A goal based on the RDA or AI set for vitamins, minerals, macronutrients, and acceptable intake ranges for macronutrients for various age/gender groups. Adequacy of intake relates to meeting the individual's requirement for that nutrient. [1]

Nutrient-Dense Foods: Nutrient-dense foods are those that provide substantial amounts of vitamins and minerals and relatively fewer calories.

Ounce-Equivalent: In the grains food group, the amount of a food counted as equal to a one-ounce slice of bread; in the meat, poultry, fish, dry beans, eggs, and nuts food group, the amount of food counted as equal to one ounce of cooked meat, poultry, or fish.

n-6 PUFAs: Linoleic acid, one of the n-6 fatty acids, is required, but cannot be synthesized by humans, and therefore, is considered essential in the diet. Primary sources are liquid vegetable oils, including soybean oil, corn oil, and safflower oil.

n-3 PUFAs: The n-3 fatty acid a-linolenic acid is required because it is not synthesized by humans, and therefore, is considered essential in the diet. It is obtained from plant sources, including soybean oil, canola oil, walnuts, and flaxseed. Eicosapentaenoic acid (EPA) and docosahexaenoic acid (DHA) are long chain n-3 fatty acids that are contained in fish and shellfish.

Pathogen: Any microorganism that can cause or is capable of causing disease.

Phytochemicals: Substances found in edible fruits and vegetables that may be ingested by humans daily in gram quantities, and that exhibit a potential for modulating the human metabolism in a manner favorable for reducing the risk of cancer. [1]

Polyunsaturated Fatty Acids (PUFA): Polyunsaturated fatty acids have two or more double bonds and may be of two types, based on the position of the first double bond.

Portion Size: The amount of a food consumed in one eating occasion.

Probability of Adequacy: The probability that a given nutrient intake is adequate for an individual can be calculated if the requirement distribution is known. If this distribution is approximately normal, it is defined by the Estimated Average Requirement (EAR) and its standard deviation. [1]

Recommended Dietary Allowance (RDA): The dietary intake level that is sufficient to meet the nutrient requirement of nearly all (97 to 98 percent) healthy individuals in a particular life stage and gender group.

Resistance Exercise: Anaerobic training, including weight training, weight machine use, and resistance band workouts. Resistance training will increase strength, muscular endurance, and muscle size. Running and jogging are not resistance exercise.

Salmonellosis: An infection caused by bacteria called *Salmonella*. Most persons infected with *Salmonella* develop diarrhea, fever, and abdominal cramps 12 to 72 hours after infection. The illness usually lasts 4 to 7 days, and most people recover without treatment. Salmonellosis is prevented by cooking poultry, ground beef, and eggs thoroughly before eating and not eating or drinking foods containing raw eggs or raw unpasteurized milk. [1]

Saturated Fatty Acids: Saturated fatty acids have no double bonds. They primarily come from animal products such as meat and dairy products. In general, animal fats are solid at room temperature.

Sedentary Behaviors: In scientific literature, sedentary is often defined in terms of little or no physical activity during leisure time. A sedentary lifestyle is a lifestyle characterized by little or no physical activity.

Serving Size: A standardized amount of a food, such as a cup or an ounce, used in providing dietary guidance or in making comparisons among similar foods.

Simple Carbohydrates: Sugars composed of a single sugar molecule (monosaccharide) or two joined sugar molecules (a disaccharide), such as glucose, fructose, lactose, and sucrose. Simple carbohydrates include white and brown sugar, fruit sugar, corn syrup, molasses, honey, and candy. [1]

Structured Exercise: Physical activity performed in a planned manner for enhancing health and/or fitness. [1]

Tolerable Upper Intake Level (UL): The highest average daily nutrient intake level likely to pose no risk of adverse health affects for nearly all individuals in a particular life stage and gender group. As intake increases above the UL, the potential risk of adverse health affects increases.

***Trans* fatty acids:** *Trans* fatty acids, or *trans* fats, are unsaturated fatty acids that contain at least one non-conjugated double bond in the *trans* configuration. Sources of *trans* fatty acids include hydrogenated/

partially hydrogenated vegetable oils that are used to make shortening and commercially prepared baked goods, snack foods, fried foods, and margarine. *Trans* fatty acids also are present in foods that come from ruminant animals (e.g., cattle and sheep). Such foods include dairy products, beef, and lamb.

Vegetarian: There are several categories of vegetarians, all of whom avoid meat and/or animal products. The vegan or total vegetarian diet includes only foods from plants: fruits, vegetables, legumes (dried beans and peas), grains, seeds, and nuts. The lactovegetarian diet includes plant foods plus cheese and other dairy products. The ovo-lactovegetarian (or lacto-ovovegetarian) diet also includes eggs. Semi-vegetarians do not eat red meat, but include chicken and fish with plant foods, dairy products, and eggs.

Vigorous Physical Activity: Any activity that burns more than 7 kcal/min, or the equivalent of 6 or more metabolic equivalents (MET), and results in achieving 74 to 88 percent of peak heart rate. An estimate of a person's peak heart rate can be obtained by subtracting the person's age from 220. Examples of vigorous physical activity include jogging, mowing the lawn with a non-motorized push mower, chopping wood, participating in high impact aerobic dancing, swimming continuous laps, or bicycling uphill. Vigorous-intensity physical activity may be intense enough to represent a substantial challenge to an individual, and results in a significant increase in heart and breathing rate.

Weight-Bearing Exercise: Any activity one performs that works bones and muscles against gravity including walking, running, hiking, dancing, gymnastics, and soccer.

Whole Grains: Foods made from the entire grain seed, usually called the kernel, which consists of the bran, germ, and endosperm. If the kernel has been cracked, crushed, or flaked, it must retain nearly the same relative proportions of bran, germ, and endosperm as the original grain in order to be called whole grain.

Chapter 68

Finding Useful Nutrition Information Online

Tips for Searching the Internet for Nutrition Information

When searching on the Internet, try using directory sites of respected organizations, rather than doing blind searches with a search engine. Ask yourself the following questions.

Who operates the site?

Is the site run by the government, a university, or a reputable medical or health-related association (e.g., American Medical Association, American Diabetes Association, American Heart Association, National Institutes of Health, National Academies of Science, or U.S. Food and Drug Administration)? Is the information written or reviewed by qualified health professionals, experts in the field, academia, government, or the medical community?

What is the purpose of the site?

Is the purpose of the site to objectively educate the public or just to sell a product? Be aware of practitioners or organizations whose main interest is in marketing products, either directly, or through sites with which they are linked. Commercial sites should clearly distinguish

Excerpted from "Tips for the Savvy Supplement User: Making Informed Decisions and Evaluating Information," *Dietary Supplements*, January 2002, U.S. Food and Drug Administration (FDA).

scientific information from advertisements. Most nonprofit and government sites contain no advertising, and access to the site and materials offered are usually free.

What is the source of the information and does it have any references?

Has the study been reviewed by recognized scientific experts and published in reputable peer-reviewed scientific journals, like the *New England Journal of Medicine*? Does the information say "some studies show..." or does it state where the study is listed so that you can check the authenticity of the references? For example, can the study be found in the National Library of Medicine's database of literature citations (PubMed link—http://www.ncbi.nlm.nih.gov/PubMed).

Is the information current?

Check the date when the material was posted or updated. Often new research or other findings are not reflected in old material, (e.g., side effects or interactions with other products or new evidence that might have changed earlier thinking). Ideally, health and medical sites should be updated frequently.

How reliable is the Internet or e-mail solicitation?

While the Internet is a rich source of health information, it is also an easy vehicle for spreading myths, hoaxes, and rumors about alleged news, studies, products, or findings. To avoid falling prey to such hoaxes, be skeptical and watch out for overly emphatic language with UPPERCASE LETTERS and lots of exclamation points!!!! Beware of such phrases such as: "This is not a hoax" or "Send this to everyone you know."

Ask yourself: Does it sound too good to be true?

Do the claims for the product seem exaggerated or unrealistic? Are there simplistic conclusions being drawn from a complex study to sell a product? While the Web can be a valuable source of accurate, reliable information, it also has a wealth of misinformation that may not be obvious. Learn to distinguish hype from evidence-based science. Nonsensical lingo can sound very convincing. Also, be skeptical about anecdotal information from persons who have no formal training in nutrition or botanicals, or from personal testimonials (e.g., from store employees, friends, or online chat rooms and message boards) about incredible benefits or results obtained from using a product. Question these people on their training and knowledge in nutrition or medicine.

Think Twice about Chasing the Latest Headline

Sound health advice is generally based on a body of research, not a single study. Be wary of results claiming a "quick fix" that depart from previous research and scientific beliefs. Keep in mind science does not proceed by dramatic breakthroughs, but by taking many small steps, slowly building towards a consensus. Furthermore, news stories, about the latest scientific study, especially those on television or radio, are often too brief to include important details that may apply to you or allow you to make an informed decision.

Online Nutrition Information

The following websites and search engines provide reliable diet and nutrition information, resources, and Internet links for further research.

American Dietetic Association
Website: http://www.eatright.org

American Institute for Cancer Research
Website: http://www.aicr.org

Center for Science in the Public Interest
Website: http://www.cspinet.org

Dietary Guidelines for Americans
Website: http://www.healthierus.gov/dietaryguidelines

Federal Trade Commission
Website: http://ftc.gov

Food and Nutrition Information Center
Website: http://www.nal.usda.gov/fnic

Food, Nutrition, and Consumer Services
Website: http://www.fns.usda.gov

Go Ask Alice!
Website: http://www.goaskalice.columbia.edu

Healthfinder
Website: http://www.healthfinder.gov

Healthier US.Gov
Website: http://www.healthierus.gov

International Food Information Council
Website: http://www.ific.org

Mayo Clinic Healthy Living Center
Website: http://www.mayoclinic.com/findinformation/
healthylivingcenter/index.cfm

MedWatch
Website: http://www.fda.gov/medwatch

MyPyramid Food Guidance Plan
Website: http://www.mypyramid.gov

National Agricultural Library
Website: http://www.nal.usda.gov

National Center for Biotechnology Information
Website: http://www.ncbi.nlm.nih.gov/entrez/query.fcgi

National Heart, Lung, and Blood Institute
Website: http://www.nhlbi.nih.gov

National Library of Medicine
Website: http://www.medlineplus.gov

National Nutrient Database
Website: http://www.nal.usda.gov/fnic/foodcomp

Nemours Foundation
Website: http://www.kidshealth.org
Website: http://www.teenshealth.org

Partnership for Healthy Weight Management
Website: http://www.consumer.gov/weightloss

U.S. Department of Agriculture
Website: http://www.usda.gov

U.S. Department of Health and Human Services
Website: http://www.dhhs.gov

U.S. Food and Drug Administration
Website: http://www.fda.gov

Vegetarian Resource Group
Website: http://www.vrg.org

WebMD
Website: http://www.webmd.com

Weight-Control Information Network
Website: http://win.niddk.nih.gov

Chapter 69

Nutrition Resource List for Consumers

General Nutrition Books

Duyff, Roberta. *American Dietetic Association's Complete Food and Nutrition Guide, 2ⁿᵈ Edition*. Wiley, 2002. ISBN: 0471229245.

Duyff, Roberta Larson. *ADA 365 Days of Healthy Eating*. Wiley, 2003. ISBN: 0471442216.

American Dietetic Association. *ADA Pocket Supermarket Guide, 3ʳᵈ edition*. Wiley, 2005. ISBN: 0880914076.

Pennington, Jean and Douglass, Judith. *Bowes & Church's Food Values of Portions Commonly Used, 18ᵗʰ edition, Revised*. Lippincott, 2004. ISBN: 0781744296.

O'Neil, Carolyn, and Webb, Denise. *The Dish on Eating Healthy and Being Fabulous*. Atria Books, 2004. ISBN: 0743476883.

Peeke, Pamela. *Fight Fat after Forty*. Penguin Books, 2000. ISBN: 014100181.

The Johns Hopkins Medical Guide to Health after 50. Medletter Associates, 2003. ISBN: 0929661737.

Information in this chapter was compiled from "Eating Smart: A Nutrition Resource List for Consumers," U.S. Department of Agriculture (USDA), May 2005; and "General Nutrition Resources List for Seniors," USDA, October 2002.

Humphrey, James Harry. *Living Longer and Livelier: Guidelines for Older Adults*. Kroshka Books, 2000. ISBN: 1560727454.

Creagen, Edward T. *Mayo Clinic on Health and Aging: Answers to Help You Make the Most of the Rest of Your Life*. Mayo Foundation for Medical Education and Research, 2001. ISBN: 1893005070.

Rinzler, Carol Ann. *Nutrition For Dummies, 3rd edition*. Wiley, 2003. ISBN: 0764540823.

Jacobson, Michael F. and Hurley, Jayne. *Restaurant Confidential*. Workman Publishing Company, 2002. ISBN: 0761100350.

Nelson, Miriam E. and Knipe, Judy. *Strong Women Eat Well: Nutritional Strategies for a Healthy Body and Mind*. Putnam, 2001. ISBN: 0399147403.

Katz, David L. and Gonzalez, Maura H. *The Way to Eat*. Sourcebooks, 2004. ISBN: 1570719837.

Cookbooks

ADA, Food and Culinary DPG, and Napier, Kristine. *ADA Cooking Healthy Across America*. Wiley, 2005. ISBN: 0471474304.

American Heart Association. *American Heart Association Meals in Minutes Cookbook*. Crown Publishing Group, 2002. ISBN: 0609809776.

Wesler, Cathy A. *The Complete Cooking Light Cookbook*. Oxmoor House, 2000. ISBN: 084871945X.

Cain, Anne Chappell. *Cooking Light 5-Ingredient, 15-Minute Cookbook*. Oxmoor House, 1999. ISBN: 0848718526.

Cleveland Clinic Foundation. *Creative Cooking for Renal Diabetic Diets*. Senay Publishing, ISBN: 0941511014.

Cleveland Clinic Foundation. *Creative Cooking for Renal Diets*. Senay Publishing. ISBN: 0941511006.

Stanley, Kathleen. *Diabetic Cooking for Seniors*. McGraw-Hill/Contemporary Distributed Products, 2001. ISBN: 1580400736.

Eds. Margolis, Simeon, and Wilder, Lora Brown. *St. Johns Hopkins Cookbook Library: Recipes for a Healthy Heart*. Medletter Associates, 2003. ISBN: 092966177X.

Carroll, John Phillip. *The Mayo Clinic Williams-Sonoma Cookbook: Simple Solutions for Eating Well.* Time Life Custom Publishing, 2001. ISBN: 0737020687.

American Institute for Cancer Research. *The New American Plate Cookbook Recipes for a Healthy Weight and Healthy Life.* University of California Press, 2005. ISBN: 0520242343.

Glick, Ruth and Baggett, Nancy. *One Pot Meals for People with Diabetes.* McGraw-Hill/Contemporary Distributed Products, 2002. ISBN: 1580400663.

Peters, Mardy. *The Renal Gourmet.* Emenar, Inc. ISBN: 096417300X.

Newsletters and Magazines

American Institute for Cancer Research Newsletter. American Institute for Cancer Research, 1759 R Street NW, Washington, DC 20009; 800-843-8114 (in Washington, D.C. 202-328-7744). Website: http://www.aicr.org/publications/news.lasso.

Cooking Light Magazine. Cooking Light Customer Service, 2100 Lakeshore Dr., Birmingham, AL 35209; 205-445-6000. E-mail: cookinglight @customersvc.com. Website: http://www.cookinglight.com/cooking.

Dr. Irene's Nutrition Tidbits Newsletter. E-mail newsletter. Website: http://drirene.healthandage.com/qa3.htm.

EatingWell Magazine. Eating Well, Inc., 823A Ferry Rd., Charlotte, VT 05445; 802-425-5700. Website: http://www.eatingwell.com.

Environmental Nutrition Newsletter. Free online trial available prior to opening a paid subscription. Website: http://www.environmental nutrition.com.

FDA Consumer. Available free of charge online at http://www.fda.gov/ fdac; or in print by paid subscription from: Superintendent of Documents, P.O. Box 371954, Pittsburgh, PA 15250; 202-512-1800.

Feeding Kids Newsletter. Free E-mail newsletter. Website: http:// nutritionforkids.com/Feeding_Kids.htm.

Food Reflections Newsletter. University of Nebraska Cooperative Extension. Free E-mail newsletter. Website: http://lancaster.unl.edu/food/ foodtalk.htm.

Harvard Health Publications. Harvard University. Purchase subscriptions online. Website: http://www.health.harvard.edu/newsletters.

Nutrition Action Healthletter. Center for Science in the Public Interest. Open a paid subscription online at http://www.cspinet.org/nah, or by mail: Ordering Information, 1875 Connecticut Ave., N.W., Suite 300, Washington, DC 20009; E-mail: circ@cspinet.org.

Nutrition and Your Child. USDA/Agricultural Research Service Children's Nutrition Research Center at Baylor College of Medicine. Available free in PDF format on the Website at http://www.kidsnutrition .org/consumer/nyc/index.htm.

Nutrition Spotlight. Free online newsletter. Website: http://www.oznet .ksu.edu/dp_fnut/spotlight/welcome.htm.

Tufts Health and Nutrition Letter. Tufts University. Purchase a subscription online or write: P.O. Box 420235, Palm Coast, FL 32142; 800-274-7581. E-mail: nyhealthletter@tufts.edu. Website: http://health letter.tufts.edu.

University of California at Berkeley Wellness Letter. University of California Berkeley Wellness Letter Subscription Department, P.O. Box 420148, Palm Coast, FL 32142; 800-829-9170. Website: http:// www.berkeleywellness.com/index.php.

Chapter 70

Directory of Nutrition Information Sources

Government Agencies and Organizations

Administration on Aging
Washington, DC 20201
Phone: 202-619-0724
Fax: 202-357-3560
Website: http://www.aoa.gov
E-mail: aoainfo@aoa.gov

Center for Food Safety and Applied Nutrition (CFSAN)
Food and Drug Administration
5100 Paint Branch Pkwy.
College Park, MD 20740-3835
Toll-Free: 888-723-3366
Website: http://
www.cfsan.fda.gov

Center for Nutrition Policy and Promotion (CNPP)
3101 Park Center Dr., Rm. 1034
Alexandria, VA 22302-1594
Website: http://
www.mypyramid.gov
E-mail: support@cnpp.usda.gov

Centers for Disease Control and Prevention (CDC)
1600 Clifton Rd.
Atlanta, GA 30333
Toll-Free: 800-311-3435
Phone: 404-639-3534
Website: http://www.cdc.gov

Resources in this chapter were compiled from several sources deemed reliable. All contact information was verified and updated in August 2005.

Eldercare Locator
Administration on Aging
330 Independence Ave. S.W.
Washington, DC 20201
Toll-Free: 800-677-1116
Phone: 202-619-7501
Website: http://
www.eldercare.gov
E-mail:
eldercarelocator@spherix.com

FDA MedWatch
5600 Fishers Lane, HFD-410
Rockville, MD 20857
Toll-Free: 800-332-1088
Fax: 301-827-7241
Website: http://www.fda.gov/
medwatch

Federal Trade Commission (FTC)
600 Pennsylvania Ave., N.W.
Washington, DC 20580
Toll-Free: 877-382-4357
Website: http://www.ftc.gov

Food and Nutrition Information Center
USDA Agriculture Research Service
10301 Baltimore Ave.
Beltsville, MD 20705-2351
Phone: 301-504-5719
Fax: 301-504-6409
TTY: 301-504-6856
Website: http://
www.nal.usda.gov/fnic
E-mail: fnic@nal.usda.gov

Food, Nutrition, and Consumer Services
3101 Park Center Dr.
Alexandria, VA 22302
Toll-Free: 800-221-5689
Phone: 703-305-2286
Website: http://www.fns.usda.gov
E-mail: FSPHQ-
WEB@fns.usda.gov

Food Safety and Inspection Service
1400 Independence Ave., S.W.
Room 2932-S
Washington, DC 20250-3700
Toll-Free: 800-535-4555
Toll-Free TTY: 800-256-7072
Website: http://www.fsis.usda.gov
E-mail: fsis@usda.gov

Healthier US.Gov
U.S. Department of Health and Human Services
200 Independence Ave., S.W.
Washington, DC 20201
Toll-Free: 877-696-6775
Phone: 202-619-6775
Website: http://
www.healthierus.gov

Milk Matters Calcium Education Campaign
31 Center Dr., Room 2A32
Bethesda, MD 20892-2425
Toll-Free: 800-370-2943
Phone: 301-496-5133
Fax: 301-496-7101
Website: http://
www.nichd.nih.gov/milk
E-mail:
NICHDMilkMatters@nail.nih.gov

National Center for Complementary and Alternative Medicine (NCCAM) Clearinghouse
P.O. Box 7923
Gaithersburg, MD 20898-7923
Toll-Free: 888-644-6226
International: 301-519-3153
Toll-Free Fax: 866-464-3616
Fax-on-Demand Service: 888-644-6226
Toll-Free TTY: 866-464-3615
Website: http://nccam.nih.gov
E-mail: info@nccam.nih.gov

National Diabetes Information Clearinghouse
1 Information Way
Bethesda, MD 20892-3560
Toll-Free: 800-860-8747
Fax: 703-738-4929
Website: http://
diabetes.niddk.nih.gov
E-mail: ndic@info.niddk.nih.gov

National Digestive Diseases Information Clearinghouse
2 Information Way
Bethesda, MD 20892-3570
Toll-Free: 800-891-5389
Fax: 703-738-4929
Website: http://
digestive.niddk.nih.gov
E-mail:
nddic@info.niddk.nih.gov

National Heart, Lung, and Blood Institute (NHLBI)
P.O. Box 30105
Bethesda, MD 20824-0105
Toll-Free: 800-575-9355
Phone: 301-592-8573
Fax: 301-592-8563
TTY: 240-629-3255
Website: http://
www.nhlbi.nih.gov
E-mail: nhlbiinfo@nhlbi.nih.gov

National Institute of Child Health and Human Development (NICHD)
P.O. Box 3006
Rockville, MD 20847
Toll-Free: 800-370-2943
Fax: 301-984-1473
Toll-Free TTY: 888-320-6942
Website: http://
www.nichd.nih.gov
E-mail: NICHDInformation
ResourceCenter@mail.nih.gov

National Institute of Diabetes and Digestive and Kidney Diseases (NIDDK)
Information Clearinghouse
5 Information Way
Bethesda, MD 20892-3560
Toll-Free: 800-860-8747
Phone: 301-654-3810
Website: http://
www.niddk.nih.gov

National Institute on Aging (NIA)
Bldg. 31, Room 5C27
31 Center Dr., MSC 2292
Bethesda, MD 20892
Toll-Free: 800-222-2225
Phone: 301-496-1752
Fax: 301-496-1072
Toll-Free TTY: 800-222-4225
Website: http://www.nia.nih.gov

National Kidney and Urologic Diseases Information Clearinghouse
3 Information Way
Bethesda, MD 20892-3580
Toll-Free: 800-891-5390
Fax: 703-738-4929
Website: http://
kidney.niddk.nih.gov

Office of Dietary Supplements (ODS)
Room 3B01, MSC 7517
6100 Executive Blvd.
Bethesda, MD 20892-7515
Phone: 301-435-2920
Fax: 301-480-1845
Website: http://dietary-
supplements.info.nih.gov
E-mail: ods@nih.gov

U.S. Department of Agriculture (USDA)
1400 Independence Ave., S.W.
Washington, DC 20250
Website: http://www.usda.gov

U.S. Department of Health and Human Services (HHS)
200 Independence Ave., S.W.
Washington, DC 20201
Toll-Free: 877-696-6775
Phone: 202-619-6775
Website: http://www.hhs.gov

U.S. Environmental Protection Agency (EPA)
Fish Advisory Program
1200 Pennsylvania Ave., N.W.
Washington, DC 20460
Website: http://www.epa.gov/ost/
fish

U.S. Food and Drug Administration (FDA)
5600 Fishers Lane
Rockville, MD 20857
Toll-Free: 888-463-6332
Website: http://www.fda.gov

Weight-Control Information Network (WIN)
1 Win Way
Bethesda, MD 20892-3665
Toll-Free: 877-946-4627
Phone: 202-828-1025
Fax: 202-828-1028
Website: http://
win.niddk.nih.gov
E-mail: win@info.niddk.nih.gov

Private and Nonprofit Organizations

American Academy of Allergy, Asthma, and Immunology
555 E. Wells St., Suite 1100
Milwaukee, WI 53202-3823
Toll-Free: 800-822-2762
Phone: 414-272-6071
Website: http://www.aaaai.org
E-mail: info@aaaai.org

American Association of Diabetes Educators
100 W. Monroe, Suite 400
Chicago, IL 60603
Toll-Free: 800-338-3633
Fax: 312-424-2427
Website: http://www.aadenet.org
E-mail: aade@aadenet.org

American Association of Kidney Patients
3503 E. Frontage Rd., Ste. 315
Tampa, FL 33607
Toll-Free: 800-749-2257
Fax: 813-636-8122
Website: http://www.aakp.org
E-mail: info@aakp.org

American Celiac Society
59 Crystal Ave.
West Orange, NJ 07052
Phone: 504-737-3293
Fax: 973-669-8808
E-mail:
amerceliacsoc@onebox.com

American College of Allergy, Asthma and Immunology
85 W. Algonquin Rd.
Suite 550
Arlington Heights, IL 60005
Phone: 847-427-1200
Fax: 847-427-1294
Website: http://www.acaai.org
E-mail: mail @acaai.org

American Diabetes Association
1701 N. Beauregard St.
Alexandria, VA 22311
Toll-Free: 800-342-2383
Website: http://www.diabetes.org
E-mail: askADA@diabetes.org

American Dietetic Association (ADA)
120 S. Riverside Plaza
Suite 2000
Chicago, IL 60606-6995
Toll-Free: 800-877-1600
Fax: 312-899-4899
Website: http://
www.eatright.org/Public
E-mail: hotline@eatright.org

American Heart Association
7272 Greenville Ave.
Dallas, TX 75231
Toll-Free: 800-242-8721
Website: http://
www.americanheart.org

American Institute for Cancer Research
1759 R Street N.W.
Washington, DC 20009
Toll-Free: 800-843-8114
Phone: 202-328-7744
Fax: 202-328-7226
Website: http://www.aicr.org
E-mail: aicrweb@aicr.org

Asthma and Allergy Foundation of America
1233 20th Street, N.W.
Suite 402
Washington, DC 20036
Toll-Free: 800-727-8462
Phone: 202-466-7643
Fax: 202-466-8940
Website: http://www.aafa.org
E-mail: info@aafa.org

Celiac Disease Foundation
13251 Ventura Blvd., #1
Studio City, CA 91604
Phone: 818-990-2354
Fax: 818-990-2379
Website: http://www.celiac.org
E-mail: cdf@celiac.org

Celiac Sprue Association/USA Inc.
P.O. Box 31700
Omaha, NE 68131-0700
Toll-Free: 877-272-4272
Phone: 402-558-0600
Fax: 402-558-1347
Website: http://
www.csaceliacs.org
E-mail: celiacs@csaceliacs.org

Cystic Fibrosis Foundation
6931 Arlington Rd.
Bethesda, MD 20814
Toll-Free: 800-FIGHT CF (344-4823)
Phone: 301-951-4422
Fax: 301-951-6378
Website: http://www.cff.org
E-mail: info@cff.org

Food Allergy and Anaphylaxis Network (FAAN)
11781 Lee Jackson Hwy.
Suite 160
Fairfax, VA 22033
Toll-Free: 800-929-4040
Fax: 703-691-2713
Website: http://
www.foodallergy.org
E-mail: faan@foodallergy.org

Gluten Intolerance Group (GIG) of North America
15110 10th Ave. S.W., Suite A
Seattle, WA 98166
Phone: 206-246-6652
Fax: 206-246-6531
Website: http://www.gluten.net
E-mail: info@gluten.net

Institute of Food Technologists
525 W. Van Buren, Suite 1000
Chicago, IL 60607
Toll-Free: 800-438-3663
Phone: 312-782-8424
Fax: 312-782-8348
Website: http://www.ift.org/cms
E-mail: info@ift.org

International Food Information Council Foundation
1100 Connecticut Ave., N.W.
Suite 430
Washington, DC 20036
Phone: 202-296-6540
Fax: 202-296-6547
Website: http://www.ific.org
E-mail: foodinfo@ific.org

International Foundation for Functional Gastrointestinal Disorders (IFFGD)
P.O. Box 170864
Milwaukee, WI 53217
Toll-Free: 888-964-2001
Phone: 414-964-1799
Fax: 414-964-7176
Website: http://www.iffgd.org
E-mail: iffgd@iffgd.org

National Kidney Foundation
30 East 33rd St.
New York, NY 10016
Toll-Free: 800-622-9010
Phone: 212-889-2210
Fax: 212-689-9261
Website: http://www.kidney.org
E-mail: info@kidney.org

Index

Index

Health Reference Series
COMPLETE CATALOG

List price $87 per volume. **School and library price $78 per volume.**

Adolescent Health Sourcebook

Basic Consumer Health Information about Common Medical, Mental, and Emotional Concerns in Adolescents, Including Facts about Acne, Body Piercing, Mononucleosis, Nutrition, Eating Disorders, Stress, Depression, Behavior Problems, Peer Pressure, Violence, Gangs, Drug Use, Puberty, Sexuality, Pregnancy, Learning Disabilities, and More

Along with a Glossary of Terms and Other Resources for Further Help and Information

Edited by Chad T. Kimball. 658 pages. 2002. 0-7808-0248-9.

"It is written in clear, nontechnical language aimed at general readers. . . . Recommended for public libraries, community colleges, and other agencies serving health care consumers."
— *American Reference Books Annual, 2003*

"Recommended for school and public libraries. Parents and professionals dealing with teens will appreciate the easy-to-follow format and the clearly written text. This could become a 'must have' for every high school teacher." — *E-Streams, Jan '03*

"A good starting point for information related to common medical, mental, and emotional concerns of adolescents." — *School Library Journal, Nov '02*

"This book provides accurate information in an easy to access format. It addresses topics that parents and caregivers might not be aware of and provides practical, useable information." — *Doody's Health Sciences Book Review Journal, Sep-Oct '02*

"Recommended reference source."
— *Booklist, American Library Association, Sep '02*

AIDS Sourcebook, 3rd Edition

Basic Consumer Health Information about Acquired Immune Deficiency Syndrome (AIDS) and Human Immunodeficiency Virus (HIV) Infection, Including Facts about Transmission, Prevention, Diagnosis, Treatment, Opportunistic Infections, and Other Complications, with a Section for Women and Children, Including Details about Associated Gynecological Concerns, Pregnancy, and Pediatric Care

Along with Updated Statistical Information, Reports on Current Research Initiatives, a Glossary, and Directories of Internet, Hotline, and Other Resources

Edited by Dawn D. Matthews. 664 pages. 2003. 0-7808-0631-X.

ALSO AVAILABLE: *AIDS Sourcebook, 1st Edition.* Edited by Karen Bellenir and Peter D. Dresser. 831 pages. 1995. 0-7808-0031-1.

AIDS Sourcebook, 2nd Edition. Edited by Karen Bellenir. 751 pages. 1999. 0-7808-0225-X.

"The 3rd edition of the *AIDS Sourcebook*, part of Omnigraphics' *Health Reference Series*, is a welcome update. . . . This resource is highly recommended for academic and public libraries."
— *American Reference Books Annual, 2004*

"Excellent sourcebook. This continues to be a highly recommended book. There is no other book that provides as much information as this book provides."
— *AIDS Book Review Journal, Dec-Jan 2000*

"Recommended reference source."
— *Booklist, American Library Association, Dec '99*

"A solid text for college-level health libraries."
— *The Bookwatch, Aug '99*

Cited in *Reference Sources for Small and Medium-Sized Libraries, American Library Association, 1999*

Alcoholism Sourcebook

Basic Consumer Health Information about the Physical and Mental Consequences of Alcohol Abuse, Including Liver Disease, Pancreatitis, Wernicke-Korsakoff Syndrome (Alcoholic Dementia), Fetal Alcohol Syndrome, Heart Disease, Kidney Disorders, Gastrointestinal Problems, and Immune System Compromise and Featuring Facts about Addiction, Detoxification, Alcohol Withdrawal, Recovery, and the Maintenance of Sobriety

Along with a Glossary and Directories of Resources for Further Help and Information

Edited by Karen Bellenir. 613 pages. 2000. 0-7808-0325-6.

"This title is one of the few reference works on alcoholism for general readers. For some readers this will be a welcome complement to the many self-help books on the market. Recommended for collections serving general readers and consumer health collections."
— *E-Streams, Mar '01*

"This book is an excellent choice for public and academic libraries."
— *American Reference Books Annual, 2001*

"Recommended reference source."
— *Booklist, American Library Association, Dec '00*

"Presents a wealth of information on alcohol use and abuse and its effects on the body and mind, treatment, and prevention." — *SciTech Book News, Dec '00*

"Important new health guide which packs in the latest consumer information about the problems of alcoholism." — *Reviewer's Bookwatch, Nov '00*

SEE ALSO *Drug Abuse Sourcebook, Substance Abuse Sourcebook*

607

Allergies Sourcebook, 2nd Edition

Basic Consumer Health Information about Allergic Disorders, Triggers, Reactions, and Related Symptoms, Including Anaphylaxis, Rhinitis, Sinusitis, Asthma, Dermatitis, Conjunctivitis, and Multiple Chemical Sensitivity

Along with Tips on Diagnosis, Prevention, and Treatment, Statistical Data, a Glossary, and a Directory of Sources for Further Help and Information

Edited by Annemarie S. Muth. 598 pages. 2002. 0-7808-0376-0.

ALSO AVAILABLE: *Allergies Sourcebook, 1st Edition.* Edited by Allan R. Cook. 611 pages. 1997. 0-7808-0036-2.

"This book brings a great deal of useful material together. . . . This is an excellent addition to public and consumer health library collections."
— *American Reference Books Annual, 2003*

"This second edition would be useful to laypersons with little or advanced knowledge of the subject matter. This book would also serve as a resource for nursing and other health care professions students. It would be useful in public, academic, and hospital libraries with consumer health collections." — *E-Streams, Jul '02*

■

Alternative Medicine Sourcebook, 2nd Edition

Basic Consumer Health Information about Alternative and Complementary Medical Practices, Including Acupuncture, Chiropractic, Herbal Medicine, Homeopathy, Naturopathic Medicine, Mind-Body Interventions, Ayurveda, and Other Non-Western Medical Traditions

Along with Facts about such Specific Therapies as Massage Therapy, Aromatherapy, Qigong, Hypnosis, Prayer, Dance, and Art Therapies, a Glossary, and Resources for Further Information

Edited by Dawn D. Matthews. 618 pages. 2002. 0-7808-0605-0.

ALSO AVAILABLE: *Alternative Medicine Sourcebook, 1st Edition.* Edited by Allan R. Cook. 737 pages. 1999. 0-7808-0200-4.

"Recommended for public, high school, and academic libraries that have consumer health collections. Hospital libraries that also serve the public will find this to be a useful resource." — *E-Streams, Feb '03*

"Recommended reference source."
— *Booklist, American Library Association, Jan '03*

"An important alternate health reference."
— *MBR Bookwatch, Oct '02*

"A great addition to the reference collection of every type of library." — *American Reference Books Annual, 2000*

Alzheimer's Disease Sourcebook, 3rd Edition

Basic Consumer Health Information about Alzheimer's Disease, Other Dementias, and Related Disorders, Including Multi-Infarct Dementia, AIDS Dementia Complex, Dementia with Lewy Bodies, Huntington's Disease, Wernicke-Korsakoff Syndrome (Alcohol-Reated Dementia), Delirium, and Confusional States

Along with Information for People Newly Diagnosed with Alzheimer's Disease and Caregivers, Reports Detailing Current Research Efforts in Prevention, Diagnosis, and Treatment, Facts about Long-Term Care Issues, and Listings of Sources for Additional Information

Edited by Karen Bellenir. 645 pages. 2003. 0-7808-0666-2.

ALSO AVAILABLE: *Alzheimer's, Stroke & 29 Other Neurological Disorders Sourcebook, 1st Edition.* Edited by Frank E. Bair. 579 pages. 1993. 1-55888-748-2.

ALSO AVAILABLE: *Alzheimer's Disease Sourcebook, 2nd Edition.* Edited by Karen Bellenir. 524 pages. 1999. 0-7808-0223-3.

"This very informative and valuable tool will be a great addition to any library serving consumers, students and health care workers."
— *American Reference Books Annual, 2004*

"This is a valuable resource for people affected by dementias such as Alzheimer's. It is easy to navigate and includes important information and resources."
— *Doody's Review Service, Feb. 2004*

"Recommended reference source."
— *Booklist, American Library Association, Oct '99*

SEE ALSO *Brain Disorders Sourcebook*

■

Arthritis Sourcebook, 2nd Edition

Basic Consumer Health Information about Osteoarthritis, Rheumatoid Arthritis, Other Rheumatic Disorders, Infectious Forms of Arthritis, and Diseases with Symptoms Linked to Arthritis, Featuring Facts about Diagnosis, Pain Management, and Surgical Therapies

Along with Coping Strategies, Research Updates, a Glossary, and Resources for Additional Help and Information

Edited by Amy L. Sutton. 593 pages. 2004. 0-7808-0667-0.

ALSO AVAILABLE: *Arthritis Sourcebook, 1st Edition.* Edited by Allan R. Cook. 550 pages. 1998. 0-7808-0201-2.

". . . accessible to the layperson."
— *Reference and Research Book News, Feb '99*

■

Asthma Sourcebook

Basic Consumer Health Information about Asthma, Including Symptoms, Traditional and Nontraditional Remedies, Treatment Advances, Quality-of-Life Aids,

Medical Research Updates, and the Role of Allergies, Exercise, Age, the Environment, and Genetics in the Development of Asthma

Along with Statistical Data, a Glossary, and Directories of Support Groups, and Other Resources for Further Information

Edited by Annemarie S. Muth. 628 pages. 2000. 0-7808-0381-7.

"A worthwhile reference acquisition for public libraries and academic medical libraries whose readers desire a quick introduction to the wide range of asthma information." — *Choice, Association of College & Research Libraries, Jun '01*

"Recommended reference source."
— *Booklist, American Library Association, Feb '01*

"Highly recommended." — *The Bookwatch, Jan '01*

"There is much good information for patients and their families who deal with asthma daily."
— *American Medical Writers Association Journal, Winter '01*

"This informative text is recommended for consumer health collections in public, secondary school, community college libraries and the libraries of universities with a large undergraduate population."
— *American Reference Books Annual, 2001*

▪

Attention Deficit Disorder Sourcebook

Basic Consumer Health Information about Attention Deficit/Hyperactivity Disorder in Children and Adults, Including Facts about Causes, Symptoms, Diagnostic Criteria, and Treatment Options Such as Medications, Behavior Therapy, Coaching, and Homeopathy

Along with Reports on Current Research Initiatives, Legal Issues, and Government Regulations, and Featuring a Glossary of Related Terms, Internet Resources, and a List of Additional Reading Material

Edited by Dawn D. Matthews. 470 pages. 2002. 0-7808-0624-7.

"Recommended reference source."
— *Booklist, American Library Association, Jan '03*

"This book is recommended for all school libraries and the reference or consumer health sections of public libraries." — *American Reference Books Annual, 2003*

▪

Back & Neck Sourcebook, 2nd Edition

Basic Consumer Health Information about Spinal Pain, Spinal Cord Injuries, and Related Disorders, Such as Degenerative Disk Disease, Osteoarthritis, Scoliosis, Sciatica, Spina Bifida, and Spinal Stenosis, and Featuring Facts about Maintaining Spinal Health, Self-Care, Pain Management, Rehabilitative Care, Chiropractic Care, Spinal Surgeries, and Complementary Therapies

Along with Suggestions for Preventing Back and Neck Pain, a Glossary of Related Terms, and a Directory of Resources

Edited by Amy L. Sutton. 633 pages. 2004. 0-7808-0738-3

ALSO AVAILABLE: Back & Neck Disorders Sourcebook, 1st Edition. Edited by Karen Bellenir. 548 pages. 1997. 0-7808-0202-0.

"The strength of this work is its basic, easy-to-read format. Recommended."
— *Reference and User Services Quarterly, American Library Association, Winter '97*

▪

Blood & Circulatory Disorders Sourcebook, 2nd Edition

Basic Consumer Health Information about the Blood and Circulatory System and Related Disorders, Such as Anemia and Other Hemoglobin Diseases, Cancer of the Blood and Associated Bone Marrow Disorders, Clotting and Bleeding Problems, and Conditions That Affect the Veins, Blood Vessels, and Arteries, Including Facts about the Donation and Transplantation of Bone Marrow, Stem Cells, and Blood and Tips for Keeping the Blood and Circulatory System Healthy

Along with a Glossary of Related Terms and Resources for Additional Help and Information

Edited by Amy L. Sutton. 659 pages. 2005. 0-7808-0746-4.

ALSO AVAILABLE: Blood and Circulatory Disorders Sourcebook, 1st Edition. Edited by Karen Bellenir and Linda M. Shin. 554 pages. 1998. 0-7808-0203-9.

"Recommended reference source."
— *Booklist, American Library Association, Feb '99*

"An important reference sourcebook written in simple language for everyday, non-technical users. "
— *Reviewer's Bookwatch, Jan '99*

▪

Brain Disorders Sourcebook, 2nd Edition

Basic Consumer Health Information about Acquired and Traumatic Brain Injuries, Infections of the Brain, Epilepsy and Seizure Disorders, Cerebral Palsy, and Degenerative Neurological Disorders, Including Amyotrophic Lateral Sclerosis (ALS), Dementias, Multiple Sclerosis, and More

Along with Information on the Brain's Structure and Function, Treatment and Rehabilitation Options, Reports on Current Research Initiatives, a Glossary of Terms Related to Brain Disorders and Injuries, and a Directory of Sources for Further Help and Information

Edited by Sandra J. Judd. 625 pages. 2005. 0-7808-0744-8.

ALSO AVAILABLE: Brain Disorders Sourcebook, 1st Edition. Edited by Karen Bellenir. 481 pages. 1999. 0-7808-0229-2.

"Belongs on the shelves of any library with a consumer health collection." — *E-Streams, Mar '00*

SEE ALSO *Alzheimer's Disease Sourcebook*

∎

Breast Cancer Sourcebook, 2nd Edition

Basic Consumer Health Information about Breast Cancer, Including Facts about Risk Factors, Prevention, Screening and Diagnostic Methods, Treatment Options, Complementary and Alternative Therapies, Post-Treatment Concerns, Clinical Trials, Special Risk Populations, and New Developments in Breast Cancer Research

Along with Breast Cancer Statistics, a Glossary of Related Terms, and a Directory of Resources for Additional Help and Information

Edited by Sandra J. Judd. 595 pages. 2004. 0-7808-0668-9.

ALSO AVAILABLE: *Breast Cancer Sourcebook, 1st Edition.* Edited by Edward J. Prucha and Karen Bellenir. 580 pages. 2001. 0-7808-0244-6.

"It would be a useful reference book in a library or on loan to women in a support group."
—*Cancer Forum, Mar '03*

"Recommended reference source."
—*Booklist, American Library Association, Jan '02*

"This reference source is highly recommended. It is quite informative, comprehensive and detailed in nature, and yet it offers practical advice in easy-to-read language. It could be thought of as the 'bible' of breast cancer for the consumer." —*E-Streams, Jan '02*

"The broad range of topics covered in lay language make the *Breast Cancer Sourcebook* an excellent addition to public and consumer health library collections."
—*American Reference Books Annual 2002*

"From the pros and cons of different screening methods and results to treatment options, *Breast Cancer Sourcebook* provides the latest information on the subject."
—*Library Bookwatch, Dec '01*

"This thoroughgoing, very readable reference covers all aspects of breast health and cancer.... Readers will find much to consider here. Recommended for all public and patient health collections."
—*Library Journal, Sep '01*

SEE ALSO *Cancer Sourcebook for Women, Women's Health Concerns Sourcebook*

∎

Breastfeeding Sourcebook

Basic Consumer Health Information about the Benefits of Breastmilk, Preparing to Breastfeed, Breastfeeding as a Baby Grows, Nutrition, and More, Including Information on Special Situations and Concerns Such as Mastitis, Illness, Medications, Allergies, Multiple Births, Prematurity, Special Needs, and Adoption

Along with a Glossary and Resources for Additional Help and Information

Edited by Jenni Lynn Colson. 388 pages. 2002. 0-7808-0332-9.

SEE ALSO *Pregnancy & Birth Sourcebook*

"Particularly useful is the information about professional lactation services and chapters on breastfeeding when returning to work. . . . *Breastfeeding Sourcebook* will be useful for public libraries, consumer health libraries, and technical schools offering nurse assistant training, especially in areas where Internet access is problematic."
—*American Reference Books Annual, 2003*

∎

Burns Sourcebook

Basic Consumer Health Information about Various Types of Burns and Scalds, Including Flame, Heat, Cold, Electrical, Chemical, and Sun Burns

Along with Information on Short-Term and Long-Term Treatments, Tissue Reconstruction, Plastic Surgery, Prevention Suggestions, and First Aid

Edited by Allan R. Cook. 604 pages. 1999. 0-7808-0204-7.

"This is an exceptional addition to the series and is highly recommended for all consumer health collections, hospital libraries, and academic medical centers."
—*E-Streams, Mar '00*

"This key reference guide is an invaluable addition to all health care and public libraries in confronting this ongoing health issue."
—*American Reference Books Annual, 2000*

"Recommended reference source."
—*Booklist, American Library Association, Dec '99*

SEE ALSO *Skin Disorders Sourcebook*

∎

Cancer Sourcebook, 4th Edition

Basic Consumer Health Information about Major Forms and Stages of Cancer, Featuring Facts about Head and Neck Cancers, Lung Cancers, Gastrointestinal Cancers, Genitourinary Cancers, Lymphomas, Blood Cell Cancers, Endocrine Cancers, Skin Cancers, Bone Cancers, Sarcomas, and Others, and Including Information about Cancer Treatments and Therapies, Identifying and Reducing Cancer Risks, and Strategies for Coping with Cancer and the Side Effects of Treatment

Along with a Cancer Glossary, Statistical and Demographic Data, and a Directory of Sources for Additional Help and Information

Edited by Karen Bellenir. 1,119 pages. 2003. 0-7808-0633-6.

ALSO AVAILABLE: *Cancer Sourcebook, 1st Edition.* Edited by Frank E. Bair. 932 pages. 1990. 1-55888-888-8.

New Cancer Sourcebook, 2nd Edition. Edited by Allan R. Cook. 1,313 pages. 1996. 0-7808-0041-9.

Cancer Sourcebook, 3rd Edition. Edited by Edward J. Prucha. 1,069 pages. 2000. 0-7808-0227-6.

"With cancer being the second leading cause of death for Americans, a prodigious work such as this one, which locates centrally so much cancer-related information, is clearly an asset to this nation's citizens and others."
— *Journal of the National Medical Association, 2004*

"This title is recommended for health sciences and public libraries with consumer health collections."
— *E-Streams, Feb '01*

". . . can be effectively used by cancer patients and their families who are looking for answers in a language they can understand. Public and hospital libraries should have it on their shelves."
— *American Reference Books Annual, 2001*

"Recommended reference source."
— *Booklist, American Library Association, Dec '00*

Cited in *Reference Sources for Small and Medium-Sized Libraries, American Library Association, 1999*

"The amount of factual and useful information is extensive. The writing is very clear, geared to general readers. Recommended for all levels."
— *Choice, Association of College & Research Libraries, Jan '97*

SEE ALSO *Breast Cancer Sourcebook, Cancer Sourcebook for Women, Pediatric Cancer Sourcebook, Prostate Cancer Sourcebook*

■

Cancer Sourcebook for Women, 2nd Edition

Basic Consumer Health Information about Gynecologic Cancers and Related Concerns, Including Cervical Cancer, Endometrial Cancer, Gestational Trophoblastic Tumor, Ovarian Cancer, Uterine Cancer, Vaginal Cancer, Vulvar Cancer, Breast Cancer, and Common Non-Cancerous Uterine Conditions, with Facts about Cancer Risk Factors, Screening and Prevention, Treatment Options, and Reports on Current Research Initiatives

Along with a Glossary of Cancer Terms and a Directory of Resources for Additional Help and Information

Edited by Karen Bellenir. 604 pages. 2002. 0-7808-0226-8.

ALSO AVAILABLE: Cancer Sourcebook for Women, 1st Edition. Edited by Allan R. Cook and Peter D. Dresser. 524 pages. 1996. 0-7808-0076-1.

"An excellent addition to collections in public, consumer health, and women's health libraries."
— *American Reference Books Annual, 2003*

"Overall, the information is excellent, and complex topics are clearly explained. As a reference book for the consumer it is a valuable resource to assist them to make informed decisions about cancer and its treatments."
— *Cancer Forum, Nov '02*

"Highly recommended for academic and medical reference collections."
— *Library Bookwatch, Sep '02*

"This is a highly recommended book for any public or consumer library, being reader friendly and containing accurate and helpful information."
— *E-Streams, Aug '02*

"Recommended reference source."
— *Booklist, American Library Association, Jul '02*

SEE ALSO *Breast Cancer Sourcebook, Women's Health Concerns Sourcebook*

■

Cardiovascular Diseases & Disorders Sourcebook, 3rd Edition

Basic Consumer Health Information about Heart and Vascular Diseases and Disorders, Such as Angina, Heart Attacks, Arrhythmias, Cardiomyopathy, Valve Disease, Atherosclerosis, and Aneurysms, with Information about Managing Cardiovascular Risk Factors and Maintaining Heart Health, Medications and Procedures Used to Treat Cardiovascular Disorders, and Concerns of Special Significance to Women

long with Reports on Current Research Initiatives, a Glossary of Related Medical Terms, and a Directory of Sources for Further Help and Information

Edited by Sandra J. Judd. 713 pages. 2005. 0-7808-0739-1.

ALSO AVAILABLE: Heart Diseases & Disorders Sourcebook, 2nd Edition. Edited by Karen Bellenir. 612 pages. 2000. 0-7808-0238-1.

Cardiovascular Diseases & Disorders Sourcebook, 1st Edition. Edited by Karen Bellenir and Peter D. Dresser. 683 pages. 1995. 0-7808-0032-X.

"This work stands out as an imminently accessible resource for the general public. It is recommended for the reference and circulating shelves of school, public, and academic libraries."
— *American Reference Books Annual, 2001*

"Recommended reference source."
— *Booklist, American Library Association, Dec '00*

"Provides comprehensive coverage of matters related to the heart. This title is recommended for health sciences and public libraries with consumer health collections."
— *E-Streams, Oct '00*

SEE ALSO *Healthy Heart Sourcebook for Women*

■

Caregiving Sourcebook

Basic Consumer Health Information for Caregivers, Including a Profile of Caregivers, Caregiving Responsibilities and Concerns, Tips for Specific Conditions, Care Environments, and the Effects of Caregiving

Along with Facts about Legal Issues, Financial Information, and Future Planning, a Glossary, and a Listing of Additional Resources

Edited by Joyce Brennfleck Shannon. 600 pages. 2001. 0-7808-0331-0.

"Essential for most collections."
— *Library Journal, Apr 1, 2002*

"An ideal addition to the reference collection of any public library. Health sciences information professionals may also want to acquire the *Caregiving Source-*

book for their hospital or academic library for use as a ready reference tool by health care workers interested in aging and caregiving." —*E-Streams, Jan '02*

"Recommended reference source."
—*Booklist, American Library Association, Oct '01*

■

Child Abuse Sourcebook

Basic Consumer Health Information about the Physical, Sexual, and Emotional Abuse of Children, with Additional Facts about Neglect, Munchausen Syndrome by Proxy (MSBP), Shaken Baby Syndrome, and Controversial Issues Related to Child Abuse, Such as Withholding Medical Care, Corporal Punishment, and Child Maltreatment in Youth Sports, and Featuring Facts about Child Protective Services, Foster Care, Adoption, Parenting Challenges, and Other Abuse Prevention Efforts

Along with a Glossary of Related Terms and Resources for Additional Help and Information

Edited by Dawn D. Matthews. 620 pages. 2004. 0-7808-0705-7.

■

Childhood Diseases & Disorders Sourcebook

Basic Consumer Health Information about Medical Problems Often Encountered in Pre-Adolescent Children, Including Respiratory Tract Ailments, Ear Infections, Sore Throats, Disorders of the Skin and Scalp, Digestive and Genitourinary Diseases, Infectious Diseases, Inflammatory Disorders, Chronic Physical and Developmental Disorders, Allergies, and More

Along with Information about Diagnostic Tests, Common Childhood Surgeries, and Frequently Used Medications, with a Glossary of Important Terms and Resource Directory

Edited by Chad T. Kimball. 662 pages. 2003. 0-7808-0458-9.

"This is an excellent book for new parents and should be included in all health care and public libraries."
—*American Reference Books Annual, 2004*

■

Colds, Flu & Other Common Ailments Sourcebook

Basic Consumer Health Information about Common Ailments and Injuries, Including Colds, Coughs, the Flu, Sinus Problems, Headaches, Fever, Nausea and Vomiting, Menstrual Cramps, Diarrhea, Constipation, Hemorrhoids, Back Pain, Dandruff, Dry and Itchy Skin, Cuts, Scrapes, Sprains, Bruises, and More

Along with Information about Prevention, Self-Care, Choosing a Doctor, Over-the-Counter Medications, Folk Remedies, and Alternative Therapies, and Including a Glossary of Important Terms and a Directory of Resources for Further Help and Information

Edited by Chad T. Kimball. 638 pages. 2001. 0-7808-0435-X.

"A good starting point for research on common illnesses. It will be a useful addition to public and consumer health library collections."
—*American Reference Books Annual 2002*

"Will prove valuable to any library seeking to maintain a current, comprehensive reference collection of health resources. . . . Excellent reference."
—*The Bookwatch, Aug '01*

"Recommended reference source."
—*Booklist, American Library Association, July '01*

■

Communication Disorders Sourcebook

Basic Information about Deafness and Hearing Loss, Speech and Language Disorders, Voice Disorders, Balance and Vestibular Disorders, and Disorders of Smell, Taste, and Touch

Edited by Linda M. Ross. 533 pages. 1996. 0-7808-0077-X.

"This is skillfully edited and is a welcome resource for the layperson. It should be found in every public and medical library." —*Booklist Health Sciences Supplement, American Library Association, Oct '97*

■

Congenital Disorders Sourcebook

Basic Information about Disorders Acquired during Gestation, Including Spina Bifida, Hydrocephalus, Cerebral Palsy, Heart Defects, Craniofacial Abnormalities, Fetal Alcohol Syndrome, and More

Along with Current Treatment Options and Statistical Data

Edited by Karen Bellenir. 607 pages. 1997. 0-7808-0205-5.

"Recommended reference source."
—*Booklist, American Library Association, Oct '97*

SEE ALSO Pregnancy & Birth Sourcebook

■

Consumer Issues in Health Care Sourcebook

Basic Information about Health Care Fundamentals and Related Consumer Issues, Including Exams and Screening Tests, Physician Specialties, Choosing a Doctor, Using Prescription and Over-the-Counter Medications Safely, Avoiding Health Scams, Managing Common Health Risks in the Home, Care Options for Chronically or Terminally Ill Patients, and a List of Resources for Obtaining Help and Further Information

Edited by Karen Bellenir. 618 pages. 1998. 0-7808-0221-7.

"Both public and academic libraries will want to have a copy in their collection for readers who are interested in self-education on health issues."
—*American Reference Books Annual, 2000*

■

Contagious Diseases Sourcebook

Basic Consumer Health Information about Infectious Diseases Spread by Person-to-Person Contact through Direct Touch, Airborne Transmission, Sexual Contact, or Contact with Blood or Other Body Fluids, Including Hepatitis, Herpes, Influenza, Lice, Measles, Mumps, Pinworm, Ringworm, Severe Acute Respiratory Syndrome (SARS), Streptococcal Infections, Tuberculosis, and Others

Along with Facts about Disease Transmission, Antimicrobial Resistance, and Vaccines, with a Glossary and Directories of Resources for More Information

Edited by Karen Bellenir. 643 pages. 2004. 0-7808-0736-7.

■

Contagious & Non-Contagious Infectious Diseases Sourcebook

Basic Information about Contagious Diseases like Measles, Polio, Hepatitis B, and Infectious Mononucleosis, and Non-Contagious Infectious Diseases like Tetanus and Toxic Shock Syndrome, and Diseases Occurring as Secondary Infections Such as Shingles and Reye Syndrome

Along with Vaccination, Prevention, and Treatment Information, and a Section Describing Emerging Infectious Disease Threats

Edited by Karen Bellenir and Peter D. Dresser. 566 pages. 1996. 0-7808-0075-3.

■

Death & Dying Sourcebook

Basic Consumer Health Information for the Layperson about End-of-Life Care and Related Ethical and Legal Issues, Including Chief Causes of Death, Autopsies, Pain Management for the Terminally Ill, Life Support Systems, Insurance, Euthanasia, Assisted Suicide, Hospice Programs, Living Wills, Funeral Planning, Counseling, Mourning, Organ Donation, and Physician Training

Along with Statistical Data, a Glossary, and Listings of Sources for Further Help and Information

Edited by Annemarie S. Muth. 641 pages. 1999. 0-7808-0230-6.

■

Dental Care & Oral Health Sourcebook, 2nd Edition

Basic Consumer Health Information about Dental Care, Including Oral Hygiene, Dental Visits, Pain Management, Cavities, Crowns, Bridges, Dental Implants, and Fillings, and Other Oral Health Concerns, Such as Gum Disease, Bad Breath, Dry Mouth, Genetic and Developmental Abnormalities, Oral Cancers, Orthodontics, and Temporomandibular Disorders

Along with Updates on Current Research in Oral Health, a Glossary, a Directory of Dental and Oral Health Organizations, and Resources for People with Dental and Oral Health Disorders

Edited by Amy L. Sutton. 609 pages. 2003. 0-7808-0634-4.

ALSO AVAILABLE: Oral Health Sourcebook, 1st Edition. Edited by Allan R. Cook. 558 pages. 1997. 0-7808-0082-6.

■

Depression Sourcebook

Basic Consumer Health Information about Unipolar Depression, Bipolar Disorder, Postpartum Depression, Seasonal Affective Disorder, and Other Types of Depression in Children, Adolescents, Women, Men, the Elderly, and Other Selected Populations

Along with Facts about Causes, Risk Factors, Diagnostic Criteria, Treatment Options, Coping Strategies, Suicide Prevention, a Glossary, and a Directory of Sources for Additional Help and Information

Edited by Karen Belleni. 602 pages. 2002. 0-7808-0611-5.

Dermatological Disorders Sourcebook, 2nd Edition

Basic Consumer Health Information about Conditions and Disorders Affecting the Skin, Hair, and Nails, Such as Acne, Rosacea, Rashes, Dermatitis, Pigmentation Disorders, Birthmarks, Skin Cancer, Skin Injuries, Psoriasis, Scleroderma, and Hair Loss, Including Facts about Medications and Treatments for Dermatological Disorders and Tips for Maintaining Healthy Skin, Hair, and Nails

Along with Information about How Aging Affects the Skin, a Glossary of Related Terms, and a Directory of Resources for Additional Help and Information

Edited by Amy L. Sutton. 645 pages. 2005. 0-7808-0795-2.

ALSO AVAILABLE: *Skin Disorders Sourcebook, 1st Edition.* Edited by Allan R. Cook. 647 pages. 1997. 0-7808-0080-X.

"... comprehensive, easily read reference book."
—*Doody's Health Sciences Book Reviews, Oct '97*

Diabetes Sourcebook, 3rd Edition

Basic Consumer Health Information about Type 1 Diabetes (Insulin-Dependent or Juvenile-Onset Diabetes), Type 2 Diabetes (Noninsulin-Dependent or Adult-Onset Diabetes), Gestational Diabetes, Impaired Glucose Tolerance (IGT), and Related Complications, Such as Amputation, Eye Disease, Gum Disease, Nerve Damage, and End-Stage Renal Disease, Including Facts about Insulin, Oral Diabetes Medications, Blood Sugar Testing, and the Role of Exercise and Nutrition in the Control of Diabetes

Along with a Glossary and Resources for Further Help and Information

Edited by Dawn D. Matthews. 622 pages. 2003. 0-7808-0629-8.

ALSO AVAILABLE: *Diabetes Sourcebook, 1st Edition.* Edited by Karen Bellenir and Peter D. Dresser. 827 pages. 1994. 1-55888-751-2.

Diabetes Sourcebook, 2nd Edition. Edited by Karen Bellenir. 688 pages. 1998. 0-7808-0224-1.

"This edition is even more helpful than earlier versions. . . . It is a truly valuable tool for anyone seeking readable and authoritative information on diabetes."
—*American Reference Books Annual, 2004*

"An invaluable reference." —*Library Journal, May '00*

Selected as one of the 250 "Best Health Sciences Books of 1999." —*Doody's Rating Service, Mar-Apr 2000*

"Provides useful information for the general public."
—*Healthlines, University of Michigan Health Management Research Center, Sep/Oct '99*

"... provides reliable mainstream medical information ... belongs on the shelves of any library with a consumer health collection." —*E-Streams, Sep '99*

"Recommended reference source."
—*Booklist, American Library Association, Feb '99*

Diet & Nutrition Sourcebook, 3rd Edition

Basic Consumer Health Information about Dietary Guidelines and the Food Guidance System, Recommended Daily Nutrient Intakes, Serving Proportions, Weight Control, Vitamins and Supplements, Nutrition Issues for Different Life Stages and Lifestyles, and the Needs of People with Specific Medical Concerns, Including Cancer, Celiac Disease, Diabetes, Eating Disorders, Food Allergies, and Cardiovascular Disease

Along with Facts about Federal Nutrition Support Programs, a Glossary of Nutrition and Dietary Terms, and Directories of Additional Resources for More Information about Nutrition

Edited by Joyce Brennfleck Shannon. 633 pages. 2006. 0-7808-0800-2.

ALSO AVAILABLE: *Diet & Nutrition Sourcebook, 1st Edition.* Edited by Dan R. Harris. 662 pages. 1996. 0-7808-0084-2.

Diet & Nutrition Sourcebook, 2nd Edition. Edited by Karen Bellenir. 650 pages. 1999. 0-7808-0228-4.

"This book is an excellent source of basic diet and nutrition information." —*Booklist Health Sciences Supplement, American Library Association, Dec '00*

"This reference document should be in any public library, but it would be a very good guide for beginning students in the health sciences. If the other books in this publisher's series are as good as this, they should all be in the health sciences collections."
—*American Reference Books Annual, 2000*

"This book is an excellent general nutrition reference for consumers who desire to take an active role in their health care for prevention. Consumers of all ages who select this book can feel confident they are receiving current and accurate information." —*Journal of Nutrition for the Elderly, Vol. 19, No. 4, '00*

"Recommended reference source."
—*Booklist, American Library Association, Dec '99*

SEE ALSO Digestive Diseases & Disorders Sourcebook, Eating Disorders Sourcebook, Gastrointestinal Diseases & Disorders Sourcebook, Vegetarian Sourcebook

Digestive Diseases & Disorders Sourcebook

Basic Consumer Health Information about Diseases and Disorders that Impact the Upper and Lower Digestive System, Including Celiac Disease, Constipation, Crohn's Disease, Cyclic Vomiting Syndrome, Diarrhea, Diverticulosis and Diverticulitis, Gallstones, Heartburn, Hemorrhoids, Hernias, Indigestion (Dyspepsia), Irritable Bowel Syndrome, Lactose Intolerance, Ulcers, and More

Along with Information about Medications and Other Treatments, Tips for Maintaining a Healthy Digestive Tract, a Glossary, and Directory of Digestive Diseases Organizations

Edited by Karen Bellenir. 335 pages. 2000. 0-7808-0327-2.

"This title would be an excellent addition to all public or patient-research libraries."
—*American Reference Books Annual, 2001*

"This title is recommended for public, hospital, and health sciences libraries with consumer health collections." — *E-Streams, Jul-Aug '00*

"Recommended reference source."
—*Booklist, American Library Association, May '00*

SEE ALSO *Diet & Nutrition Sourcebook, Eating Disorders Sourcebook, Gastrointestinal Diseases & Disorders Sourcebook*

∎

Disabilities Sourcebook

Basic Consumer Health Information about Physical and Psychiatric Disabilities, Including Descriptions of Major Causes of Disability, Assistive and Adaptive Aids, Workplace Issues, and Accessibility Concerns

Along with Information about the Americans with Disabilities Act, a Glossary, and Resources for Additional Help and Information

Edited by Dawn D. Matthews. 616 pages. 2000. 0-7808-0389-2.

"It is a must for libraries with a consumer health section." — *American Reference Books Annual 2002*

"A much needed addition to the Omnigraphics *Health Reference Series*. A current reference work to provide people with disabilities, their families, caregivers or those who work with them, a broad range of information in one volume, has not been available until now.... It is recommended for all public and academic library reference collections." — *E-Streams, May '01*

"An excellent source book in easy-to-read format covering many current topics; highly recommended for all libraries." — *Choice, Association of College and Research Libraries, Jan '01*

"Recommended reference source."
—*Booklist, American Library Association, Jul '00*

∎

Domestic Violence Sourcebook, 2nd Edition

Basic Consumer Health Information about the Causes and Consequences of Abusive Relationships, Including Physical Violence, Sexual Assault, Battery, Stalking, and Emotional Abuse, and Facts about the Effects of Violence on Women, Men, Young Adults, and the Elderly, with Reports about Domestic Violence in Selected Populations, and Featuring Facts about Medical Care, Victim Assistance and Protection, Prevention Strategies, Mental Health Services, and Legal Issues

Along with a Glossary of Related Terms and Resources for Additional Help and Information

Edited by Dawn D. Matthews. 628 pages. 2004. 0-7808-0669-7.

ALSO AVAILABLE: *Domestic Violence & Child Abuse Sourcebook, 1st Edition.* Edited by Helene Henderson. 1,064 pages. 2001. 0-7808-0235-7.

"Interested lay persons should find the book extremely beneficial.... A copy of *Domestic Violence and Child Abuse Sourcebook* should be in every public library in the United States."
— *Social Science & Medicine, No. 56, 2003*

"This is important information. The Web has many resources but this sourcebook fills an important societal need. I am not aware of any other resources of this type." — *Doody's Review Service, Sep '01*

"Recommended for all libraries, scholars, and practitioners." — *Choice, Association of College & Research Libraries, Jul '01*

"Recommended reference source."
— *Booklist, American Library Association, Apr '01*

"Important pick for college-level health reference libraries." — *The Bookwatch, Mar '01*

"Because this problem is so widespread and because this book includes a lot of issues within one volume, this work is recommended for all public libraries."
—*American Reference Books Annual, 2001*

∎

Drug Abuse Sourcebook, 2nd Edition

Basic Consumer Health Information about Illicit Substances of Abuse and the Misuse of Prescription and Over-the-Counter Medications, Including Depressants, Hallucinogens, Inhalants, Marijuana, Stimulants, and Anabolic Steroids

Along with Facts about Related Health Risks, Treatment Programs, Prevention Programs, a Glossary of Abuse and Addiction Terms, a Glossary of Drug-Related Street Terms, and a Directory of Resources for More Information

Edited by Catherine Ginther. 607 pages. 2004. 0-7808-0740-5.

ALSO AVAILABLE: *Drug Abuse Sourcebook, 1st Edition.* Edited by Karen Bellenir. 629 pages. 2000. 0-7808-0242-X.

"Containing a wealth of information.... This resource belongs in libraries that serve a lower-division undergraduate or community college clientele as well as the general public." — *Choice, Association of College and Research Libraries, Jun '01*

"Recommended reference source."
— *Booklist, American Library Association, Feb '01*

"Highly recommended." — *The Bookwatch, Jan '01*

"Even though there is a plethora of books on drug abuse, this volume is recommended for school, public, and college libraries."
—*American Reference Books Annual, 2001*

SEE ALSO *Alcoholism Sourcebook, Substance Abuse Sourcebook*

Ear, Nose & Throat Disorders Sourcebook

Basic Information about Disorders of the Ears, Nose, Sinus Cavities, Pharynx, and Larynx, Including Ear Infections, Tinnitus, Vestibular Disorders, Allergic and Non-Allergic Rhinitis, Sore Throats, Tonsillitis, and Cancers That Affect the Ears, Nose, Sinuses, and Throat

Along with Reports on Current Research Initiatives, a Glossary of Related Medical Terms, and a Directory of Sources for Further Help and Information

Edited by Karen Bellenir and Linda M. Shin. 576 pages. 1998. 0-7808-0206-3.

"Overall, this sourcebook is helpful for the consumer seeking information on ENT issues. It is recommended for public libraries."
—*American Reference Books Annual, 1999*

"Recommended reference source."
—*Booklist, American Library Association, Dec '98*

■

Eating Disorders Sourcebook

Basic Consumer Health Information about Eating Disorders, Including Information about Anorexia Nervosa, Bulimia Nervosa, Binge Eating, Body Dysmorphic Disorder, Pica, Laxative Abuse, and Night Eating Syndrome

Along with Information about Causes, Adverse Effects, and Treatment and Prevention Issues, and Featuring a Section on Concerns Specific to Children and Adolescents, a Glossary, and Resources for Further Help and Information

Edited by Dawn D. Matthews. 322 pages. 2001. 0-7808-0335-3.

"Recommended for health science libraries that are open to the public, as well as hospital libraries. This book is a good resource for the consumer who is concerned about eating disorders." — *E-Streams, Mar '02*

"This volume is another convenient collection of excerpted articles. Recommended for school and public library patrons; lower-division undergraduates; and two-year technical program students." — *Choice, Association of College & Research Libraries, Jan '02*

"Recommended reference source." — *Booklist, American Library Association, Oct '01*

SEE ALSO *Diet & Nutrition Sourcebook, Digestive Diseases & Disorders Sourcebook, Gastrointestinal Diseases & Disorders Sourcebook*

■

Emergency Medical Services Sourcebook

Basic Consumer Health Information about Preventing, Preparing for, and Managing Emergency Situations, When and Who to Call for Help, What to Expect in the Emergency Room, the Emergency Medical Team, Patient Issues, and Current Topics in Emergency Medicine

Along with Statistical Data, a Glossary, and Sources of Additional Help and Information

Edited by Jenni Lynn Colson. 494 pages. 2002. 0-7808-0420-1.

"Handy and convenient for home, public, school, and college libraries. Recommended."
— *Choice, Association of College and Research Libraries, Apr '03*

"This reference can provide the consumer with answers to most questions about emergency care in the United States, or it will direct them to a resource where the answer can be found."
—*American Reference Books Annual, 2003*

"Recommended reference source."
— *Booklist, American Library Association, Feb '03*

■

Endocrine & Metabolic Disorders Sourcebook

Basic Information for the Layperson about Pancreatic and Insulin-Related Disorders Such as Pancreatitis, Diabetes, and Hypoglycemia; Adrenal Gland Disorders Such as Cushing's Syndrome, Addison's Disease, and Congenital Adrenal Hyperplasia; Pituitary Gland Disorders Such as Growth Hormone Deficiency, Acromegaly, and Pituitary Tumors; Thyroid Disorders Such as Hypothyroidism, Graves' Disease, Hashimoto's Disease, and Goiter; Hyperparathyroidism; and Other Diseases and Syndromes of Hormone Imbalance or Metabolic Dysfunction

Along with Reports on Current Research Initiatives

Edited by Linda M. Shin. 574 pages. 1998. 0-7808-0207-1.

"Omnigraphics has produced another needed resource for health information consumers."
—*American Reference Books Annual, 2000*

"Recommended reference source."
— *Booklist, American Library Association, Dec '98*

■

Environmental Health Sourcebook, 2nd Edition

Basic Consumer Health Information about the Environment and Its Effect on Human Health, Including the Effects of Air Pollution, Water Pollution, Hazardous Chemicals, Food Hazards, Radiation Hazards, Biological Agents, Household Hazards, Such as Radon, Asbestos, Carbon Monoxide, and Mold, and Information about Associated Diseases and Disorders, Including Cancer, Allergies, Respiratory Problems, and Skin Disorders

Along with Information about Environmental Concerns for Specific Populations, a Glossary of Related Terms, and Resources for Further Help and Information

Edited by Dawn D. Matthews. 673 pages. 2003. 0-7808-0632-8.

ALSO AVAILABLE: *Environmentally Induced Disorders Sourcebook, 1st Edition.* Edited by Allan R.

Cook. 620 pages. 1997. 0-7808-0083-4.

"This recently updated edition continues the level of quality and the reputation of the numerous other volumes in Omnigraphics' *Health Reference Series*."
— *American Reference Books Annual, 2004*

"Recommended reference source."
— *Booklist, American Library Association, Sep '98*

"This book will be a useful addition to anyone's library." — *Choice Health Sciences Supplement, Association of College and Research Libraries, May '98*

". . . a good survey of numerous environmentally induced physical disorders . . . a useful addition to anyone's library."
— *Doody's Health Sciences Book Reviews, Jan '98*

". . . provide[s] introductory information from the best authorities around. Since this volume covers topics that potentially affect everyone, it will surely be one of the most frequently consulted volumes in the *Health Reference Series*." — *Rettig on Reference, Nov '97*

Environmentally Induced Disorders Sourcebook, 1st Edition
SEE *Environmental Health Sourcebook, 2nd Edition*

Ethnic Diseases Sourcebook

Basic Consumer Health Information for Ethnic and Racial Minority Groups in the United States, Including General Health Indicators and Behaviors, Ethnic Diseases, Genetic Testing, the Impact of Chronic Diseases, Women's Health, Mental Health Issues, and Preventive Health Care Services

Along with a Glossary and a Listing of Additional Resources

Edited by Joyce Brennfleck Shannon. 664 pages. 2001. 0-7808-0336-1.

"Recommended for health sciences libraries where public health programs are a priority."
— *E-Streams, Jan '02*

"Not many books have been written on this topic to date, and the *Ethnic Diseases Sourcebook* is a strong addition to the list. It will be an important introductory resource for health consumers, students, health care personnel, and social scientists. It is recommended for public, academic, and large hospital libraries."
— *American Reference Books Annual 2002*

"Recommended reference source."
— *Booklist, American Library Association, Oct '01*

"Will prove valuable to any library seeking to maintain a current, comprehensive reference collection of health resources. . . . An excellent source of health information about genetic disorders which affect particular ethnic and racial minorities in the U.S."
— *The Bookwatch, Aug '01*

Eye Care Sourcebook, 2nd Edition

Basic Consumer Health Information about Eye Care and Eye Disorders, Including Facts about the Diagnosis, Prevention, and Treatment of Common Refractive Problems Such as Myopia, Hyperopia, Astigmatism, and Presbyopia, and Eye Diseases, Including Glaucoma, Cataract, Age-Related Macular Degeneration, and Diabetic Retinopathy

Along with a Section on Vision Correction and Refractive Surgeries, Including LASIK and LASEK, a Glossary, and Directories of Resources for Additional Help and Information

Edited by Amy L. Sutton. 543 pages. 2003. 0-7808-0635-2.

ALSO AVAILABLE: Ophthalmic Disorders Sourcebook, 1st Edition. Edited by Linda M. Ross. 631 pages. 1996. 0-7808-0081-8.

". . . a solid reference tool for eye care and a valuable addition to a collection."
— *American Reference Books Annual, 2004*

Family Planning Sourcebook

Basic Consumer Health Information about Planning for Pregnancy and Contraception, Including Traditional Methods, Barrier Methods, Hormonal Methods, Permanent Methods, Future Methods, Emergency Contraception, and Birth Control Choices for Women at Each Stage of Life

Along with Statistics, a Glossary, and Sources of Additional Information

Edited by Amy Marcaccio Keyzer. 520 pages. 2001. 0-7808-0379-5.

"Recommended for public, health, and undergraduate libraries as part of the circulating collection."
— *E-Streams, Mar '02*

"Information is presented in an unbiased, readable manner, and the sourcebook will certainly be a necessary addition to those public and high school libraries where Internet access is restricted or otherwise problematic." — *American Reference Books Annual 2002*

"Recommended reference source."
— *Booklist, American Library Association, Oct '01*

"Will prove valuable to any library seeking to maintain a current, comprehensive reference collection of health resources. . . . Excellent reference."
— *The Bookwatch, Aug '01*

SEE ALSO *Pregnancy & Birth Sourcebook*

Fitness & Exercise Sourcebook, 2nd Edition

Basic Consumer Health Information about the Fundamentals of Fitness and Exercise, Including How to Begin and Maintain a Fitness Program, Fitness as a Lifestyle, the Link between Fitness and Diet, Advice for Specific Groups of People, Exercise as It Relates to Specific Medical Conditions, and Recent Research in Fitness and Exercise

Along with a Glossary of Important Terms and Resources for Additional Help and Information

Edited by Kristen M. Gledhill. 646 pages. 2001. 0-7808-0334-5.

ALSO AVAILABLE: *Fitness & Exercise Sourcebook, 1st Edition.* Edited by Dan R. Harris. 663 pages. 1996. 0-7808-0186-5.

"This work is recommended for all general reference collections."
— *American Reference Books Annual 2002*

"Highly recommended for public, consumer, and school grades fourth through college."
— *E-Streams, Nov '01*

"Recommended reference source." — *Booklist, American Library Association, Oct '01*

"The information appears quite comprehensive and is considered reliable. . . . This second edition is a welcomed addition to the series."
— *Doody's Review Service, Sep '01*

"This reference is a valuable choice for those who desire a broad source of information on exercise, fitness, and chronic-disease prevention through a healthy lifestyle." — *American Medical Writers Association Journal, Fall '01*

"Will prove valuable to any library seeking to maintain a current, comprehensive reference collection of health resources. . . . Excellent reference."
— *The Bookwatch, Aug '01*

■

Food & Animal Borne Diseases Sourcebook

Basic Information about Diseases That Can Be Spread to Humans through the Ingestion of Contaminated Food or Water or by Contact with Infected Animals and Insects, Such as Botulism, E. Coli, Hepatitis A, Trichinosis, Lyme Disease, and Rabies

Along with Information Regarding Prevention and Treatment Methods, and Including a Special Section for International Travelers Describing Diseases Such as Cholera, Malaria, Travelers' Diarrhea, and Yellow Fever, and Offering Recommendations for Avoiding Illness

Edited by Karen Bellenir and Peter D. Dresser. 535 pages. 1995. 0-7808-0033-8.

"Targeting general readers and providing them with a single, comprehensive source of information on selected topics, this book continues, with the excellent caliber of its predecessors, to catalog topical information on health matters of general interest. Readable and thorough, this valuable resource is highly recommended for all libraries."
— *Academic Library Book Review, Summer '96*

"A comprehensive collection of authoritative information." — *Emergency Medical Services, Oct '95*

Food Safety Sourcebook

Basic Consumer Health Information about the Safe Handling of Meat, Poultry, Seafood, Eggs, Fruit Juices, and Other Food Items, and Facts about Pesticides, Drinking Water, Food Safety Overseas, and the Onset, Duration, and Symptoms of Foodborne Illnesses, Including Types of Pathogenic Bacteria, Parasitic Protozoa, Worms, Viruses, and Natural Toxins

Along with the Role of the Consumer, the Food Handler, and the Government in Food Safety; a Glossary, and Resources for Additional Help and Information

Edited by Dawn D. Matthews. 339 pages. 1999. 0-7808-0326-4.

"This book is recommended for public libraries and universities with home economic and food science programs." — *E-Streams, Nov '00*

"Recommended reference source."
— *Booklist, American Library Association, May '00*

"This book takes the complex issues of food safety and foodborne pathogens and presents them in an easily understood manner. [It does] an excellent job of covering a large and often confusing topic."
— *American Reference Books Annual, 2000*

■

Forensic Medicine Sourcebook

Basic Consumer Information for the Layperson about Forensic Medicine, Including Crime Scene Investigation, Evidence Collection and Analysis, Expert Testimony, Computer-Aided Criminal Identification, Digital Imaging in the Courtroom, DNA Profiling, Accident Reconstruction, Autopsies, Ballistics, Drugs and Explosives Detection, Latent Fingerprints, Product Tampering, and Questioned Document Examination

Along with Statistical Data, a Glossary of Forensics Terminology, and Listings of Sources for Further Help and Information

Edited by Annemarie S. Muth. 574 pages. 1999. 0-7808-0232-2.

"Given the expected widespread interest in its content and its easy to read style, this book is recommended for most public and all college and university libraries."
— *E-Streams, Feb '01*

"Recommended for public libraries."
— *Reference & User Services Quarterly, American Library Association, Spring 2000*

"Recommended reference source."
— *Booklist, American Library Association, Feb '00*

"A wealth of information, useful statistics, references are up-to-date and extremely complete. This wonderful collection of data will help students who are interested in a career in any type of forensic field. It is a great resource for attorneys who need information about types of expert witnesses needed in a particular case. It also offers useful information for fiction and nonfiction writers whose work involves a crime. A fascinating compilation. All levels." — *Choice, Association of College and Research Libraries, Jan 2000*

618

◼

Gastrointestinal Diseases & Disorders Sourcebook, 2nd Edition

Basic Consumer Health Information about the Upper and Lower Gastrointestinal (GI) Tract, Including the Esophagus, Stomach, Intestines, Rectum, Liver, and Pancreas, with Facts about Gastroesophageal Reflux Disease, Gastritis, Hernias, Ulcers, Celiac Disease, Diverticulitis, Irritable Bowel Syndrome, Hemorrhoids, Gastrointestinal Cancers, and Other Diseases and Disorders Related to the Digestive Process

Along with Information about Commonly Used Diagnostic and Surgical Procedures, Statistics, Reports on Current Research Initiatives and Clinical Trials, a Glossary, and Resources for Additional Help and Information

Edited by Sandra J. Judd. 682 pages. 2006. 0-7808-0798-7.

ALSO AVAILABLE: *Gastrointestinal Diseases & Disorders Sourcebook, 1st Edition.* Edited by Linda M. Ross. 413 pages. 1996. 0-7808-0078-8.

SEE ALSO *Diet & Nutrition Sourcebook, Digestive Diseases & Disorders, Eating Disorders Sourcebook*

◼

Genetic Disorders Sourcebook, 3rd Edition

Basic Consumer Health Information about Hereditary Diseases and Disorders, Including Facts about the Human Genome, Genetic Inheritance Patterns, Disorders Associated with Specific Genes, Such as Sickle Cell Disease, Hemophilia, and Cystic Fibrosis, Chromosome Disorders, Such as Down Syndrome, Fragile X Syndrome, and Turner Syndrome, and Complex Diseases and Disorders Resulting from the Interaction of Environmental and Genetic Factors, Such as Allergies, Cancer, and Obesity

Along with Facts about Genetic Testing, Suggestions for Parents of Children with Special Needs, Reports on Current Research Initiatives, a Glossary of Genetic Terminology, and Resources for Additional Help and Information

Edited by Karen Bellenir. 777 pages. 2004. 0-7808-0742-1.

ALSO AVAILABLE: *Genetic Disorders Sourcebook, 1st Edition.* Edited by Karen Bellenir. 642 pages. 1996. 0-7808-0034-6.

Genetic Disorders Sourcebook, 2nd Edition. Edited by Kathy Massimini. 768 pages. 2001. 0-7808-0241-1.

◼

Head Trauma Sourcebook

Basic Information for the Layperson about Open-Head and Closed-Head Injuries, Treatment Advances, Recovery, and Rehabilitation

Along with Reports on Current Research Initiatives

Edited by Karen Bellenir. 414 pages. 1997. 0-7808-0208-X.

◼

Headache Sourcebook

Basic Consumer Health Information about Migraine, Tension, Cluster, Rebound and Other Types of Headaches, with Facts about the Cause and Prevention of Headaches, the Effects of Stress and the Environment, Headaches during Pregnancy and Menopause, and Childhood Headaches

Along with a Glossary and Other Resources for Additional Help and Information

Edited by Dawn D. Matthews. 362 pages. 2002. 0-7808-0337-X.

◼

Health Insurance Sourcebook

Basic Information about Managed Care Organizations, Traditional Fee-for-Service Insurance, Insurance Portability and Pre-Existing Conditions Clauses, Medicare, Medicaid, Social Security, and Military Health Care

Along with Information about Insurance Fraud

Edited by Wendy Wilcox. 530 pages. 1997. 0-7808-0222-5.

619

Health Reference Series Cumulative Index 1999

A Comprehensive Index to the Individual Volumes of the Health Reference Series, Including a Subject Index, Name Index, Organization Index, and Publication Index

Along with a Master List of Acronyms and Abbreviations

Edited by Edward J. Prucha, Anne Holmes, and Robert Rudnick. 990 pages. 2000. 0-7808-0382-5.

"This volume will be most helpful in libraries that have a relatively complete collection of the Health Reference Series." *—American Reference Books Annual, 2001*

"Essential for collections that hold any of the numerous *Health Reference Series* titles."
— Choice, Association of College and Research Libraries, Nov '00

■

Healthy Aging Sourcebook

Basic Consumer Health Information about Maintaining Health through the Aging Process, Including Advice on Nutrition, Exercise, and Sleep, Help in Making Decisions about Midlife Issues and Retirement, and Guidance Concerning Practical and Informed Choices in Health Consumerism

Along with Data Concerning the Theories of Aging, Different Experiences in Aging by Minority Groups, and Facts about Aging Now and Aging in the Future; and Featuring a Glossary, a Guide to Consumer Help, Additional Suggested Reading, and Practical Resource Directory

Edited by Jenifer Swanson. 536 pages. 1999. 0-7808-0390-6.

"Recommended reference source."
—Booklist, American Library Association, Feb '00

SEE ALSO *Physical & Mental Issues in Aging Sourcebook*

■

Healthy Children Sourcebook

Basic Consumer Health Information about the Physical and Mental Development of Children between the Ages of 3 and 12, Including Routine Health Care, Preventative Health Services, Safety and First Aid, Healthy Sleep, Dental Care, Nutrition, and Fitness, and Featuring Parenting Tips on Such Topics as Bedwetting, Choosing Day Care, Monitoring TV and Other Media, and Establishing a Foundation for Substance Abuse Prevention

Along with a Glossary of Commonly Used Pediatric Terms and Resources for Additional Help and Information.

Edited by Chad T. Kimball. 647 pages. 2003. 0-7808-0247-0.

"It is hard to imagine that any other single resource exists that would provide such a comprehensive guide of timely information on health promotion and disease prevention for children aged 3 to 12."
— American Reference Books Annual, 2004

"The strengths of this book are many. It is clearly written, presented and structured."
—Journal of the National Medical Association, 2004

■

Healthy Heart Sourcebook for Women

Basic Consumer Health Information about Cardiac Issues Specific to Women, Including Facts about Major Risk Factors and Prevention, Treatment and Control Strategies, and Important Dietary Issues

Along with a Special Section Regarding the Pros and Cons of Hormone Replacement Therapy and Its Impact on Heart Health, and Additional Help, Including Recipes, a Glossary, and a Directory of Resources

Edited by Dawn D. Matthews. 336 pages. 2000. 0-7808-0329-9.

"A good reference source and recommended for all public, academic, medical, and hospital libraries."
—Medical Reference Services Quarterly, Summer '01

"Because of the lack of information specific to women on this topic, this book is recommended for public libraries and consumer libraries."
—American Reference Books Annual, 2001

"Contains very important information about coronary artery disease that all women should know. The information is current and presented in an easy-to-read format. The book will make a good addition to any library." *— American Medical Writers Association Journal, Summer '00*

"Important, basic reference."
— Reviewer's Bookwatch, Jul '00

SEE ALSO *Heart Diseases & Disorders Sourcebook, Women's Health Concerns Sourcebook*

■

Heart Diseases & Disorders Sourcebook, 2nd Edition

SEE *Cardiovascular Diseases & Disorders Sourcebook, 3rd Edition*

■

Hepatitis Sourcebook

Basic Consumer Health Information about Hepatitis A, Hepatitis B, Hepatitis C, and Other Forms of Hepatitis, Including Autoimmune Hepatitis, Alcoholic Hepatitis, Nonalcoholic Steatohepatitis, and Toxic Hepatitis, with Facts about Risk Factors, Screening Methods, Diagnostic Tests, and Treatment Options

Along with Information on Liver Health, Tips for People Living with Chronic Hepatitis, Reports on Current Research Initiatives, a Glossary of Terms Related to Hepatitis, and a Directory of Sources for Further Help and Information

Edited by Sandra J. Judd. 597 pages. 2005. 0-7808-0749-9.

Household Safety Sourcebook

Basic Consumer Health Information about Household Safety, Including Information about Poisons, Chemicals, Fire, and Water Hazards in the Home

Along with Advice about the Safe Use of Home Maintenance Equipment, Choosing Toys and Nursery Furniture, Holiday and Recreation Safety, a Glossary, and Resources for Further Help and Information

Edited by Dawn D. Matthews. 606 pages. 2002. 0-7808-0338-8.

"This work will be useful in public libraries with large consumer health and wellness departments."
— *American Reference Books Annual, 2003*

"As a sourcebook on household safety this book meets its mark. It is encyclopedic in scope and covers a wide range of safety issues that are commonly seen in the home." — *E-Streams, Jul '02*

Hypertension Sourcebook

Basic Consumer Health Information about the Causes, Diagnosis, and Treatment of High Blood Pressure, with Facts about Consequences, Complications, and Co-Occurring Disorders, Such as Coronary Heart Disease, Diabetes, Stroke, Kidney Disease, and Hypertensive Retinopathy, and Issues in Blood Pressure Control, Including Dietary Choices, Stress Management, and Medications

Along with Reports on Current Research Initiatives and Clinical Trials, a Glossary, and Resources for Additional Help and Information

Edited by Dawn D. Matthews and Karen Bellenir. 613 pages. 2004. 0-7808-0674-3.

Immune System Disorders Sourcebook, 2nd Edition

Basic Consumer Health Information about Disorders of the Immune System, Including Immune System Function and Response, Diagnosis of Immune Disorders, Information about Inherited Immune Disease, Acquired Immune Disease, and Autoimmune Diseases, Including Primary Immune Deficiency, Acquired Immunodeficiency Syndrome (AIDS), Lupus, Multiple Sclerosis, Type 1 Diabetes, Rheumatoid Arthritis, and Graves Disease

Along with Treatments, Tips for Coping with Immune Disorders, a Glossary, and a Directory of Additional Resources

Edited by Joyce Brennfleck Shannon. 671 pages. 2005. 0-7808-0748-0.

ALSO AVAILABLE: *Immune System Disorders Sourcebook.* Edited by Allan R. Cook. 608 pages. 1997. 0-7808-0209-8.

Infant & Toddler Health Sourcebook

Basic Consumer Health Information about the Physical and Mental Development of Newborns, Infants, and Toddlers, Including Neonatal Concerns, Nutrition Recommendations, Immunization Schedules, Common Pediatric Disorders, Assessments and Milestones, Safety Tips, and Advice for Parents and Other Caregivers

Along with a Glossary of Terms and Resource Listings for Additional Help

Edited by Jenifer Swanson. 585 pages. 2000. 0-7808-0246-2.

"As a reference for the general public, this would be useful in any library." — *E-Streams, May '01*

"Recommended reference source."
— *Booklist, American Library Association, Feb '01*

"This is a good source for general use."
— *American Reference Books Annual, 2001*

Infectious Diseases Sourcebook

Basic Consumer Health Information about Non-Contagious Bacterial, Viral, Prion, Fungal, and Parasitic Diseases Spread by Food and Water, Insects and Animals, or Environmental Contact, Including Botulism, E. Coli, Encephalitis, Legionnaires' Disease, Lyme Disease, Malaria, Plague, Rabies, Salmonella, Tetanus, and Others, and Facts about Newly Emerging Diseases, Such as Hantavirus, Mad Cow Disease, Monkeypox, and West Nile Virus

Along with Information about Preventing Disease Transmission, the Threat of Bioterrorism, and Current Research Initiatives, with a Glossary and Directory of Resources for More Information

Edited by Karen Bellenir. 634 pages. 2004. 0-7808-0675-1.

Injury & Trauma Sourcebook

Basic Consumer Health Information about the Impact of Injury, the Diagnosis and Treatment of Common and Traumatic Injuries, Emergency Care, and Specific Injuries Related to Home, Community, Workplace, Transportation, and Recreation

Along with Guidelines for Injury Prevention, a Glossary, and a Directory of Additional Resources

Edited by Joyce Brennfleck Shannon. 696 pages. 2002. 0-7808-0421-X.

"This publication is the most comprehensive work of its kind about injury and trauma."
— *American Reference Books Annual, 2003*

"This sourcebook provides concise, easily readable, basic health information about injuries. . . . This book is well organized and an easy to use reference resource suitable for hospital, health sciences and public libraries with consumer health collections."
— *E-Streams, Nov '02*

Kidney & Urinary Tract Diseases & Disorders Sourcebook, 1st Edition

SEE Urinary Tract *&* Kidney Diseases *&* Disorders Sourcebook, 2nd Edition

Learning Disabilities Sourcebook, 2nd Edition

Basic Consumer Health Information about Learning Disabilities, Including Dyslexia, Developmental Speech and Language Disabilities, Non-Verbal Learning Disorders, Developmental Arithmetic Disorder, Developmental Writing Disorder, and Other Conditions That Impede Learning Such as Attention Deficit/ Hyperactivity Disorder, Brain Injury, Hearing Impairment, Klinefelter Syndrome, Dyspraxia, and Tourette Syndrome

Along with Facts about Educational Issues and Assistive Technology, Coping Strategies, a Glossary of Related Terms, and Resources for Further Help and Information

Edited by Dawn D. Matthews. 621 pages. 2003. 0-7808-0626-3.

ALSO AVAILABLE: *Learning Disabilities Sourcebook, 1st Edition.* Edited by Linda M. Shin. 579 pages. 1998. 0-7808-0210-1.

"The second edition of *Learning Disabilities Sourcebook* far surpasses the earlier edition in that it is more focused on information that will be useful as a consumer health resource." — *American Reference Books Annual, 2004*

"Teachers as well as consumers will find this an essential guide to understanding various syndromes and their latest treatments. [An] invaluable reference for public and school library collections alike." — *Library Bookwatch, Apr '03*

Named "Outstanding Reference Book of 1999." — *New York Public Library, Feb 2000*

"An excellent candidate for inclusion in a public library reference section. It's a great source of information. Teachers will also find the book useful. Definitely worth reading." — *Journal of Adolescent & Adult Literacy, Feb 2000*

"Readable . . . provides a solid base of information regarding successful techniques used with individuals who have learning disabilities, as well as practical suggestions for educators and family members. Clear lan-

Leukemia Sourcebook

Basic Consumer Health Information about Adult and Childhood Leukemias, Including Acute Lymphocytic Leukemia (ALL), Chronic Lymphocytic Leukemia (CLL), Acute Myelogenous Leukemia (AML), Chronic Myelogenous Leukemia (CML), and Hairy Cell Leukemia, and Treatments Such as Chemotherapy, Radiation Therapy, Peripheral Blood Stem Cell and Marrow Transplantation, and Immunotherapy

Along with Tips for Life During and After Treatment, a Glossary, and Directories of Additional Resources

Edited by Joyce Brennfleck Shannon. 587 pages. 2003. 0-7808-0627-1.

"Unlike other medical books for the layperson, . . . the language does not talk down to the reader. . . . This volume is highly recommended for all libraries." — *American Reference Books Annual, 2004*

Liver Disorders Sourcebook

Basic Consumer Health Information about the Liver and How It Works; Liver Diseases, Including Cancer, Cirrhosis, Hepatitis, and Toxic and Drug Related Diseases; Tips for Maintaining a Healthy Liver; Laboratory Tests, Radiology Tests, and Facts about Liver Transplantation

Along with a Section on Support Groups, a Glossary, and Resource Listings

Edited by Joyce Brennfleck Shannon. 591 pages. 2000. 0-7808-0383-3.

"A valuable resource." — *American Reference Books Annual, 2001*

"This title is recommended for health sciences and public libraries with consumer health collections." — *E-Streams, Oct '00*

"Recommended reference source." — *Booklist, American Library Association, Jun '00*

Lung Disorders Sourcebook

Basic Consumer Health Information about Emphysema, Pneumonia, Tuberculosis, Asthma, Cystic Fibrosis, and Other Lung Disorders, Including Facts about Diagnostic Procedures, Treatment Strategies, Disease Prevention Efforts, and Such Risk Factors as Smoking, Air Pollution, and Exposure to Asbestos, Radon, and Other Agents

Along with a Glossary and Resources for Additional Help and Information

Edited by Dawn D. Matthews. 678 pages. 2002. 0-7808-0339-6.

"This title is a great addition for public and school libraries because it provides concise health information on the lungs."
— American Reference Books Annual, 2003

"Highly recommended for academic and medical reference collections." — Library Bookwatch, Sep '02

■

Medical Tests Sourcebook, 2nd Edition

Basic Consumer Health Information about Medical Tests, Including Age-Specific Health Tests, Important Health Screenings and Exams, Home-Use Tests, Blood and Specimen Tests, Electrical Tests, Scope Tests, Genetic Testing, and Imaging Tests, Such as X-Rays, Ultrasound, Computed Tomography, Magnetic Resonance Imaging, Angiography, and Nuclear Medicine

Along with a Glossary and Directory of Additional Resources

Edited by Joyce Brennfleck Shannon. 654 pages. 2004. 0-7808-0670-0.

ALSO AVAILABLE: Medical Tests, 1st Edition. Edited by Joyce Brennfleck Shannon. 691 pages. 1999. 0-7808-0243-8.

"Recommended for hospital and health sciences libraries with consumer health collections."
— E-Streams, Mar '00

"This is an overall excellent reference with a wealth of general knowledge that may aid those who are reluctant to get vital tests performed."
— Today's Librarian, Jan 2000

"A valuable reference guide."
— American Reference Books Annual, 2000

■

Men's Health Concerns Sourcebook, 2nd Edition

Basic Consumer Health Information about the Medical and Mental Concerns of Men, Including Theories about the Shorter Male Lifespan, the Leading Causes of Death and Disability, Physical Concerns of Special Significance to Men, Reproductive and Sexual Concerns, Sexually Transmitted Diseases, Men's Mental and Emotional Health, and Lifestyle Choices That Affect Wellness, Such as Nutrition, Fitness, and Substance Use

Along with a Glossary of Related Terms and a Directory of Organizational Resources in Men's Health

Edited by Robert Aquinas McNally. 644 pages. 2004. 0-7808-0671-9.

ALSO AVAILABLE: Men's Health Concerns Sourcebook, 1st Edition. Edited by Allan R. Cook. 738 pages. 1998. 0-7808-0212-8.

"This comprehensive resource and the series are highly recommended."
— American Reference Books Annual, 2000

"Recommended reference source."
— Booklist, American Library Association, Dec '98

■

Mental Health Disorders Sourcebook, 3rd Edition

Basic Consumer Health Information about Mental and Emotional Health and Mental Illness, Including Facts about Depression, Bipolar Disorder, and Other Mood Disorders, Phobias, Post-Traumatic Stress Disorder (PTSD), Obsessive-Compulsive Disorder, and Other Anxiety Disorders, Impulse Control Disorders, Eating Disorders, Personality Disorders, and Psychotic Disorders, Including Schizophrenia and Dissociative Disorders

Along with Statistical Information, a Special Section Concerning Mental Health Issues in Children and Adolescents, a Glossary, and Directories of Resources for Additional Help and Information

Edited by Karen Bellenir. 661 pages. 2005. 0-7808-0747-2.

ALSO AVAILABLE: Mental Health Disorders Sourcebook, 1st Edition. Edited by Karen Bellenir. 548 pages. 1995. 0-7808-0040-0.

ALSO AVAILABLE: Mental Health Disorders Sourcebook, 2nd Edition. Edited by Karen Bellenir. 605 pages. 2000. 0-7808-0240-3.

"Well organized and well written."
— American Reference Books Annual, 2001

"Recommended reference source."
— Booklist, American Library Association, Jun '00

■

Mental Retardation Sourcebook

Basic Consumer Health Information about Mental Retardation and Its Causes, Including Down Syndrome, Fetal Alcohol Syndrome, Fragile X Syndrome, Genetic Conditions, Injury, and Environmental Sources

Along with Preventive Strategies, Parenting Issues, Educational Implications, Health Care Needs, Employment and Economic Matters, Legal Issues, a Glossary, and a Resource Listing for Additional Help and Information

Edited by Joyce Brennfleck Shannon. 642 pages. 2000. 0-7808-0377-9.

"Public libraries will find the book useful for reference and as a beginning research point for students, parents, and caregivers."
— American Reference Books Annual, 2001

"The strength of this work is that it compiles many basic fact sheets and addresses for further information in one volume. It is intended and suitable for the general public. This sourcebook is relevant to any collection providing health information to the general public."
— E-Streams, Nov '00

"From preventing retardation to parenting and family challenges, this covers health, social and legal issues and will prove an invaluable overview."
— Reviewer's Bookwatch, Jul '00

Movement Disorders Sourcebook

Basic Consumer Health Information about Neurological Movement Disorders, Including Essential Tremor, Parkinson's Disease, Dystonia, Cerebral Palsy, Huntington's Disease, Myasthenia Gravis, Multiple Sclerosis, and Other Early-Onset and Adult-Onset Movement Disorders, Their Symptoms and Causes, Diagnostic Tests, and Treatments

Along with Mobility and Assistive Technology Information, a Glossary, and a Directory of Additional Resources

Edited by Joyce Brennfleck Shannon. 655 pages. 2003. 0-7808-0628-X.

". . . a good resource for consumers and recommended for public, community college and undergraduate libraries."
— American Reference Books Annual, 2004

Muscular Dystrophy Sourcebook

Basic Consumer Health Information about Congenital, Childhood-Onset, and Adult-Onset Forms of Muscular Dystrophy, Such as Duchenne, Becker, Emery-Dreifuss, Distal, Limb-Girdle, Facioscapulohumeral (FSHD), Myotonic, and Ophthalmoplegic Muscular Dystrophies, Including Facts about Diagnostic Tests, Medical and Physical Therapies, Management of Co-Occurring Conditions, and Parenting Guidelines

Along with Practical Tips for Home Care, a Glossary, and Directories of Additional Resources

Edited by Joyce Brennfleck Shannon. 577 pages. 2004. 0-7808-0676-X.

Obesity Sourcebook

Basic Consumer Health Information about Diseases and Other Problems Associated with Obesity, and Including Facts about Risk Factors, Prevention Issues, and Management Approaches

Along with Statistical and Demographic Data, Information about Special Populations, Research Updates, a Glossary, and Source Listings for Further Help and Information

Edited by Wilma Caldwell and Chad T. Kimball. 376 pages. 2001. 0-7808-0333-7.

"The book synthesizes the reliable medical literature on obesity into one easy-to-read and useful resource for the general public."
— American Reference Books Annual 2002

"This is a very useful resource book for the lay public."
—Doody's Review Service, Nov '01

"Well suited for the health reference collection of a public library or an academic health science library that serves the general population." —E-Streams, Sep '01

"Recommended reference source."
—Booklist, American Library Association, Apr '01

" Recommended pick both for specialty health library collections and any general consumer health reference collection." — The Bookwatch, Apr '01

Ophthalmic Disorders Sourcebook, 1st Edition

SEE Eye Care Sourcebook, 2nd Edition

Oral Health Sourcebook

SEE Dental Care & Oral Health Sourcebook, 2nd Ed.

Osteoporosis Sourcebook

Basic Consumer Health Information about Primary and Secondary Osteoporosis and Juvenile Osteoporosis and Related Conditions, Including Fibrous Dysplasia, Gaucher Disease, Hyperthyroidism, Hypophosphatasia, Myeloma, Osteopetrosis, Osteogenesis Imperfecta, and Paget's Disease

Along with Information about Risk Factors, Treatments, Traditional and Non-Traditional Pain Management, a Glossary of Related Terms, and a Directory of Resources

Edited by Allan R. Cook. 584 pages. 2001. 0-7808-0239-X.

"This would be a book to be kept in a staff or patient library. The targeted audience is the layperson, but the therapist who needs a quick bit of information on a particular topic will also find the book useful."
— Physical Therapy, Jan '02

"This resource is recommended as a great reference source for public, health, and academic libraries, and is another triumph for the editors of Omnigraphics."
— American Reference Books Annual 2002

"Recommended for all public libraries and general health collections, especially those supporting patient education or consumer health programs."
— E-Streams, Nov '01

"Will prove valuable to any library seeking to maintain a current, comprehensive reference collection of health resources. . . . From prevention to treatment and associated conditions, this provides an excellent survey."
— The Bookwatch, Aug '01

"Recommended reference source."
— Booklist, American Library Association, July '01

SEE ALSO Women's Health Concerns Sourcebook

Pain Sourcebook, 2nd Edition

Basic Consumer Health Information about Specific Forms of Acute and Chronic Pain, Including Muscle and Skeletal Pain, Nerve Pain, Cancer Pain, and Disorders Characterized by Pain, Such as Fibromyalgia, Shingles, Angina, Arthritis, and Headaches

Along with Information about Pain Medications and Management Techniques, Complementary and Alternative Pain Relief Options, Tips for People Living with Chronic Pain, a Glossary, and a Directory of Sources for Further Information

Edited by Karen Bellenir. 670 pages. 2002. 0-7808-0612-3.

ALSO AVAILABLE: *Pain Sourcebook, 1st Edition.* Edited by Allan R. Cook. 667 pages. 1997. 0-7808-0213-6.

"A source of valuable information. . . . This book offers help to nonmedical people who need information about pain and pain management. It is also an excellent reference for those who participate in patient education."
— *Doody's Review Service, Sep '02*

"The text is readable, easily understood, and well indexed. This excellent volume belongs in all patient education libraries, consumer health sections of public libraries, and many personal collections."
— *American Reference Books Annual, 1999*

"A beneficial reference." — *Booklist Health Sciences Supplement, American Library Association, Oct '98*

"The information is basic in terms of scholarship and is appropriate for general readers. Written in journalistic style . . . intended for non-professionals. Quite thorough in its coverage of different pain conditions and summarizes the latest clinical information regarding pain treatment." — *Choice, Association of College and Research Libraries, Jun '98*

"Recommended reference source."
— *Booklist, American Library Association, Mar '98*

■

Pediatric Cancer Sourcebook

Basic Consumer Health Information about Leukemias, Brain Tumors, Sarcomas, Lymphomas, and Other Cancers in Infants, Children, and Adolescents, Including Descriptions of Cancers, Treatments, and Coping Strategies

Along with Suggestions for Parents, Caregivers, and Concerned Relatives, a Glossary of Cancer Terms, and Resource Listings

Edited by Edward J. Prucha. 587 pages. 1999. 0-7808-0245-4.

"An excellent source of information. Recommended for public, hospital, and health science libraries with consumer health collections." — *E-Streams, Jun '00*

"Recommended reference source."
— *Booklist, American Library Association, Feb '00*

"A valuable addition to all libraries specializing in health services and many public libraries."
— *American Reference Books Annual, 2000*

■

Physical & Mental Issues in Aging Sourcebook

Basic Consumer Health Information on Physical and Mental Disorders Associated with the Aging Process, Including Concerns about Cardiovascular Disease, Pulmonary Disease, Oral Health, Digestive Disorders, Musculoskeletal and Skin Disorders, Metabolic Changes, Sexual and Reproductive Issues, and Changes in Vision, Hearing, and Other Senses

Along with Data about Longevity and Causes of Death, Information on Acute and Chronic Pain, Descriptions of Mental Concerns, a Glossary of Terms, and Resource Listings for Additional Help

Edited by Jenifer Swanson. 660 pages. 1999. 0-7808-0233-0.

"This is a treasure of health information for the layperson." — *Choice Health Sciences Supplement, Association of College & Research Libraries, May 2000*

"Recommended for public libraries."
— *American Reference Books Annual, 2000*

"Recommended reference source."
— *Booklist, American Library Association, Oct '99*

SEE ALSO *Healthy Aging Sourcebook*

■

Podiatry Sourcebook

Basic Consumer Health Information about Foot Conditions, Diseases, and Injuries, Including Bunions, Corns, Calluses, Athlete's Foot, Plantar Warts, Hammertoes and Clawtoes, Clubfoot, Heel Pain, Gout, and More

Along with Facts about Foot Care, Disease Prevention, Foot Safety, Choosing a Foot Care Specialist, a Glossary of Terms, and Resource Listings for Additional Information

Edited by M. Lisa Weatherford. 380 pages. 2001. 0-7808-0215-2.

"Recommended reference source."
— *Booklist, American Library Association, Feb '02*

"There is a lot of information presented here on a topic that is usually only covered sparingly in most larger comprehensive medical encyclopedias."
— *American Reference Books Annual 2002*

■

Pregnancy & Birth Sourcebook, 2nd Edition

Basic Consumer Health Information about Conception and Pregnancy, Including Facts about Fertility, Infertility, Pregnancy Symptoms and Complications, Fetal Growth and Development, Labor, Delivery, and the Postpartum Period, as Well as Information about Maintaining Health and Wellness during Pregnancy and Caring for a Newborn

Along with Information about Public Health Assistance for Low-Income Pregnant Women, a Glossary, and Directories of Agencies and Organizations Providing Help and Support

Edited by Amy L. Sutton. 626 pages. 2004. 0-7808-0672-7.

ALSO AVAILABLE: *Pregnancy & Birth Sourcebook, 1st Edition.* Edited by Heather E. Aldred. 737 pages. 1997. 0-7808-0216-0.

"A well-organized handbook. Recommended."
— *Choice, Association of College and Research Libraries, Apr '98*

"Recommended reference source."
— *Booklist, American Library Association, Mar '98*

"Recommended for public libraries."
— *American Reference Books Annual, 1998*

SEE ALSO *Congenital Disorders Sourcebook, Family Planning Sourcebook*

Prostate Cancer Sourcebook

Basic Consumer Health Information about Prostate Cancer, Including Information about the Associated Risk Factors, Detection, Diagnosis, and Treatment of Prostate Cancer

Along with Information on Non-Malignant Prostate Conditions, and Featuring a Section Listing Support and Treatment Centers and a Glossary of Related Terms

Edited by Dawn D. Matthews. 358 pages. 2001. 0-7808-0324-8.

"Recommended reference source."
— *Booklist, American Library Association, Jan '02*

"A valuable resource for health care consumers seeking information on the subject. . . .All text is written in a clear, easy-to-understand language that avoids technical jargon. Any library that collects consumer health resources would strengthen their collection with the addition of the *Prostate Cancer Sourcebook*."
— *American Reference Books Annual 2002*

Prostate & Urological Disorders Sourcebook

Basic Consumer Health Information about Urogenital and Sexual Disorders in Men, Including Prostate and Other Andrological Cancers, Prostatitis, Benign Prostatic Hyperplasia, Testicular and Penile Trauma, Cryptorchidism, Peyronie Disease, Erectile Dysfunction, and Male Factor Infertility, and Facts about Commonly Used Tests and Procedures, Such as Prostatectomy, Vasectomy, Vasectomy Reversal, Penile Implants, and Semen Analysis

Along with a Glossary of Andrological Terms and a Directory of Resources for Additional Information

Edited by Karen Bellenir. 631 pages. 2005. 0-7808-0797-9.

Public Health Sourcebook

Basic Information about Government Health Agencies, Including National Health Statistics and Trends, Healthy People 2000 Program Goals and Objectives, the Centers for Disease Control and Prevention, the Food and Drug Administration, and the National Institutes of Health

Along with Full Contact Information for Each Agency

Edited by Wendy Wilcox. 698 pages. 1998. 0-7808-0220-9.

"Recommended reference source."
— *Booklist, American Library Association, Sep '98*

"This consumer guide provides welcome assistance in navigating the maze of federal health agencies and their data on public health concerns."
— *SciTech Book News, Sep '98*

Reconstructive & Cosmetic Surgery Sourcebook

Basic Consumer Health Information on Cosmetic and Reconstructive Plastic Surgery, Including Statistical Information about Different Surgical Procedures, Things to Consider Prior to Surgery, Plastic Surgery Techniques and Tools, Emotional and Psychological Considerations, and Procedure-Specific Information

Along with a Glossary of Terms and a Listing of Resources for Additional Help and Information

Edited by M. Lisa Weatherford. 374 pages. 2001. 0-7808-0214-4.

"An excellent reference that addresses cosmetic and medically necessary reconstructive surgeries. . . . The style of the prose is calm and reassuring, discussing the many positive outcomes now available due to advances in surgical techniques."
— *American Reference Books Annual 2002*

"Recommended for health science libraries that are open to the public, as well as hospital libraries that are open to the patients. This book is a good resource for the consumer interested in plastic surgery."
— *E-Streams, Dec '01*

"Recommended reference source."
— *Booklist, American Library Association, July '01*

Rehabilitation Sourcebook

Basic Consumer Health Information about Rehabilitation for People Recovering from Heart Surgery, Spinal Cord Injury, Stroke, Orthopedic Impairments, Amputation, Pulmonary Impairments, Traumatic Injury, and More, Including Physical Therapy, Occupational Therapy, Speech/ Language Therapy, Massage Therapy, Dance Therapy, Art Therapy, and Recreational Therapy

Along with Information on Assistive and Adaptive Devices, a Glossary, and Resources for Additional Help and Information

Edited by Dawn D. Matthews. 531 pages. 1999. 0-7808-0236-5.

"This is an excellent resource for public library reference and health collections."
— *American Reference Books Annual, 2001*

"Recommended reference source."
— *Booklist, American Library Association, May '00*

Respiratory Diseases & Disorders Sourcebook

Basic Information about Respiratory Diseases and Disorders, Including Asthma, Cystic Fibrosis, Pneumonia, the Common Cold, Influenza, and Others, Featuring Facts about the Respiratory System, Statistical and Demographic Data, Treatments, Self-Help Management Suggestions, and Current Research Initiatives

Edited by Allan R. Cook and Peter D. Dresser. 771 pages. 1995. 0-7808-0037-0.

"Designed for the layperson and for patients and their families coping with respiratory illness. . . . an extensive array of information on diagnosis, treatment, management, and prevention of respiratory illnesses for the general reader." —*Choice, Association of College and Research Libraries, Jun '96*

"A highly recommended text for all collections. It is a comforting reminder of the power of knowledge that good books carry between their covers." —*Academic Library Book Review, Spring '96*

"A comprehensive collection of authoritative information presented in a nontechnical, humanitarian style for patients, families, and caregivers." —*Association of Operating Room Nurses, Sep/Oct '95*

SEE ALSO Lung Disorders Sourcebook

■

Sexually Transmitted Diseases Sourcebook, 2nd Edition

Basic Consumer Health Information about Sexually Transmitted Diseases, Including Information on the Diagnosis and Treatment of Chlamydia, Gonorrhea, Hepatitis, Herpes, HIV, Mononucleosis, Syphilis, and Others

Along with Information on Prevention, Such as Condom Use, Vaccines, and STD Education; And Featuring a Section on Issues Related to Youth and Adolescents, a Glossary, and Resources for Additional Help and Information

Edited by Dawn D. Matthews. 538 pages. 2001. 0-7808-0249-7.

ALSO AVAILABLE: Sexually Transmitted Diseases Sourcebook, 1st Edition. Edited by Linda M. Ross. 550 pages. 1997. 0-7808-0217-9.

"Recommended for consumer health collections in public libraries, and secondary school and community college libraries." —*American Reference Books Annual 2002*

"Every school and public library should have a copy of this comprehensive and user-friendly reference book." —*Choice, Association of College & Research Libraries, Sep '01*

"This is a highly recommended book. This is an especially important book for all school and public libraries." —*AIDS Book Review Journal, Jul-Aug '01*

"Recommended reference source." —*Booklist, American Library Association, Apr '01*

"Recommended pick both for specialty health library collections and any general consumer health reference collection." —*The Bookwatch, Apr '01*

■

Skin Disorders Sourcebook, 1st Edition

SEE Dermatological Disorders Sourcebook, 2nd Edition

Sleep Disorders Sourcebook, 2nd Edition

Basic Consumer Health Information about Sleep and Sleep Disorders, Including Insomnia, Sleep Apnea, Restless Legs Syndrome, Narcolepsy, Parasomnias, and Other Health Problems That Affect Sleep, Plus Facts about Diagnostic Procedures, Treatment Strategies, Sleep Medications, and Tips for Improving Sleep Quality

Along with a Glossary of Related Terms and Resources for Additional Help and Information

Edited by Amy L. Sutton. 567 pages. 2005. 0-7808-0745-6.

ALSO AVAILABLE: Sleep Disorders Sourcebook, 1st Edition. Edited by Jenifer Swanson. 439 pages. 1998. 0-7808-0234-9.

"This text will complement any home or medical library. It is user-friendly and ideal for the adult reader." —*American Reference Books Annual, 2000*

"A useful resource that provides accurate, relevant, and accessible information on sleep to the general public. Health care providers who deal with sleep disorders patients may also find it helpful in being prepared to answer some of the questions patients ask." —*Respiratory Care, Jul '99*

"Recommended reference source." —*Booklist, American Library Association, Feb '99*

■

Smoking Concerns Sourcebook

Basic Consumer Health Information about Nicotine Addiction and Smoking Cessation, Featuring Facts about the Health Effects of Tobacco Use, Including Lung and Other Cancers, Heart Disease, Stroke, and Respiratory Disorders, Such as Emphysema and Chronic Bronchitis

Along with Information about Smoking Prevention Programs, Suggestions for Achieving and Maintaining a Smoke-Free Lifestyle, Statistics about Tobacco Use, Reports on Current Research Initiatives, a Glossary of Related Terms, and Directories of Resources for Additional Help and Information

Edited by Karen Bellenir. 621 pages. 2004. 0-7808-0323-X.

■

Sports Injuries Sourcebook, 2nd Edition

Basic Consumer Health Information about the Diagnosis, Treatment, and Rehabilitation of Common Sports-Related Injuries in Children and Adults

Along with Suggestions for Conditioning and Training, Information and Prevention Tips for Injuries Frequently Associated with Specific Sports and Special Populations, a Glossary, and a Directory of Additional Resources

Edited by Joyce Brennfleck Shannon. 614 pages. 2002. 0-7808-0604-2.

ALSO AVAILABLE: Sports Injuries Sourcebook, 1st Edition. Edited by Heather E. Aldred. 624 pages. 1999. 0-7808-0218-7.

"This is an excellent reference for consumers and it is recommended for public, community college, and undergraduate libraries."
— *American Reference Books Annual, 2003*

"Recommended reference source."
— *Booklist, American Library Association, Feb '03*

■

Stress-Related Disorders Sourcebook

Basic Consumer Health Information about Stress and Stress-Related Disorders, Including Stress Origins and Signals, Environmental Stress at Work and Home, Mental and Emotional Stress Associated with Depression, Post-Traumatic Stress Disorder, Panic Disorder, Suicide, and the Physical Effects of Stress on the Cardiovascular, Immune, and Nervous Systems

Along with Stress Management Techniques, a Glossary, and a Listing of Additional Resources

Edited by Joyce Brennfleck Shannon. 610 pages. 2002. 0-7808-0560-7.

"Well written for a general readership, the *Stress-Related Disorders Sourcebook* is a useful addition to the health reference literature."
— *American Reference Books Annual, 2003*

"I am impressed by the amount of information. It offers a thorough overview of the causes and consequences of stress for the layperson. . . . A well-done and thorough reference guide for professionals and nonprofessionals alike." — *Doody's Review Service, Dec '02*

■

Stroke Sourcebook

Basic Consumer Health Information about Stroke, Including Ischemic, Hemorrhagic, Transient Ischemic Attack (TIA), and Pediatric Stroke, Stroke Triggers and Risks, Diagnostic Tests, Treatments, and Rehabilitation Information

Along with Stroke Prevention Guidelines, Legal and Financial Information, a Glossary, and a Directory of Additional Resources

Edited by Joyce Brennfleck Shannon. 606 pages. 2003. 0-7808-0630-1.

"This volume is highly recommended and should be in every medical, hospital, and public library."
— *American Reference Books Annual, 2004*

■

Substance Abuse Sourcebook

Basic Health-Related Information about the Abuse of Legal and Illegal Substances Such as Alcohol, Tobacco, Prescription Drugs, Marijuana, Cocaine, and Heroin; and Including Facts about Substance Abuse Prevention Strategies, Intervention Methods, Treatment and Recovery Programs, and a Section Addressing the Special Problems Related to Substance Abuse during Pregnancy

Edited by Karen Bellenir. 573 pages. 1996. 0-7808-0038-9.

"A valuable addition to any health reference section. Highly recommended."
— *The Book Report, Mar/Apr '97*

". . . a comprehensive collection of substance abuse information that's both highly readable and compact. Families and caregivers of substance abusers will find the information enlightening and helpful, while teachers, social workers and journalists should benefit from the concise format. Recommended."
— *Drug Abuse Update, Winter '96/'97*

SEE ALSO Alcoholism Sourcebook, Drug Abuse Sourcebook

■

Surgery Sourcebook

Basic Consumer Health Information about Inpatient and Outpatient Surgeries, Including Cardiac, Vascular, Orthopedic, Ocular, Reconstructive, Cosmetic, Gynecologic, and Ear, Nose, and Throat Procedures and More

Along with Information about Operating Room Policies and Instruments, Laser Surgery Techniques, Hospital Errors, Statistical Data, a Glossary, and Listings of Sources for Further Help and Information

Edited by Annemarie S. Muth and Karen Bellenir. 596 pages. 2002. 0-7808-0380-9.

"Large public libraries and medical libraries would benefit from this material in their reference collections."
— *American Reference Books Annual, 2004*

"Invaluable reference for public and school library collections alike." — *Library Bookwatch, Apr '03*

■

Thyroid Disorders Sourcebook

Basic Consumer Health Information about Disorders of the Thyroid and Parathyroid Glands, Including Hypothyroidism, Hyperthyroidism, Graves Disease, Hashimoto Thyroiditis, Thyroid Cancer, and Parathyroid Disorders, Featuring Facts about Symptoms, Risk Factors, Tests, and Treatments

Along with Information about the Effects of Thyroid Imbalance on Other Body Systems, Environmental Factors That Affect the Thyroid Gland, a Glossary, and a Directory of Additional Resources

Edited by Joyce Brennfleck Shannon. 599 pages. 2005. 0-7808-0745-6.

■

Transplantation Sourcebook

Basic Consumer Health Information about Organ and Tissue Transplantation, Including Physical and Financial Preparations, Procedures and Issues Relating to Specific Solid Organ and Tissue Transplants, Rehabilitation, Pediatric Transplant Information, the Future of Transplantation, and Organ and Tissue Donation

Along with a Glossary and Listings of Additional Resources

Edited by Joyce Brennfleck Shannon. 628 pages. 2002. 0-7808-0322-1.

"Along with these advances [in transplantation technology] have come a number of daunting questions for potential transplant patients, their families, and their health care providers. This reference text is the best single tool to address many of these questions. . . . It will be a much-needed addition to the reference collections in health care, academic, and large public libraries."
— *American Reference Books Annual, 2003*

"Recommended for libraries with an interest in offering consumer health information." — *E-Streams, Jul '02*

"This is a unique and valuable resource for patients facing transplantation and their families."
— *Doody's Review Service, Jun '02*

Traveler's Health Sourcebook

Basic Consumer Health Information for Travelers, Including Physical and Medical Preparations, Transportation Health and Safety, Essential Information about Food and Water, Sun Exposure, Insect and Snake Bites, Camping and Wilderness Medicine, and Travel with Physical or Medical Disabilities

Along with International Travel Tips, Vaccination Recommendations, Geographical Health Issues, Disease Risks, a Glossary, and a Listing of Additional Resources

Edited by Joyce Brennfleck Shannon. 613 pages. 2000. 0-7808-0384-1.

"Recommended reference source."
— *Booklist, American Library Association, Feb '01*

"This book is recommended for any public library, any travel collection, and especially any collection for the physically disabled."
— *American Reference Books Annual, 2001*

Urinary Tract & Kidney Diseases & Disorders Sourcebook, 2nd Edition

Basic Consumer Health Information about the Urinary System, Including the Bladder, Urethra, Ureters, and Kidneys, with Facts about Urinary Tract Infections, Incontinence, Congenital Disorders, Kidney Stones, Cancers of the Urinary Tract and Kidneys, Kidney Failure, Dialysis, and Kidney Transplantation

Along with Statistical and Demographic Information, Reports on Current Research in Kidney and Urologic Health, a Summary of Commonly Used Diagnostic Tests, a Glossary of Related Terms, and a Directory of Resources for Additional Help and Information

Edited by Ivy L. Alexander. 649 pages. 2005. 0-7808-0750-2.

ALSO AVAILABLE: *Kidney & Urinary Tract Diseases & Disorders Sourcebook, 1st Ed.* Edited by Linda M. Ross. 602 pages. 1997. 0-7808-0079-6.

Vegetarian Sourcebook

Basic Consumer Health Information about Vegetarian Diets, Lifestyle, and Philosophy, Including Definitions of Vegetarianism and Veganism, Tips about Adopting Vegetarianism, Creating a Vegetarian Pantry, and Meeting Nutritional Needs of Vegetarians, with Facts Regarding Vegetarianism's Effect on Pregnant and Lactating Women, Children, Athletes, and Senior Citizens

Along with a Glossary of Commonly Used Vegetarian Terms and Resources for Additional Help and Information

Edited by Chad T. Kimball. 360 pages. 2002. 0-7808-0439-2.

"Organizes into one concise volume the answers to the most common questions concerning vegetarian diets and lifestyles. This title is recommended for public and secondary school libraries." — *E-Streams, Apr '03*

"Invaluable reference for public and school library collections alike." — *Library Bookwatch, Apr '03*

"The articles in this volume are easy to read and come from authoritative sources. The book does not necessarily support the vegetarian diet but instead provides the pros and cons of this important decision. The *Vegetarian Sourcebook* is recommended for public libraries and consumer health libraries."
— *American Reference Books Annual, 2003*

Women's Health Concerns Sourcebook, 2nd Edition

Basic Consumer Health Information about the Medical and Mental Concerns of Women, Including Maintaining Health and Wellness, Gynecological Concerns, Breast Health, Sexuality and Reproductive Issues, Menopause, Cancer in Women, the Leading Causes of Death and Disability among Women, Physical Concerns of Special Significance to Women, and Women's Mental and Emotional Health

Along with a Glossary of Related Terms and Directories of Resources for Additional Help and Information

Edited by Amy L. Sutton. 748 pages. 2004. 0-7808-0673-5.

ALSO AVAILABLE: *Women's Health Concerns Sourcebook, 1st Edition.* Edited by Heather E. Aldred. 567 pages. 1997. 0-7808-0219-5.

"Handy compilation. There is an impressive range of diseases, devices, disorders, procedures, and other physical and emotional issues covered . . . well organized, illustrated, and indexed." — *Choice, Association of College and Research Libraries, Jan '98*

SEE ALSO *Breast Cancer Sourcebook, Cancer Sourcebook for Women, Healthy Heart Sourcebook for Women, Osteoporosis Sourcebook*

Workplace Health & Safety Sourcebook

Basic Consumer Health Information about Workplace Health and Safety, Including the Effect of Workplace Hazards on the Lungs, Skin, Heart, Ears, Eyes, Brain,

Reproductive Organs, Musculoskeletal System, and Other Organs and Body Parts

Along with Information about Occupational Cancer, Personal Protective Equipment, Toxic and Hazardous Chemicals, Child Labor, Stress, and Workplace Violence

Edited by Chad T. Kimball. 626 pages. 2000. 0-7808-0231-4.

"As a reference for the general public, this would be useful in any library."   —*E-Streams, Jun '01*

"Provides helpful information for primary care physicians and other caregivers interested in occupational medicine. . . . General readers; professionals."
  — *Choice, Association of College & Research Libraries, May '01*

"Recommended reference source."
  —*Booklist, American Library Association, Feb '01*

"Highly recommended."   — *The Bookwatch, Jan '01*

■

Worldwide Health Sourcebook

Basic Information about Global Health Issues, Including Malnutrition, Reproductive Health, Disease Dispersion and Prevention, Emerging Diseases, Risky Health Behaviors, and the Leading Causes of Death

Along with Global Health Concerns for Children, Women, and the Elderly, Mental Health Issues, Research and Technology Advancements, and Economic, Environmental, and Political Health Implications, a Glossary, and a Resource Listing for Additional Help and Information

Edited by Joyce Brennfleck Shannon. 614 pages. 2001. 0-7808-0330-2.

"Named an Outstanding Academic Title." —*Choice, Association of College & Research Libraries, Jan '02*

"Yet another handy but also unique compilation in the extensive Health Reference Series, this is a useful work because many of the international publications reprinted or excerpted are not readily available. Highly recommended."   —*Choice, Association of College & Research Libraries, Nov '01*

"Recommended reference source."
  —*Booklist, American Library Association, Oct '01*

Teen Health Series

Helping Young Adults Understand, Manage, and Avoid Serious Illness

List price $65 per volume. **School and library price $58 per volume.**

Alcohol Information for Teens
Health Tips about Alcohol and Alcoholism

Including Facts about Underage Drinking, Preventing Teen Alcohol Use, Alcohol's Effects on the Brain and the Body, Alcohol Abuse Treatment, Help for Children of Alcoholics, and More

Edited by Joyce Brennfleck Shannon. 370 pages. 2005. 0-7808-0741-3.

Allergy Information for Teens
Health Tips about Allergic Reactions Such as Anaphylaxis, Respiratory Problems, and Rashes

Including Facts about Identifying and Managing Allergies to Food, Pollen, Mold, Animals, Chemicals, Drugs, and Other Substances

Edited by Karen Bellenir. 400 pages. 2006. 0-7808-0799-5.

Asthma Information for Teens
Health Tips about Managing Asthma and Related Concerns

Including Facts about Asthma Causes, Triggers, Symptoms, Diagnosis, and Treatment

Edited by Karen Bellenir. 386 pages. 2005. 0-7808-0770-7.

"It is so clearly written and well organized that even hesitant readers will be able to find the facts they need, whether for reports or personal information. . . . A succinct but complete resource."
— *School Library Journal, Sep '05*

Cancer Information for Teens
Health Tips about Cancer Awareness, Prevention, Diagnosis, and Treatment

Including Facts about Frequently Occurring Cancers, Cancer Risk Factors, and Coping Strategies for Teens Fighting Cancer or Dealing with Cancer in Friends or Family Members

Edited by Wilma R. Caldwell. 428 pages. 2004. 0-7808-0678-6.

"Recommended for school libraries, or consumer libraries that see a lot of use by teens."
— *E-Streams, May 2005*

"A valuable educational tool."
— *American Reference Books Annual, 2005*

"Young adults and their parents alike will find this new addition to the *Teen Health Series* an important reference to cancer in teens."
— *Children's Bookwatch, February 2005*

Diet Information for Teens
Health Tips about Diet and Nutrition

Including Facts about Nutrients, Dietary Guidelines, Breakfasts, School Lunches, Snacks, Party Food, Weight Control, Eating Disorders, and More

Edited by Karen Bellenir. 399 pages. 2001. 0-7808-0441-4.

"Full of helpful insights and facts throughout the book. . . . An excellent resource to be placed in public libraries or even in personal collections."
— *American Reference Books Annual 2002*

"Recommended for middle and high school libraries and media centers as well as academic libraries that educate future teachers of teenagers. It is also a suitable addition to health science libraries that serve patrons who are interested in teen health promotion and education."
— *E-Streams, Oct '01*

"This comprehensive book would be beneficial to collections that need information about nutrition, dietary guidelines, meal planning, and weight control. . . . This reference is so easy to use that its purchase is recommended."
— *The Book Report, Sep-Oct '01*

"This book is written in an easy to understand format describing issues that many teens face every day, and then provides thoughtful explanations so that teens can make informed decisions. This is an interesting book that provides important facts and information for today's teens."
— *Doody's Health Sciences Book Review Journal, Jul-Aug '01*

"A comprehensive compendium of diet and nutrition. The information is presented in a straightforward, plain-spoken manner. This title will be useful to those working on reports on a variety of topics, as well as to general readers concerned about their dietary health."
— *School Library Journal, Jun '01*

Drug Information for Teens

Health Tips about the Physical and Mental Effects of Substance Abuse

Including Facts about Alcohol, Anabolic Steroids, Club Drugs, Cocaine, Depressants, Hallucinogens, Herbal Products, Inhalants, Marijuana, Narcotics, Stimulants, Tobacco, and More

Edited by Karen Bellenir. 452 pages. 2002. 0-7808-0444-9.

"A clearly written resource for general readers and researchers alike." — *School Library Journal*

"The chapters are quick to make a connection to their teenage reading audience. The prose is straightforward and the book lends itself to spot reading. It should be useful both for practical information and for research, and it is suitable for public and school libraries."
— *American Reference Books Annual, 2003*

"Recommended reference source."
— *Booklist, American Library Association, Feb '03*

"This is an excellent resource for teens and their parents. Education about drugs and substances is key to discouraging teen drug abuse and this book provides this much needed information in a way that is interesting and factual." — *Doody's Review Service, Dec '02*

Eating Disorders Information for Teens

Health Tips about Anorexia, Bulimia, Binge Eating, and Other Eating Disorders

Including Information on the Causes, Prevention, and Treatment of Eating Disorders, and Such Other Issues as Maintaining Healthy Eating and Exercise Habits

Edited by Sandra Augustyn Lawton. 337 pages. 2005. 0-7808-0783-9.

Fitness Information for Teens

Health Tips about Exercise, Physical Well-Being, and Health Maintenance

Including Facts about Aerobic and Anaerobic Conditioning, Stretching, Body Shape and Body Image, Sports Training, Nutrition, and Activities for Non-Athletes

Edited by Karen Bellenir. 425 pages. 2004. 0-7808-0679-4.

"This book will be a great addition to any public, junior high, senior high, or secondary school library."
— *American Reference Books Annual, 2005*

Learning Disabilities Information for Teens

Health Tips about Academic Skills Disorders and Other Disabilities That Affect Learning

Including Information about Common Signs of Learning Disabilities, School Issues, Learning to Live with a Learning Disability, and Other Related Issues

Edited by Sandra Augustyn Lawton. 337 pages. 2005. 0-7808-0796-0.

Mental Health Information for Teens

Health Tips about Mental Health and Mental Illness

Including Facts about Anxiety, Depression, Suicide, Eating Disorders, Obsessive-Compulsive Disorders, Panic Attacks, Phobias, Schizophrenia, and More

Edited by Karen Bellenir. 406 pages. 2001. 0-7808-0442-2.

"In both language and approach, this user-friendly entry in the *Teen Health Series* is on target for teens needing information on mental health concerns." — *Booklist, American Library Association, Jan '02*

"Readers will find the material accessible and informative, with the shaded notes, facts, and embedded glossary insets adding appropriately to the already interesting and succinct presentation."
—*School Library Journal, Jan '02*

"This title is highly recommended for any library that serves adolescents and parents/caregivers of adolescents." — *E-Streams, Jan '02*

"Recommended for high school libraries and young adult collections in public libraries. Both health professionals and teenagers will find this book useful."
— *American Reference Books Annual 2002*

"This is a nice book written to enlighten the society, primarily teenagers, about common teen mental health issues. It is highly recommended to teachers and parents as well as adolescents."
— *Doody's Review Service, Dec '01*

Sexual Health Information for Teens

Health Tips about Sexual Development, Human Reproduction, and Sexually Transmitted Diseases

Including Facts about Puberty, Reproductive Health, Chlamydia, Human Papillomavirus, Pelvic Inflammatory Disease, Herpes, AIDS, Contraception, Pregnancy, and More

Edited by Deborah A. Stanley. 391 pages. 2003. 0-7808-0445-7.

"This work should be included in all high school libraries and many larger public libraries.... highly recommended."
— *American Reference Books Annual 2004*

"Sexual Health approaches its subject with appropriate seriousness and offers easily accessible advice and information." — *School Library Journal, Feb. 2004*

Skin Health
Information for Teens

Health Tips about Dermatological Concerns and Skin Cancer Risks

Including Facts about Acne, Warts, Hives, and Other Conditions and Lifestyle Choices, Such as Tanning, Tattooing, and Piercing, That Affect the Skin, Nails, Scalp, and Hair

Edited by Robert Aquinas McNally. 429 pages. 2003. 0-7808-0446-5.

"This volume, as with others in the series, will be a useful addition to school and public library collections."
— *American Reference Books Annual 2004*

"This volume serves as a one-stop source and should be a necessity for any health collection."
— *Library Media Connection*

Sports Injuries
Information for Teens

Health Tips about Sports Injuries and Injury Protection

Including Facts about Specific Injuries, Emergency Treatment, Rehabilitation, Sports Safety, Competition Stress, Fitness, Sports Nutrition, Steroid Risks, and More

Edited by Joyce Brennfleck Shannon. 405 pages. 2003. 0-7808-0447-3.

"This work will be useful in the young adult collections of public libraries as well as high school libraries."
— *American Reference Books Annual 2004*

Suicide Information for Teens

Health Tips about Suicide Causes and Prevention

Including Facts about Depression, Risk Factors, Getting Help, Survivor Support, and More

Edited by Joyce Brennfleck Shannon. 368 pages. 2005. 0-7808-0737-5.

Health Reference Series